# HUMAN DENTOFACIAL GROWTH

by

DENYS H. GOOSE

and

JOHN APPLETON

School of Dental Surgery
University of Liverpool

PERGAMON PRESS

OXFORD · NEW YORK · TORONTO · SYDNEY · PARIS · FRANKFURT

| | |
|---|---|
| U.K. | Pergamon Press Ltd., Headington Hill Hall, Oxford OX3 0BW, England |
| U.S.A. | Pergamon Press Inc., Maxwell House, Fairview Park, Elmsford, New York 10523, U.S.A. |
| CANADA | Pergamon Press Canada Ltd., Suite 104, 150 Consumers Rd., Willowdale, Ontario M2J 1P9, Canada |
| AUSTRALIA | Pergamon Press (Aust.) Pty. Ltd., P.O. Box 544, Potts Point, N.S.W. 2011, Australia |
| FRANCE | Pergamon Press SARL, 24 rue des Ecoles, 75240 Paris, Cedex 05, France |
| FEDERAL REPUBLIC OF GERMANY | Pergamon Press GmbH, 6242 Kronberg-Taunus, Hammerweg 6, Federal Republic of Germany |



First edition 1982

Library of Congress Cataloging in Publication Data
Goose, Denys H.
Human dentofacial growth.
Bibliography: p.
1. Face—Growth. 2. Dentition. 3. Skull—Growth.
I. Appleton, John. II. Title. [DNLM: 1. Cephalometry.
2. Maxillofacial development. 3. Tooth—Growth and development. WU 101 G678h]
QM535.G66 1982 612'.92 81-17895 AACR2

**British Library Cataloguing in Publication Data**
Goose, Denys H.
Human Dentofacial growth.
1. Facial bones—Growth
I. Title II. Appleton, John
612'.75 QM535

ISBN 0-08-026394-1 (Hardcover)
ISBN 0-08-026393-3 (Flexicover)

*Printed in Great Britain by A. Wheaton & Co. Ltd., Exeter*

Yvonne B Martin 8-95
24 June 82

# HUMAN DENTOFACIAL GROWTH

**Other Pergamon publications of related interest**

**BOOKS**

BERKOVITZ *et al.*
The Periodontal Ligament in Health and Disease

PERRYMAN
Oral Physiology and Occlusion

TYLDESLEY
Oral Diagnosis, 2nd Edition

**JOURNAL**

ARCHIVES OF ORAL BIOLOGY*

**Free specimen copy available on request*

*To the*
*late Professor J. H. Scott of Belfast*
*who did so much to stimulate interest and promote*
*research in the subject of craniofacial growth*

# *Preface*

For some years it has been evident that, in spite of the level of knowledge achieved in their preclinical years, students are unable to recall and relate facts to their later clinical training.

This problem applies in particular in relation to the difficult subjects of development and growth which are so necessary as a background to the study of Orthodontics and Paedodontics. We have, therefore, written this text specifically to help dental students master these subjects in their preclinical course with the knowledge that they will also be useful at a later stage of their careers. Thus the relevance of clinical problems is particularly stressed.

It is intended that the book will also be of value to those studying for the Primary Fellowship in Dentistry and for the Diploma in Orthodontics. For this purpose the bibliography is designed to help direct more advanced reading.

# *Acknowledgements*

We would like to thank the following for permission to use some of their material. Professor H. C. Anderson, Department of Pathology and Oncology, University of Kansas Medical Center, College of Health Sciences and Hospital, Kansas City, and Ciba Foundation Symp. 11, Elsevier/North Holland Biomedical Press, Amsterdam for Fig. 2.11; Mr P. D. Bird, Liverpool A.H.A.(T) for Fig. 9.10; Professor A. Björk, Royal Dental College, Copenhagen and *American Journal of Orthodontics* for Figs. 7.9 and 7.10; Dr B. H. Broadbent and Dr W. H. Golden in *Bolton Standards of Dentofacial Developmental Growth* 1975 and C. V. Mosby, St Louis, U.S.A. for Fig. 7.8; Mr P. G. Bush, Liverpool A.H.A.(T) for Figs. 4.7, 4.8 and 4.9; Dr H. M-L. Carty, Department of Radiodiagnosis, University of Liverpool for Fig. 9.9; Mr J. Cunningham, School of Dental Surgery, University of Liverpool for Figs. 9.4 and 9.5; Editor of the *British Dental Journal* from 'Structure and function in mandibular joint' by L. A. Rees (1954), vol. 96, pp. 125-133 (Figs. 6.3, 6.4, 6.5 and 6.9): Messrs Lippincott, Harper and Row, Philadelphia, U.S.A. for Fig. 2.4 from 'Chemical structure of tendon, cartilage, dentine and bone matrix' by G. Herring in *Clinical Orthopaedics,* vol. 60 (1968); Professor A. Lundstrom, Karolinska Institutet, School of Dentistry, Stockholm, and *Dental Practitioner* for Table 9.1; Professor C. F. A. Moorrees, Forsyth Dental Institute, Boston, U.S.A. and *Journal of the Canadian Dental Association* for Figs. 9.13 and 9.14; Professor C. F. A. Moorrees and Dr J. A. McNamara, ed. *Biology of Occlusal Development,* Center for Human Growth and Development, University of Michigan, U.S.A. for Fig. 9.7; Dr E. B. Nery, Dental Research Section, Medical Center, Veterans Administration, Wood, U.S.A. and *Archives of Oral Biology,* Pergamon Press, Oxford for Figs. 8.3, 8.4 and 8.5; Professor J. W. Osborn, Department of Oral Biology, University of Alberta, Edmonton, Canada and Academic Press, London for Figs. 8.9(a) and 8.9(b) from *Development, Function and Evolution of Teeth,* ed. P. M. Butler and K. A. Joysey, 1978; Professor J. W. Osborn and Springer Verlag Heidelberg (*Calcified Tissue Research,* 1970) for Fig. 8.22; Professor J. M. Tanner, Institute of Child Health, University of London, and Castlemead Publications, Hertford for Fig. 1.4 (chart No. 14A) and also Open Books Publishing, London for Fig. 1.6; the Controller of Her Majesty's Stationery Office for part of Table 83 from the Report on Children's Dental Health in England and Wales 1973, produced by the Social Survey Division of the Office of Population Censuses and Surveys; Dr D. G. Woodside and colleagues and the editor of the Third International Orthodontic Congress, Crosby Lockwood Staples, London for Figs. 7.11 and 7.12; Dr T. H. M. Wynne, Liverpool A.H.A.(T) for Fig.s 1.1, 3.1, 3.2, 4.3, 4.10, 4.11 and 4.12.

Especial thanks are due to Mr D. E. J. Bowden, MDS, DDO, FDS, Consultant Orthodontist to the Cheshire A.H.A. for his Chapter 'Cephalometrics and Facial Growth', and to Mr P. H. Goose, MA, BSc, ARCS, for his Statistical Appendix.

We are very grateful for the help with illustrations from Mr P. Alebone, Grosvenor Museum, Chester, Mr and Mrs. S. Rudge, Dental Department, Royal Infirmary, Chester, and for photographs from Mr J. S. Bailie, School of Dental Surgery, University of Liverpool.

Our very deepest thanks are due for the invaluable secretarial assistance provided by Mrs K. Higgins, Mrs N. Carruthers and Mrs K. Taylor; without their help we would not been able to carry out this project.

# *Contents*

# CHAPTER 1

# *Principles of Human Growth*

For the study of the early stages of human development it is necessary to rely on material provided by either natural or induced abortions; however, for the later stages it is possible to study prematurely born infants of different ages, assuming that their growth pattern would have been the same if they had remained in the uterus until full term.

## PRENATAL GROWTH

Fertilization is followed, in a successful case, by cell division of the fertilized egg, firstly floating free in the tubes and uterine cavity and later implanted in the wall of the uterus. At this stage it is known as a blastocyst and may consist of about 150 cells. It develops as an embryo from this period up to 8 weeks and the main outlines of the child are established with their appropriate systems. By this stage it is referred to as a foetus (Fig. 1.1) and growth proceeds rapidly, particularly in the early stages, there being a slowing down towards the end of pregnancy followed normally by a speeding up again after birth.

Gestational age is calculated from the beginning of the last menstrual period of the mother, and the normal length of pregnancy is between 38 and 42 weeks. Before 38 weeks is now regarded as preterm, and those at 42 weeks or later post-term. Of course, fertilization is usually 2 weeks later and therefore these ages are not strictly correct but are more convenient to use clinically and may be referred to as postmenstrual age. Dates can be confused, however, by menstrual bleeding occurring even after fertilization, or a lack of periods if pregnancy follows shortly after the birth of a previous infant.

Prematurity used to be used as a definition of all babies below 2500 g at birth, but this confuses two different groups; the first being preterm babies, that is, those born before 38 weeks who would therefore be expected to be small and whose weight may be compared with standards by means of growth charts which have been constructed for this purpose. The second group are those called "small for dates", that is they are below the weights expected at their gestation period. For example, one below 2500 g born at 40 weeks would be "small for dates"; it would, of course, be possible to be both preterm and "small for dates". This distinction is important, as purely preterm babies can be expected to catch up their growth postnatally, even if born very young,

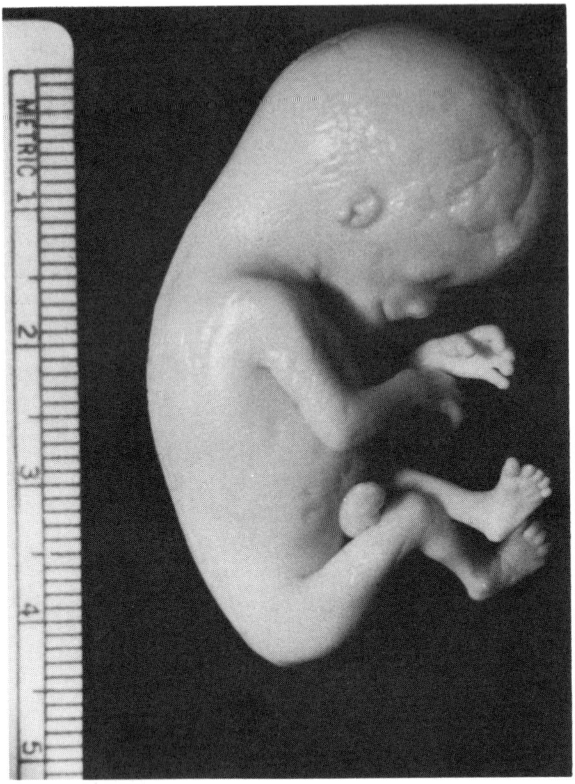


Fig. 1.1. Human foetus of nearly 10 weeks (by kind permission of Dr T. H. M. Wynne, Liverpool A.H.A.(T)).

with appropriate medical care. In general "small for dates" babies have more problems and may not catch up growth so easily. The causes of this condition are not altogether understood, but disorders of the placenta, toxaemia or hypertension in the mother, maternal smoking during pregnancy, and abnormalities of the foetus itself may all be contributing reasons.

## POSTNATAL GROWTH

There are two ways of studying growth both of which lead to the construction of growth curves by which comparison may be made with other data.

### Cross-sectional Studies

These are obtained by measuring a number of children of different ages, finding mean (or average) values for each age and joining up the means to produce a curve. Such are those in the studies already referred to, with respect to the weights of preterm infants, and they serve a useful purpose in seeing whether a particular child is some way from the average for his gestational age. Another example is provided by Meredith (1971) in which he reviewed the head circumferences of children at birth and later ages for various racial groups and found certain pronounced differences.

It is easy to see what is meant by the average or mean value, but in addition, for the purpose of comparing one value with another in order to detect a difference in a statistical sense, it is necessary to have a measure of the way in which results "scatter" around the mean. Figure 1.2 shows this for some measurements of jaws. It will be evident that the mean value here (40 mm) is in the centre of the distribution and that the probability of the occurrence of any particular value or more is given by the appropriate area under the curve, for example for 45 mm or more, the shaded area. This question and how to apply it to tests of significance are dealt with more fully in the Statistical Appendix.

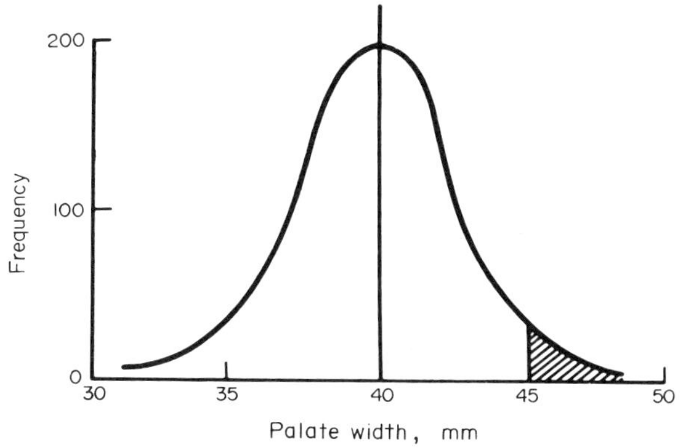


Fig. 1.2. Frequency distribution of palate widths of a group of men. The mean value is 40 mm and the shaded area represents the proportion having a value of 45 mm or more.

To facilitate comparison of, for example, a given baby's weight with those of published standards, the latter are normally given in terms of centiles (these are shown in a different connection in Fig. 1.4). In a sample of babies 50 per cent will be below a certain weight, and this value is therefore called the 50th centile. At one extreme, those below the 3rd centile will constitute only 3 per cent of babies in the sample. Similarly, only 3 per cent will be above the 97 per cent centile and other centiles between have similar meanings. It will be apparent that the 50th centile is the same as the mean in a normal distribution, similarly the 3rd and 97th centile correspond approximately to the outer limits of plus or minus 2 standard deviations, or the 5 per cent probability level (see Statistical Appendix).

Although cross-sectional studies are easy to carry out and provide valuable data, as has been shown, they do not give all the information one may require. For example, one cannot tell how quickly a child will be likely to grow between, say, 6 and 7 years of age, since the values provided are means of different groups of children. Nor will the shape of a growth curve produced from cross-sectional data be correct at puberty, since children arrive at this stage at different ages and the increased velocity of growth associated with puberty will therefore be averaged out and not appear so markedly as it does for individuals.

### Longitudinal Studies

These are achieved by measuring individual children repeatedly during their growth. The most common measurements used are height and weight, although many others have also been carried out, for example head circumference, sitting height and skinfold thickness (for assessment of body fat).

The curve produced by joining successive points of a boy's height from birth* to adulthood is called a distance curve (Fig. 1.3) and will show rapid growth up until about 2 year, then a steady increase in height up to about 13 years, and thereafter an acceleration known as the adolescent or pubertal "spurt" for a short period, then a slowing down until adult stature is achieved.

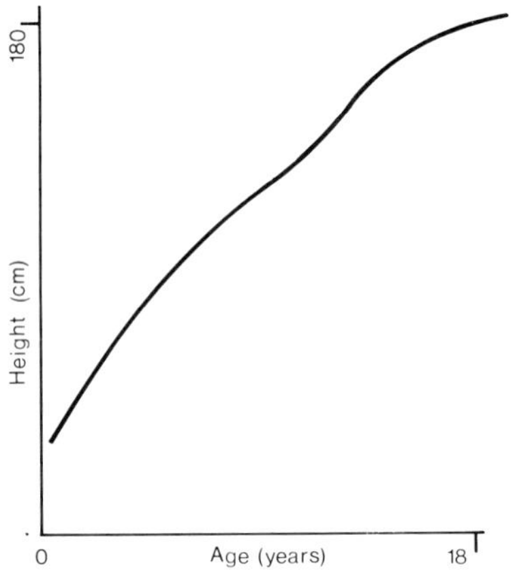


Fig. 1.3. Smoothed curve obtained by joining up the heights of a boy at different ages.

More revealing than the distance curve is one showing the velocity of growth, giving the increase in height per unit of time. It is unlikely to be possible to measure a child at exact intervals of a year and, in fact, this would not be satisfactory during rapid growth where the rate changes more frequently, so it is best to convert ages in days and months into decimals (for which tables are available). The growth achieved between certain dates can then be divided by the decimal figure obtained by subtracting the first date

* Up to the age of 2, a child is more conveniently measured lying down.

from the last giving the velocity in cm/year. Children's growth rate varies within the year and it used to be thought it was regularly seasonal, being fastest in spring. However, recently doubt has been cast on the general truth of this for all children.

In the case of girls (Fig 1.4, Castlemead Publications) it can be seen by looking at the 50th centile that the rapid infantile growth falls in rate at about 2 years of age and then proceeds more slowly until about 10.5 years when it rises to a maximum of something like 8 cm/year at the age of 12 years and thereafter falling away sharply. This maximum is very important and is known as the peak height velocity (PHV).

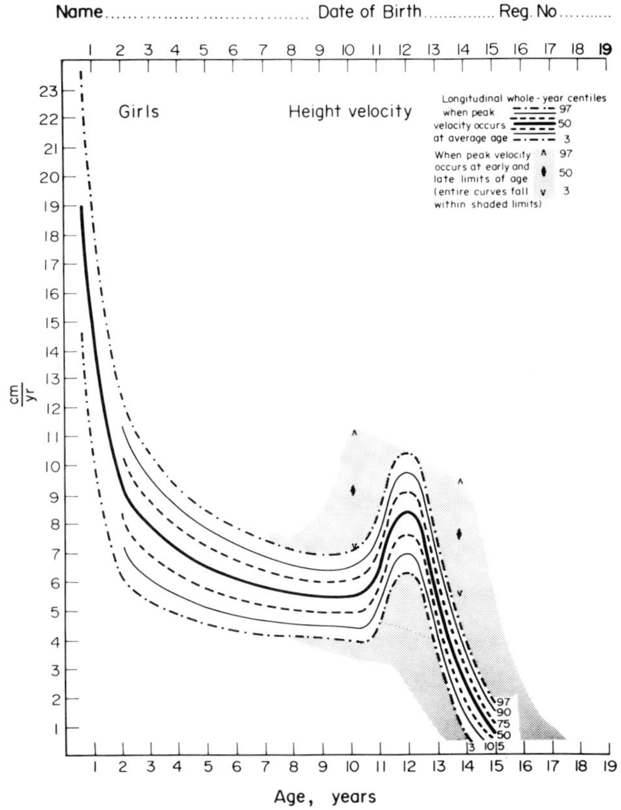


Fig. 1.4. Height velocity curve of girls in the United Kingdom (by kind permission of Professor J. M. Tanner, Institute of Child Health, University of London, and Castlemead Publications, Hertford; Chart No. 14A).

Boys are different both in timing and velocity. At birth they grow slightly faster but become equal at 7 months, and then girls grow faster until about 4 years. After this they are almost the same until adolescence which in boys is later by about 2 years, both for the peak height velocity and the start of the spurt of growth. The magnitude of the peak is higher too normally.

It is easy to construct individual curves such as that of a particular child, but more difficult to produce satisfactory standards for comparison. This is because the adolescent spurt of growth occurs at different ages for different children and thus the peak height velocity will be averaged out at a lower figure and over a wider area if all the data are used without any correction.

### Standards

Tanner *et al.* (1966) have produced combined graphs of cross-sectional and longitudinal standards so that both sorts of comparisons may be made. These were obtained from several investigations carried out in different periods and places in the United Kingdom, some being cross-sectional, some longitudinal and some mixed. This gave them the possibility of constructing velocity curves at each age, but allowance had to be made for the phase difference at puberty in order to get the correct shape of growth curve that is shown by individual children.

If a child is being followed longitudinally, it may be seen on a distance curve whether he adheres to a more or less fixed centile or not. For example, a hypothyroid child may be found to be below the 3rd centile, but then after treatment with thyroid hormone will catch up and cross the centiles diagonally and move into a normal position. Alternatively an early maturing boy might be in one of the upper centiles up to about 15 years when he begins to slow down, and so his final stature might be relatively small compared with others who matured later and he would move down to a lower centile.

Velocity curves are more valuable in picking out pathological cases than distance ones, and it should be noted that whereas it is possible to remain in the same centile for distance curves, individuals are bound to change on velocity curves since to remain, say, at the 97 centile would imply an eventually very tall adult. The shaded areas in these curves (Fig. 1.4) are to allow for the early or late maturer.

There have been many efforts to find a mathematical curve which would represent the growth process in man. For the early part of growth a straight line curve may be made from the equation $y = a + bt + c \log t$. The age is given by $t$ and $a$, $b$ and $c$ are constants; the fitting process involves calculating the values of the constants for each child.* The mean value of these constants can then be used to obtain a curve representing the group of children.

At adolescence the S-shaped Gompertz curve $Y = P + K \exp[-\exp(a\text{-}bt)]$ could describe growth; $Y$ is stature, $t$ is age, $P$ the lower asymptote or stature at the beginning of the adolescent spurt, $K$ the gain in stature during

* A simple explanation of the theory lying behind such equations is dealt with under Regression Analysis in the Statistical Appendix.

adolescence, $a$ is a constant of integration and $b$ a constant representing the rate at which the proportion $(Y - P)/K$ is increasing to equal powers of itself (Marshall 1977).

There is hope, however, that eventually the whole growth curve may be described in one formula and, of course, it is important, if this is so, that the constants should be seen to have some biological meaning.

### Growth of Other Characters

Although body weight also shows the same pattern as height and standardized graphs are available similar to those of height, other systems or organs do not. Most obvious is the reproductive system which has most of its growth at puberty and this will be referred to later on, in more detail, under the subject of maturation.

The brain and, therefore the head, grows rapidly in early childhood and by about 1 year it has reached nearly 50 per cent of its adult weight. At birth the head looks proportionately much larger compared with the rest of the body than in an adult and this is part of an overall gradient of maturity from head via trunk to legs. Figure 1.5 shows a boy of about 3 and the disproportionate size of the cranial part of the head is well seen.

Very early measurements of the head from a growth point of view are misleading because some of the increase in circumference in the postnatal period is due to recovery from moulding during birth. Thus measurements must be taken some days after birth to realistically compare with later ones. Up to the age of 18 the circumference of the head increases approximately 20 cm and half of this has been achieved by about 9 months and three-quarters by the end of the second year.

The face, on the other hand, continues to grow for a much longer period, and thus the appearance of the child alters as he grows older.

The eyes, for example, in a baby appear large, but with the later increase of the midface look relatively smaller in an adult. Similarly the young child's nose lacks prominence, looking wide and flattened and the nasal floor is not far from the inferior orbital rim. However, development of the nasal cavities and increased vertical development of the face alters this towards the adult pattern. In addition the nose itself becomes more prominent.

The mandible appears small with a poorly developed chin and a wide mandibular angle, but during growth in normal cases the lower jaw catches up. It may, however, not do so with a resulting malocclusion.

Even at puberty, changes may still occur particularly in the male, the forehead becoming more prominent, facial muscles more developed and the profile straighter with a more prominent chin.

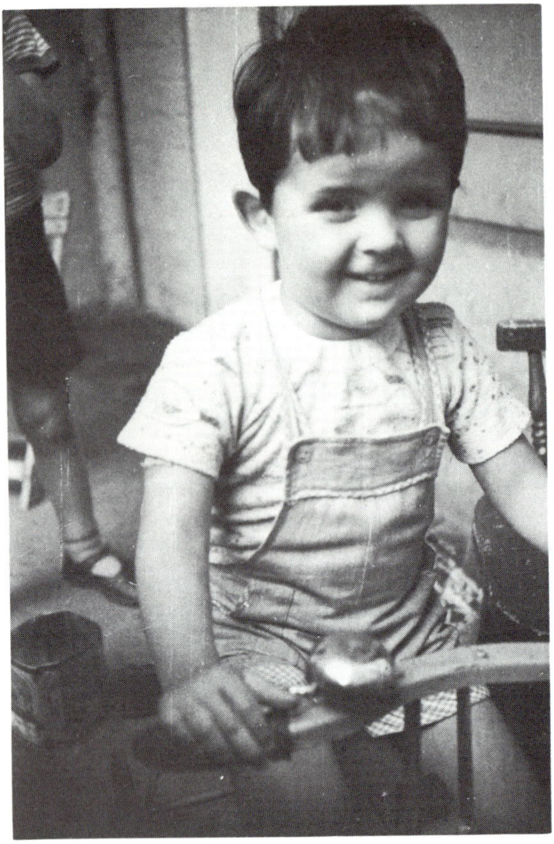

Fig. 1.5. Boy aged about 3 years. Note the smallness of his face compared with his head.

**Maturation**

Although the postnatal growth pattern, as has been described for stature, is similar for all normal children, there is a considerable variation in the rate at which they pass through the changes at puberty and in the age of commencement and completion of these changes. For example, everyone is aware of the small boy at school who is left behind in growth, his classmates becoming taller and stronger, their voices breaking, and exhibiting other pubertal changes. Later he too will follow these stages, but meanwhile it can be a psychologically disturbing period. These differences in rate of development or maturation have been referred to as the tempo of growth, some children being fast and others slow.

In order to be able to measure maturity one needs a scale and all individuals need to reach a recognizably constant end point. Thus height, for example, is not suitable because although easily measured not everyone reaches the same numerical end point, their final adult height. Stature can, of course, be used retrospectively, for example, to see when a given individual reached 50 per cent of his adult height, but is obviously no use during growth.

Before continuing with this discussion it will be necessary to look at the events during puberty in more detail and then to consider two methods of assessing maturity, skeletal and dental.

### Puberty

This is the period when there is maturation of the gonads, development of secondary sexual characteristics and an acceleration of somatic growth. Much of the quantitative information and the interrelationships of the various events at puberty were carefully documented by Tanner in his classic work *Growth at Adolescence* in 1962.

*Males.* Testicular enlargement is usually the first sign of puberty, along with changes in scrotal skin colour and texture, on average at about 11.5 years. Next the penis enlarges, beginning on the average at about 12½; pubic hair appears around the same time. However, these events are very variable in time, the range for example of the start of penis enlargement being from 10½ to 14½ years (Fig. 1.6.). Its completion usually occurs about 14½, but may be as early in some boys as 12½ and in others as late as 16½. In other words some boys will not have started this phase before others have completed it. The sequence of events, however, is much less variable than the age at which they occur.

The commencement of the adolescent growth spurt, which has already been discussed under growth curves, begins on average about a year after the first testicular enlargement, reaching the peak height velocity after about another year.

Axillary hair usually appears after pubic hair has almost reached its final stage and facial hair somewhat later. Breaking of the voice, due to the growth spurt of the larynx and increased length of vocal cords, occurs rather late in puberty, and as it may be rather gradual anyway it is not a very revealing criterion of puberty.

For clinical work rating scales have been devised for successive steps of growth of the penis and scrotum; the testes can be measured by comparison with a standard (the Prader orchidometer). Pubic hair too can be rated through five stages (Fig. 1.6).

*Females.* Girls are in advance of boys in their pubertal changes as they have been seen to be already, with the start of their growth spurt and peak height velocity.

Usually breast development is the first sign, showing as a breast bud or elevation of breast and papilla with slight enlargement of the areolar area. This occurs on an average of about 11 years with a range from 9 to 13 years. Pubic hair usually appears later, but can appear before the breast bud stage.

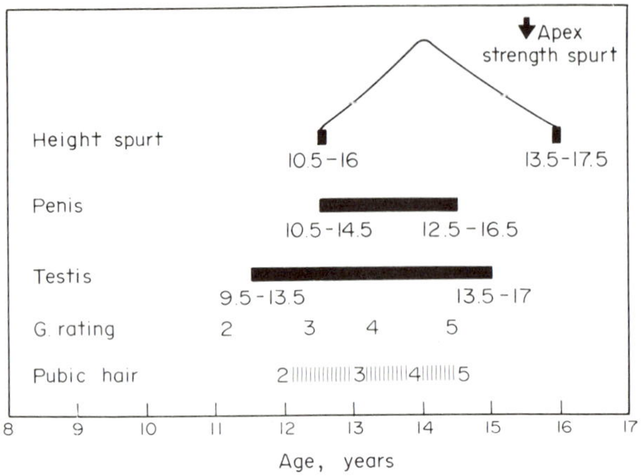


Fig. 1.6. Events at puberty in boys (From *Foetus into Man*, 1978, by kind permission of Professor J. M. Tanner, Institute of Child Health, University of London and Open Books Publishing, London).

Menarche, or the first menstrual period, is much later, being at about 13 years in populations in northern or central Europe (and girls of European descent in North America). The standard deviation of age at menarche is about 1 year in most populations so the range ± two standard deviations, 11-15 years, will include 95 per cent of girls. Most girls at the menarche have breast development advanced, but a few are still at the earlier stages. However, there is a closer relationship of menarche with height velocity; the majority of girls start to menstruate at the time of deceleration of height growth.

As has been seen, there is a sex difference in age of about 2 years in the time of peak height velocity, girls being earlier. However, there is only a difference of about 9 months in the first appearance of pubic hair, and the first appearance of breast predates the first change in testis size even less. Thus the adolescent growth spurt in girls is placed earlier in the sequence of changes than in boys.

### Skeletal Development

In development, the skeleton passes through a variety of stages which can readily be calibrated by radiographic means, since the cartilaginous areas are converted into radiopaque bone during ossification and the end result is the completely mature, fully calcified skeleton of the adult.

Although any part of the skeleton might be followed in its ossification pattern, in practice the one principally concentrated on is that of the hand and wrist, and this provides the lower ends of the radius and ulna, the carpals, the metacarpals and phalanges of the digits.

One method, which has been in use for some time, is typified by the Greulich and Pyle Atlas (1959). This presents, in a series of radiographic pictures, the degree of skeletal development found to be representative of groups of healthy American children at successive chronological ages. The radiographs used were those of white children born in the United States, of North European ancestry, in Cleveland, Ohio.

The atlas consists of about thirty standards each of boys and girls separately, thought to be typical of children at different stages. These were selected from about a hundred films of children at each age and sex which were arranged in order of relative skeletal status, that is from least to most mature. The film chosen as the standard was the one most nearly representative of the central tendency of that particular array, being normally at the midpoint of the hundred films.

To use the atlas one attempts to match a given child's radiograph with one of the plates in the atlas; his or her skeletal age will then be that of the standard chosen.

There are one or two difficulties arising when using this method. The first is that it is somewhat subjective and it may also present difficulties when some bones indicate a more advanced age than others and therefore the radiograph to be investigated does not exactly fit any one standard plate. In addition the children who formed the standards were from rather well-off U.S. families who may be more advanced in development than other groups with which they may be compared. More recently a revised atlas has been produced by Pyle, Waterhouse and Greulich (1971) for the U.S. National Health Examination Survey in which only male standards are used, the female equivalent being calculated by tables. In this each bone is also separately assessed and given a bone age.

Another approach has been to assess each bone separately into stages of development from A (lack of appearance) to I (fully formed), for the radius, hamate, trapezium, metacarpals and phalanges (or to H for the ulna and rest of carpals) by Tanner *et al.* (1975). Each bone is then allotted a weighted score designed to minimize the differences between different bones and to give an overall maturity figure when summed (from 0 to 1000).

As there are correlations between different bones, for example the five finger bones, digits 2 and 4 are not examined. Three scores can be obtained, the RUS (radius, ulna and short finger bones), carpal score and TW2, a twenty bone score using half of the RUS plus half of the carpal weights.

Although this method is complicated and time-consuming it has the advantage of ending up with an accurate numerical score representing the development of the child investigated. This can then be looked at again further on during development and progress assessed which can be useful, for example, in children receiving growth hormone treatment.

Skeletal maturation assessment in children may help to predict their adult height, and this can be useful for abnormally small or large children who may be self-conscious about it. It has also been used for girls wishing to go to ballet schools and therefore needing to be within certain limits of height.

Unfortunately, however, there has been found to be little accurate predictive value in ossification events in hand-wrist radiographs and the timing of the adolescent growth spurt. Such a relationship might have been useful in giving a clue as to whether certain forms of orthodontic treatment might be started during a period of rapid growth.

**Dental Development**

Teeth fulfil the criteria for a measure of maturity since they can be counted and eventually they all erupt, with the exceptions of those impacted or missing. In general, eruption of teeth alone has been used as the method of assessing dental maturity, although it would be better, but more time-consuming, to use radiographic evidence of crown and root formation as well. This, however, has been done too infrequently to provide much comparative data, although Demirjian and Levesque (1980) present some interesting results of their examination of over 5000 radiographs from a homogeneous French-Canadian population of children.

Using eight stages of crown and root development, they found that for the first three stages there is no sex differences in mineralization, but at stage D (completion of crown) girls are more advanced and for subsequent stages too. They argue that this sort of data is useful in predicting the time of tooth emergence which they find follows stage F (attainment of three-quarters root length) for mandibular teeth. More detail about the eruption of teeth and of their mineralization will be presented in later chapters.

The problem of analysing data from tooth eruption is to present the results in a useful way for comparison with other data. There is some variation in opinion as to what constitutes an erupted tooth, but most investigators consider it erupted as soon as any part of it has appeared in the mouth. Tables merely giving the number of teeth erupted at different ages are not very helpful as there is considerable variability in the sequence of eruption.

It is better to find the mean age of eruption of each tooth and then conventional statistical means are available for making comparisons between different populations or, of course, between the sexes. However, the mean age of eruption is not easy to ascertain if data is collected cross-sectionally.

The deciduous dentition is probably not very helpful in maturity studies as its eruption lasts only a matter of 18 months or so and can be considerably disturbed by events at birth, for example "small for dates" babies have delayed eruption. In underdeveloped countries, where birth certificates may not be available, the number of deciduous teeth present has sometimes been used to estimate age, but it is doubtful whether this can be justified except in very general terms.

The emergence of permanent teeth covers a much wider range of age and shows clear sex and ethnic group differences. However, there is considerable variation in the order of eruption as had been stated, which may confuse the issue.

Although the deciduous dentition shows very little sex difference in eruption, in the permanent dentition girls are ahead of boys in all cases. There is some evidence for earlier eruption in children from better class homes or environments.

People of New Guinea and Africans in Africa and the United States appear to have the most advanced eruption.

On the whole, however, dental development has not been used enough to judge its value in assessing physiological maturity and there appears to be only a relatively low correlation with skeletal age.

## FACTORS INFLUENCING GROWTH

Both hereditary and environmental influences are involved in growth, but it is artificial to put them in opposite camps as there is always an interaction between them. For example, in a recent study of over 46,000 participants in a national programme in the United States, Garn and Keating (1980) found birth size, maternal weight and maternal stature the most important determinates of later size.

However, it is true to say some characters such as blood groups are nearer to the genes than others, such as height or weight. Similarly in tooth size, tooth germs develop for only a limited period in a rather protected environment and thus are less susceptible to unfavourable influences than, for example, jaws which go on developing into puberty and can more easily be upset by diseases, abnormal function and, of course, surgical interference in the shape of dental extractions.

Nevertheless, it will be convenient to discuss these factors under the following broad headings, bearing in mind there will be some overlapping between sections.

(a) Endocrinal control
(b) Multifactorial inheritance
(c) Racial difference
(d) Nutrition
(e) Diseases
(f) Socio-economic factors
(g) Secular trend ?

*Endocrinal control.* In this brief section it will be impossible to do anything other than mention some of the more obvious factors influencing the growth process and to say that the overall control of endocrines is a rather complex subject involving the central nervous system as well.

Growth hormone (GH) which is produced by the pituitary is essential for normal growth. At present it is obtained from human glands and can be given to children lacking it. Their subsequent growth can then be monitored on a standard growth chart to see when they catch up to within normal limits.

It seems that GH is necessary to stimulate the production of a further group of hormones, the somatomedins, which are produced mainly by the liver but also at other sites. These, in turn, act on the growing cartilage cells in long bones.

Thyroxine, which can be produced synthetically, is necessary from early foetal life and is particularly required for the nervous system. Thus early treatment is required in babies found to be deficient in it in order to avoid damage to their brains. Children at a later age who develop a deficiency of thyroxine may not suffer such damage, but will show slow growth and delayed maturity. Treatment in time, however, will allow their growth to catch up to within normal limits.

The hormonal events in puberty are difficult to study; however, it is known that at the beginning of puberty there is an increased secretion of follicle stimulating hormone (FSH) and luteinizing hormone (LH) of the pituitary. Oestrogens are then produced in girls which cause the growth of breasts, vagina and uterus and eventually menstruation. Testosterone in boys is produced under the influence of LH and causes the growth of penis, prostate and seminal vesicles, FSH being involved in testicular growth and spermatogenesis.

The adolescent growth spurt appears to require GH as well as androgens. In boys testosterone is the main agent, but in girls adrenal androgens are responsible.

*Multifactorial inheritance*. It is generally accepted that characters such as stature are inherited multifactorially, that is to say a large number of genes all acting in a small and additive way are involved. Thus no typical mendelian ratios are observed in the offspring, but rather there is a possibility of any value, between certain limits, being achieved.

In multifactorial inheritance it is still, however, possible to show likenesses between parents and children, not by conventional genetic ratios but by the use of correlation coefficients. This coefficient can take any value between 1 to -1, 0 implying no correlation or relationship at all, 1 perfect correlation and -1 complete negative correlation, that is, when one value is high the other is low and vice versa (see Statistical Appendix for methods of calculation).

It has been shown that if many genes with small additive effects, but without dominance, are involved, then the theoretical correlation coefficient between parents and offspring would be 0.5. This has, in practice, been found to be the case for such things as height, arm span, fingerprints and tooth size. If the environment has a substantial effect, it will tend to lower correlations. For example, lower correlations than normal were found for tooth size in Chinese immigrant families whose parents had come from China or Hong Kong but whose children had been born and raised in the United Kingdom. Similarly, dominance in which a single dose of a gene gives nearly the same effect as a double dose also leads to a reduction in correlation.

If people marry others who are similar to them in a characteristic, then the parental offspring correlations for that character are increased. It is therefore necessary to check whether this so-called assortative mating occurs before attempting to calculate parent-offspring correlations.

It must, however, be admitted that it is difficult sometimes to interpret a parental offspring correlation, since some factors may be acting to increase and others to decrease it.

Twins can also be used in growth studies to estimate the relative effects of heredity and environment, although there are certain difficulties not always generally realized in using them. The zygosity has to be proved carefully by as many tests as possible to ensure one is not misclassifying the type of twin; also in some monozygotic twins one may have an advantage over the other due, perhaps, to unequal sized placentas, and this may result in intra-uterine growth retardation. Finally environmental factors also tend to be more alike in monozygotic twins. However, in general one expects monozygotic twins to be much more alike than dizygotic. For example, correlation coefficients as high as 0.9 have been found for monozygotic twins.

It has been suggested that sex linkage may be important in some characteristics such as tooth size. If this is the case, sister/sister correlations will be higher than brother/brother, father/daughter higher than father/son and mother/son will exceed mother/daughter. However, not all investigators have found this effect.

Whilst it is true that height is mainly controlled in a multifactorial way, there are also major genes which affect it. Achondroplasia, for example, due to disturbance of cartilage formation results in low stature. Marfan's syndrome, on the other hand, is associated with loose jointedness, eye and cardiovascular defects and disproportionate skeletal growth giving rise to very tall thin adults. Both these conditions are due to dominant genes.

The inheritance of rate of development is rather more difficult and time-consuming to investigate than that of adult size as it is necessary to compare growth curves between parents and offspring or between sibs. In girls, however, it is relatively easy to look at the time of menarche as an index of maturity. Several authors have described fairly high correlations between the time of menarche of mothers and daughters and between sisters. It is higher still in identical twins who may have mean differences of only about 2 or 3 months. Thus it appears that rate of development, expressed as age at menarche, it also to quite an extent under genetic control.

*Racial differences.* These may be partly hereditary and partly environmental in nature, but the genetic aspect will be highlighted here as relevant environmental causes such as diet, disease and socio-economic factors are to be dealt with later on.

There is extensive data collected together for the International Biological Programme and published in *World Wide Variation in Human Growth* by Eveleth and Tanner (1976), but here it is only possible to mention a few general points from this work. It is often assumed that Asiatics are shorter than Europeans, but some of this may be due to nutrition. In order to discount this aspect, Asiatic boys and girls coming from high socio-economic groups in Hong Kong, and so not being influenced by bad environmental conditions, were found to be distinctly less tall at all ages than Europeans, but most noticeably when adult.

Differences in bodily proportions also exist; for example, the Chinese by adolescence have a proportionately larger sitting height to leg length compared with both Europeans and Africans.

Africans have slimmer hips for a given shoulder width and longer legs compared with sitting height than Europeans. In addition, the African newborn is ahead in skeletal maturity and stays ahead in this and dental maturity if nutritional factors are equal.

These sort of differences are presumably adaptive ones which have been produced over many generations of having evolved in particular environments.

*Nutrition.* Malnutrition is a potent cause of delayed growth in children as has been shown by the various wartime studies. If the period of malnutrition is relatively short, it is possible for the child to catch up and reach a normal adult stature; in other words, the tempo of growth is affected first and not necessarily the final adult size.

In the Third World, unfortunately, severe malnutrition can occur, resulting in infants with marasmus and kwashiorkor. The former is due to both proteins and calories being short, whereas with the latter it is primarily a protein deficiency. Both these conditions are very serious and need especial paediatric care if permanent change is not to occur.

More common, however, in the Western countries is malnutrition due to various problems such as "small for dates" babies who may need intravenous feeding for a period and malabsorption states, etc. Normally with good paediatric attention these problems can be overcome and should not cause long-term effects on growth, the baby usually gaining weight at an accelerated rate and catching up. It has been noted that urban children are larger and have a more rapid tempo of growth than rural ones; this is probably at least, partially, a nutritional effect.

The so-called secular trend in recent years is likely to be at least partly nutritional and is described in more detail below.

*Diseases.* In normal children minor diseases such as infectious fevers, respiratory infections and so on are not likely to have any effect on growth, although, of course, disturbances of mineralization may occur. However, in children with inadequate diets these sort of disturbances may be important and a slowing down of growth can occur. Normally, later on, there will be a catch-up in growth and the child returns to its original centile.

Apart from achondroplasia and Marfan's syndrome already mentioned, other diseases may have a profound effect on growth. Turner's syndrome, where there is a lack of a second X chromosome, results in a girl of short stature associated with webbing of the neck, facial changes and defective sexual development. Down's syndrome, which is usually due to trisomy 21, also reduces stature as well as producing other changes.

Hypothyroidism and lack of growth hormone are two well-known endocrine disturbances which result in short stature, but fortunately now, when recognized in time, treatment by the appropriate hormone causes a marked improvement, catch-up growth occurring. Recently it has been realized that a lack of growth can occur due to psychological causes; this may happen in children who are very unhappy at home and when they are hospitalized or otherwise removed from the home environment their growth starts again and no other treatment may be necessary.

*Socio-economic factors.* Children from different social groups in society vary both in size and in the speed of their growth, so first it will be necessary briefly to say how social classes may be defined. For this purpose the classification of occupations adopted by the Registrar General in the United Kingdom may be used. Class I consists of occupations which require the highest professional qualifications, usually a university degree or its equivalent. Occupations in Social Class II may also demand a professional qualification, and school teachers and many civil servants are in this group, but in addition managers and others of a similar position in industry are included. These two social groups are of a non-manual nature in general. Class III is the largest single group, and it can be subdivided into non-manual and manual. In the former are included the remaining non-manual occupations, such as foremen, shop assistants and clerical workers. The occupations in the other section are all regarded as "skilled manual". Class IV consists mostly of semi-skilled manual occupations and Class V contains the unskilled.

In the National Child Development Study, which describes a nationwide survey in the United Kingdom of children born in the first week of March 1958, there was an overall difference in height of 3.3 cm in the 7-year-olds between children from Social Classes I and II and those of unskilled labourers, the former being taller (Goldstein 1971). Some of these differences may well persist into adult life. Family size also has an effect on growth, the larger families having smaller children, although this effect is not so marked in higher socio-economic groups.

Permanent tooth eruption has been reported to occur earlier in more favoured groups; for example, in one study children in Classes I and II were found to be 3.4 months in advance on an average over those in classes below. On the other hand, if many extractions of deciduous molar teeth are preformed, this may cause earlier eruption of premolars which may mask the effect.

Another measure of maturity, the menarche, shows that there is earlier maturation in the socially better-off classes in most populations studied.

*Secular trend.* During about the last 100 years in industrialized countries there has been a trend towards children maturing earlier and growing larger than their parents. For example, in Sweden, where data is particularly complete, there is a difference equivalent to nearly 1½ years of growth between 7 to 18 years of age from 1883 to 1938. There is, however, less difference between figures from 1938 to 1968 (Ljung *et al.* 1974).

Damon (1968), in comparing generations of Harvard graduates in the United States, found that there was an increase in height of 2.63 cm between those born (on the average) in 1858 and 1888, 1.14 cm between those born 1888 and 1918 but none between the latter and those born in 1941. This suggests that the secular trend in well-off populations is ceasing, but this is not yet the case in other sections of the community.

Acceleration of growth, as shown by the fall in the age of menarche, also demonstrates this secular trend, having gone from something like 17 years of age in 1840 to the present 13 years in Western European countries. Early literary evidence, however, seems to indicate that in the Middle Ages the age of menarche was not very different from that of today and so the retardation appears to have taken place after this period.

The reasons for these changes are not entirely understood, although it is likely that better nutrition and freedom from disease in childhood are major factors. An additional mechanism in relation to size could be due to an increase in outbreeding causing hybrid vigour, and this could have been consequent on the increase of mobility of the population and therefore the choice of mates.

## BIBLIOGRAPHY

AMUNDSEN, D. W. and C. J. DIERS (1973) The age of menarche in Mediaeval Europe, *Hum. Biol.* **45**, 363.

AVERY, G. B. (1975) *Neonatology: Pathophysiology and Management of the Newborn*, Lippincott, Philadelphia.

BOWDEN, D. E. J. and D. H. GOOSE (1969) Inheritance of tooth size in Liverpool families, *J. Med. Genet.* **6**, 55.

BUCKLER, J. H. M. (1979) *A Reference Manual of Growth and Development*, Blackwells, Oxford.

CLEMENTS, E. M. B., E. DAVIES-THOMAS and K. G. PICKETT (1953) Time of eruption of permanent teeth in British children in 1947-8, *Brit. med. J.* **1,** 1421.

DEMIRJIAN, A. and G.-Y. LEVESQUE (1980) Sexual differences in dental development and prediction of emergence, *J. dent. Res.* **59,** 1110.

DAMON, A. (1968) Secular trend in height and weight within old American families at Harvard 1870-1965, *Am. J. Phys. Anthrop.* **29,** 45.

EVELETH, P. B. and J. M. TANNER (1976) *Worldwide Variation in Human Growth,* Cambridge Univ. Press, Cambridge.

FALKNER, F. and J. M. TANNER (eds.) (1978) *Human Growth 2. Postnatal Growth,* Plenum, New York and London.

GARN, S. M. and M. T. KEATING (1980) Effect of various prenatal determinants on size and growth through seven years, *Ecol. of Food and Nutrit.* **9,** 109.

GARN, S. M., A. B. LEWIS and R. S. KEREWSKY (1965) X-linked inheritance of tooth size, *J. dent. Res.* **44,** 439.

GOLDSTEIN, H. (1971) Factors influencing the height of seven-year-old children: results from the National Child Development Study, *Hum. Biol.* **43,** 92.

GREULICH, W. W. and S. I. PYLE (1959) *Radiographic Atlas of Skeletal Development of the Hand and Wrist,* 2nd ed., Stanford Univ. Press, Stanford.

HOUSTON, W. J. B., J. C. MILLER and J. M. TANNER (1979) Prediction of the timing of the adolescent growth spurt from ossification events in hand-wrist films, *Brit. J. Ortho.* **6,** 145.

LJUNG, B. O., A. BERGSTEN-BRUCEFORS and G. LINDGREN (1974) The secular trend in physical growth in Sweden, *Ann. hum. Biol.* **1,** 245.

MARSHALL, W. A. (1977) *Human Growth and its Disorders,* Academic Press, London.

MEREDITH, H. V. (1971) Human head circumference from birth to early adulthood: racial, regional and sex comparisons, *Growth,* **35,** 233.

POST, E. M. and R. A. RICHMAN (1981) A condensed table for predicting adult stature, *J. Pediat.* **98,** 440.

PYLE, S. I., A. M. WATERHOUSE and W. W. GREULICH (1971) *A Radiographic Standard of Reference for the Growing Hand and Wrist,* Case, Western Reserve Univ. Press, distributed by Year Book Med. Publ., Chicago.

SORSBY, A. (ed.) (1973) *Clinical Genetics,* 2nd ed., Butterworths, London.

TANNER, J. M. (1962) *Growth at Adolescence,* 2nd ed., Blackwells, Oxford.

TANNER, J. M. (1978) *Foetus into Man: Physical Growth from Conception to Maturity,* Open Books, London.

TANNER, J. M., R. H. WHITEHOUSE, W. A. MARSHALL, M. J. R. HEALY and H. GOLDSTEIN (1975) *Assessment of Skeletal Maturity and Prediction of Adult Height: TW 2 Method,* Academic Press, London.

TANNER, J. M., R. H. WHITEHOUSE and M. TAKAISHI (1966) Standards from birth to maturity for height, weight, height velocity and weight velocity in British children, *Arch. Dis. Child.* **41,** 454.

VAN WERING, E. R. (1981) The secular growth trend in Aruba between 1954 and 1974, *Hum. Biol.* **53,** 105.

# CHAPTER 2

## *Bone as a Tissue*

Bone is formed throughout embryonic, foetal and post-natal life by the transformation of connective tissues. Such transformation may take place directly from sheets of fibrous connective tissue to form membrane or dermal bones. This process is referred to as intramembranous ossification and a good example arc the bones of the skull vault. In embryonic skeletal development, however, most bones develop by the transformation of hyaline cartilage models into bone by endochondral ossification. This distinction only applies embryonically, since the bone finally formed by these methods cannot be distinguished. Both methods may be involved in the formation of a single bone; for example, the mandible and the cranial base. In order to fully understand the mechanisms involved in the development and growth of the orofacial skeleton, it is necessary to be conversant with the fundamental biological roles of cartilage and bone in skeletal development and growth.

### DEVELOPMENT OF BONE

The hyaline cartilage which forms the primary cartilagenous skeleton, for example Meckel's cartilage, consists of chondrocytes enclosed by a turgid yet flexible organic matrix (Fig. 2.1). These unique and specific physical properties are endowed on the organic matrix principally by the large amounts of chondroitin sulphates in combination with non-collagenous protein which has the property of retaining large numbers of water molecules. The organic matrix is not normally calcified, except when undergoing endochondral ossification, and because the tissue is avascular, metabolites must enter and leave by simple diffusion. As there are no blood vessels to occlude, cartilage can be utilized in areas of the skeleton which are subjected to pressure. There is some evidence to suggest the greater the pressure the larger the amount of chondroitin sulphates present in the matrix relative to the other principal matrix component collagen. Because metabolites enter and leave cartilage by diffusion, it can also exist without a covering vascular membrane or perichondrium. Therefore, it is ideal in areas such as articular cartilage and the surface of cartilagenous growth centres. Also, since cartilage like soft tissue has an interstitial as well as appositional mode of growth, an enclosing membrane is not necessary. Interstitial growth is possible because the matrix is not

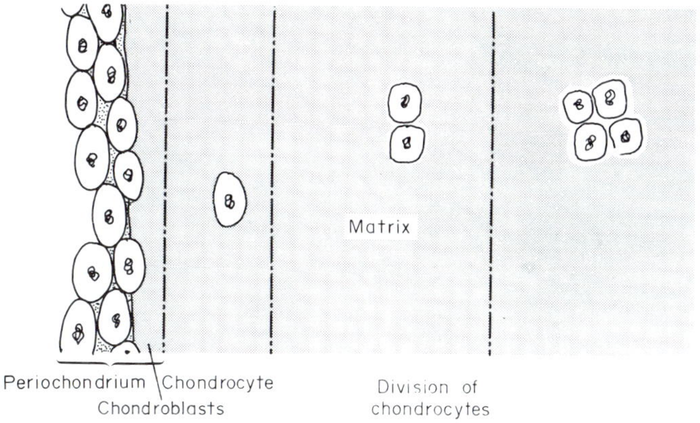


Fig. 2.1. Growth of cartilage occurs by surface deposition, as chondrocytes differentiating from the perichondrium, or interstitially by division of existing chondrocytes.

calcified and can, therefore, expand to accommodate the chrondrocytes resulting from cell division. Hence physical and biological properties of cartilage are ideal for the dual purposes of flexible support and growth necessary during skeletal development.

Because of the incorporation of mineral salts into its organic matrix, bone has the property of hardness (Fig. 2.2). Consequently diffusion of metabolites into the calcified matrix of bone, does not occur significantly and a blood supply is required. Since the bone cells become enclosed by a non-expandable calcified matrix, interstitial growth is not possible and all bone growth must be appositional, whether the method of osteogenesis is intramembranous or endochondral. A vascular covering, the periosteum, is required to produce the bone-forming cells and, therefore, allow bone growth to take place.

Cartilage can be defined specifically as a pressure-adapted tissue, but bone

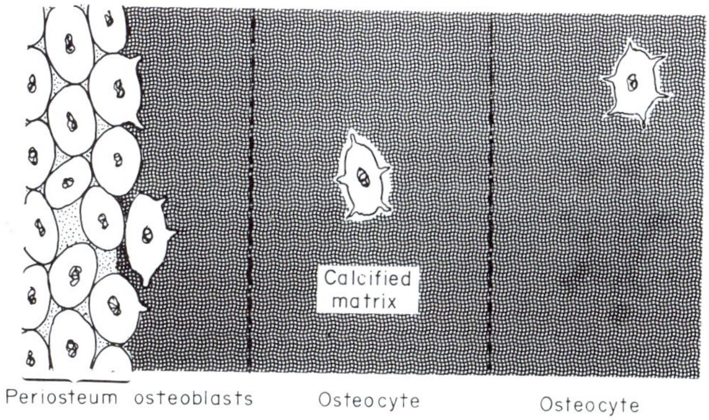


Fig. 2.2. Osteoblasts differentiate from the periosteum and become enclosed by a rigid calcified matrix. Growth must take place by surface deposition.

is a tension-adapted tissue, or more precisely the vascular periosteum of the bone, and is pressure sensitive. Pressure on the periosteum causes vascular occlusion and may produce bone resorption. Tension on the periosteum will result in the differentiation of osteoblasts from the periosteal cells and, as a result new bone will be formed.

### Calcification

Before embarking on a description of the methods of bone formation, it is necessary to appreciate some of the biochemical and physiological factors involved in calcification of bone. Indeed the same general factors may be taken into consideration when discussing the calcification of other hard tissues, for example enamel, dentine and cementum.

All hard tissue formation takes place in two phases, that is the secretion of a specific organic matrix, followed by the incorporation of mineral salts. However, the chemical nature of this inorganic phase is not yet precisely defined at all stages of hard tissue formation. There is a further problem in elucidating the mechanism by which the organic matrix becomes calcified, and as yet there is no single concept which covers all calcified tissues. Furthermore, it should be remembered that the skeleton plays an important role in calcium homeostasis. As such, the skeleton can be a sensitive indicator of hormonal imbalance, dietary deficiencies and other physiological defects in calcium and phosphorus metabolism. The latter is, however, in general outside the scope of the current text.

*The organic matrix.* About 90 per cent by weight of the organic matrix of bone is formed by the fibrous protein collagen which contributes to the tensile strength of the tissue. The organic matrix which surrounds the collagen fibres consists of protein carbohydrate complexes and lipid which constitute approximately 9.5 and 0.5 per cent respectively. Collagen is rich in the amino acids glycine, proline, hydroxyproline and hydroxylysine, the last two being found only in connective tissues. Hydroxylysine excretion in the urine, therefore, has been used as an indicator of bone turnover. There is evidence to show that the constituent amino acids of bone collagen are assembled intracellularly in association with ribosomes. Subsequently, the sub-units of collagen, tropocollagen, are transferred into vesicles and then secreted into the extracellular matrix by the vesicles fusing with the cell membrane and releasing their contents. Collagen fibrils are constructed from assemblies of tropocollagen in a particular and ordered manner so that three $\alpha_1$ polypeptide chains, in which the amino acids are in a specific sequence, each twisted into a left-hand helix around a common axis, form a triple chained rope-like structure. In cartilage the polypeptide chains are all the $\alpha_1$ type, but in bone they are two $\alpha_1$ chains and one $\alpha_2$ chain in which the amino acid sequence is different. The tropocollagen macromolecule has a molecular weight of approximately 300,000 and measures about 300 × 1.4 nM, which makes it easily resolvable in the electron microscope.

The collagen fibre is clearly recognizable in the electron microscope by its banded pattern repeated regularly at 64-nM intervals (Fig. 2.3), but there is considerable debate as to how this is achieved (Fig. 2.4). Since the bonding pattern was repeated at intervals approximately a quarter of the length of the tropocollagen macromolecule, this was thought to represent a quarter stagger arrangement. Another possible explanation suggests that the tropocollagen macromolecule has five bonding zones of 26.5 nM in length and four bonding zones 37.5 nM in length, which result in the 64 nM periodicity. Alternatively, a more radical view postulates a macromolecular micelle model in which the tropocollagen is wound into a disc-shaped structure and aligned to produce a fibril.

The stability of the fibres is maintained by hydrogen bonding between the tropocollagen units which form the triple helix. With age, stability is increased by the formation of more permanent covalent bonds. There is also some evidence to suggest that non-collagenous proteins may be involved in maintaining fibre stability.

The protein carbohydrate complexes of bone are of two types, the so-called proteoglycans and the glycoproteins. These are the substances which contribute significantly to the physical characteristics of connective tissue matrices; for example, cartilage which was mentioned earlier. Proteoglycans consist of a protein chain or core to which is attached polysaccharide side chains, glycosaminoglycans (Fig. 2.5). These glycosaminoglycans consist of regularly repeating units of two sugars. There can be sulphate groups attached to the sugars and, in fact, chondroitin sulphate, where the disaccharide unit consists of glucuronic acid and acetylgalactosamine, is predominant. The latter can be sulphated at two positions to produce chondroitin 4 sulphate and chondroitin 6 sulphate. These compounds are highly negatively charged and have been regarded as important macromolecules in the initiation of calcification in cartilage. There is also some evidence to suggest that glycoprotein may form the core to some macromolecules. Glycoproteins also contain carbohydrate covalently linked to protein. However, the carbohydrate chains are relatively short and contain a wide variety of sugars.

The amount of lipid in bone is very small and the non-polar lipids are the most abundant. Interest in lipids was stimulated by the suggestion that they are involved in the calcification process.

*The inorganic phase.* The main elemental constituents of the inorganic phase in calcified tissues are calcium, phosphate, hydroxyl ions, carbonate and water. The mineral is a basic calcium phosphate, being an apatite, hydroxyapatite $Ca_{10}(PO_4)_6OH_2$. The general formula for apatites is

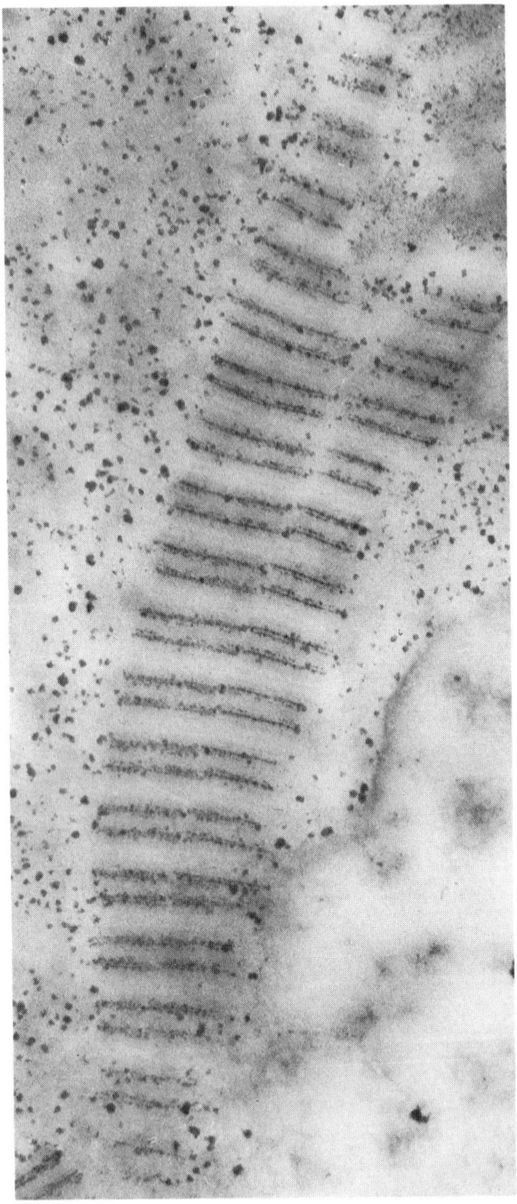

Fig. 2.3. Collagen fibre with a boundary pattern repeated at 64 nM. Calcium-binding sites on the fibres are indicated by the electron-dense particles.

$M_{10}(RO_4)X_2$. Apatites are often phosphates, and in the case of naturally occurring phosphates the dominant cation is calcium. The last element of the

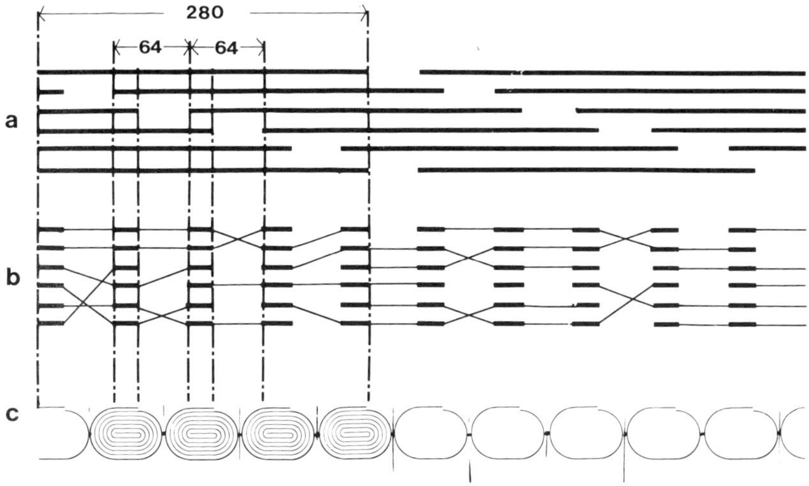


Fig. 2.4. Representation of the schemes proposed for the organization of the tropocollagen molecules into fibres; (a) quarter stagger arrangement of Hodge, (b) the aggregation scheme of Grant, (c) micelle model of Davidovits (after Herring 1968, *Clinical Orthopedics,* by kind permission Lippincott, Harper & Row).

group may be FE, $Cl_2$, Br, OH and of the phosphate apatites chlorapatite, fluoroapatite and hydroxyapatite have been most studied.

There is evidence based on X-ray analysis and electron microscopy to suggest that the mineral phase, at least in bone, is present both in the crystalline and amorphous phase, amorphous calcium phosphate. This amorphous material has no significant repetitive periodicity to give a

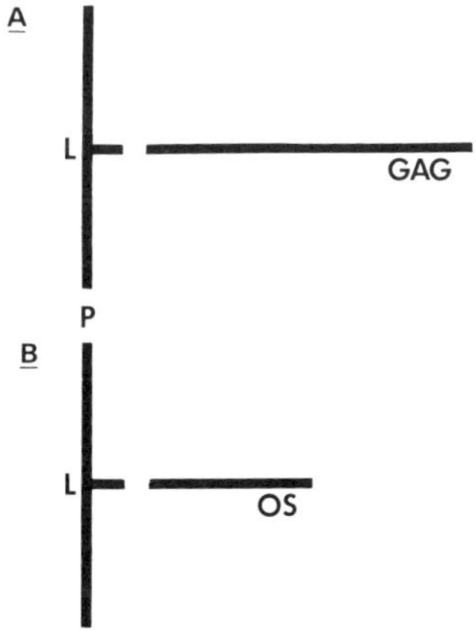


Fig. 2.5. Simplified diagram of the classes of protein carbohydrate complexes: (a) proteoglycan, (b) glycoprotein. L, covalent linkage; P, protein core; GAG, glycosaminoglycan; OS, oligosaccharide.

recognizable X-ray diffraction pattern. The presence of amorphous material was suggested initially by electron microscope studies showing non-crystalline mineral particles in bone. The X-ray diffraction studies demonstrated this indirectly and showed that the X-ray peak intensities from the apatite portion of the bone pattern were considerably less than expected if one assumes that bone mineral is entirely crystalline. There is a larger proportion of amorphous material present during the early stages of calcification in bone, but the amount decreases with age.

The amorphous material is transformed to a crystalline phase which is an apatite, probably octocalcium phosphate. This crystalline phase is progressively transformed into a final and more stable crystalline phase at physiological pH, hydroxyapatite.

The first formed crystallites in dentine, bone and cementum are very small and increase in size up to a maximum of about 5 nM × 25 nM (Fig. 2.6). Hence the mineral density of the tissue increases with the deposition of further crystallites and not by crystallite growth. The surface area presented by these crystallites, therefore, is very large and provides for various interchange reactions between the crystallites and tissue fluids. Since these crystallites are only a few unit cells in thickness, a large proportion of its ions will be at the crystallite surface.

In enamel the first formed crystallites are small but grow to a large size approximately 100 nM × 50 nM. These large crystals cannot be produced in synthetic systems under normal physiological conditions, suggesting that in enamel matrix there are specific and unique conditions promoting the growth of large crystallites (Fig. 2.6).

*The initiation of calcification.* There is considerable debate regarding the mechanism of initiation in calcified tissues. No current single theory appears completely acceptable for all calcified tissues.

One of the first important suggestions was that a mechanism exists to elevate the local concentration of calcium ions. Robison (1932) noticed that alkaline phosphatase was always present at sites of calcification and suggested that this enzyme hydrolysed phosphate esters to increase the local concentration of phosphate to the level where calcium phosphate would precipitate. The principle objections that developed to Robison's concept were that the necessary phosphate esters were never demonstrated and the alkaline phosphatase was present only in advance of the mineralizing front.

The activity product $A_{Ca} \times A_{HPO_4}$ of normal serum is about $1 \times 10^{-7}$ which is supersaturated with respect to calcium phosphate, but undersaturated with respect to hydroxyapatite. Although circulating fluids are supersaturated with respect to $Ca^{++} \times PO_4^{=}$ new crystals do not form spontaneously, that is the solution is metastable. The seeding concept suggests that a crystalline substance may, by virtue of its structure, be sufficiently

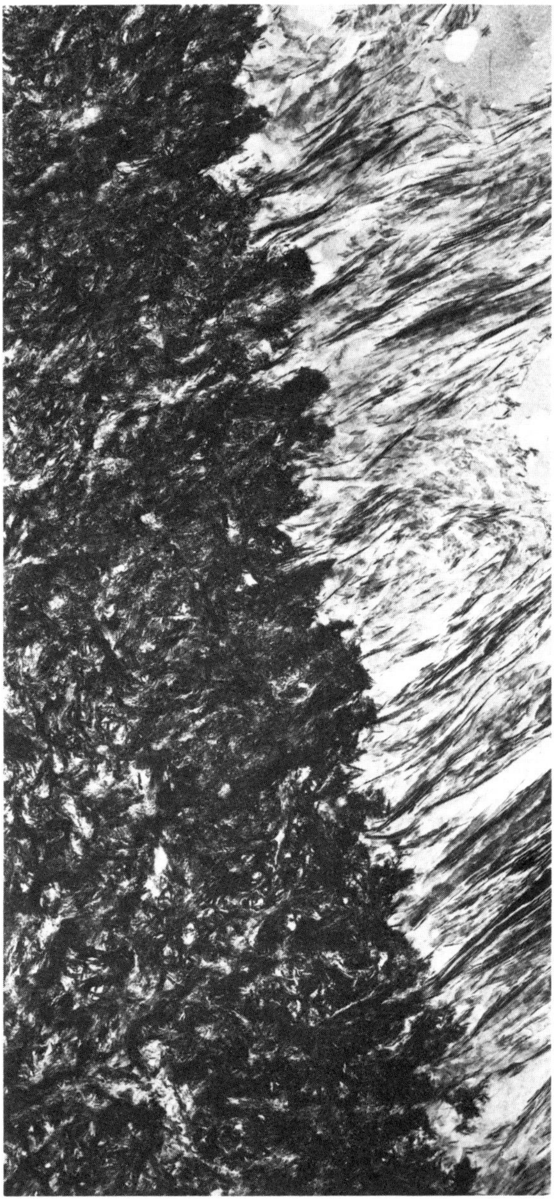

Fig. 2.6. Electron micrograph of the amelodentinal junction showing the typically small hydroxyapatite crystallites of dentine (left) and the larger crystallites of enamel (right).

similar to hydroxyapatite to induce the aggregation of calcium and phosphate ions. The body fluids which are supersaturated would then form a complete crystal by orientated growth or epitaxy. This theory overcomes the difficulty of precipitating bone salt from a solution temporarily oversaturated with calcium and phosphate ions in an area where the amount of phosphate ester is insufficient to exceed the solubility product. Thermodynamically this is more economical than precipitation, the free energy change being much smaller.

The seed may be organic and crystalline in nature, and sufficiently like hydroxyapatite for epitaxy to take place. In recent years attempts have been made to explain nucleation by collagen fibres having specific epitactic centres. Specific epitactic centres have proved difficult to identify accurately at the molecular level. However, only collagens with a 64 nM axial repeating unit are able to induce calcification *in vitro,* and collagens from tissues such as skin which do not normally calcify will only do so when solubilized or reconstituted.

Electron microscope studies show that the earliest resolvable mineral particles that can be seen are associated with the periodic banding of the collagen fibres (Fig. 2.3). Subsequently the crystals that develop are always orientated with their *C*-axis parallel to the collagen fibre.

There has always been controversy as to whether the initial calcification takes place within or on the surface of the collagen fibre. Recent work in measuring the interfibrillar space suggests that at least 63 per cent of the inorganic phase is inside the collagen fibres of bone and dentine. Since the intermolecular spaces in bone collagen are 0.6 nM but only 0.3 nM in soft tissue, phosphate ions 0.4 nM in diameter could diffuse into the collagen fibres of bone but not the collagen fibres of soft tissue. It has also been recently shown that only a small proportion of the free carboxyl groups in collagen are involved in nucleation. Therefore, though all forms of collagen may possess epitactic centres consisting of juxtaposed carboxyl groups, if these are situated within the fibres they will be accessible to diffusing ions only in hard tissue collagen.

Collagen with a 64-nM periodicity is not always present in calcifying tissues; for example, in epiphyseal or condylar growth cartilage. Calcification in cartilage may be initiated in relation to other organic macromolecules such as protein polysaccharide complexes (Fig. 2.7). There is evidence to show that preceding calcification in cartilage protein polysaccharides are degraded by proteolytic enzymes, thereby allowing apatite crystallites to develop and crystal growth to take place.

Collagen does not form part of enamel matrix in which apatite crystallites grow to become larger than crystallites in other calcified tissues. It is possible, however, that enamel matrix does not initiate calcification but collagen fibres extending through the amelodentinal junction at the beginning of hard tissue formation.

Recent work also attempts to define more clearly the role of hard tissue forming cells in the initiation and control of the calcification process. Staining of unfixed mouse calavaria for calcium and phosphate has shown that with

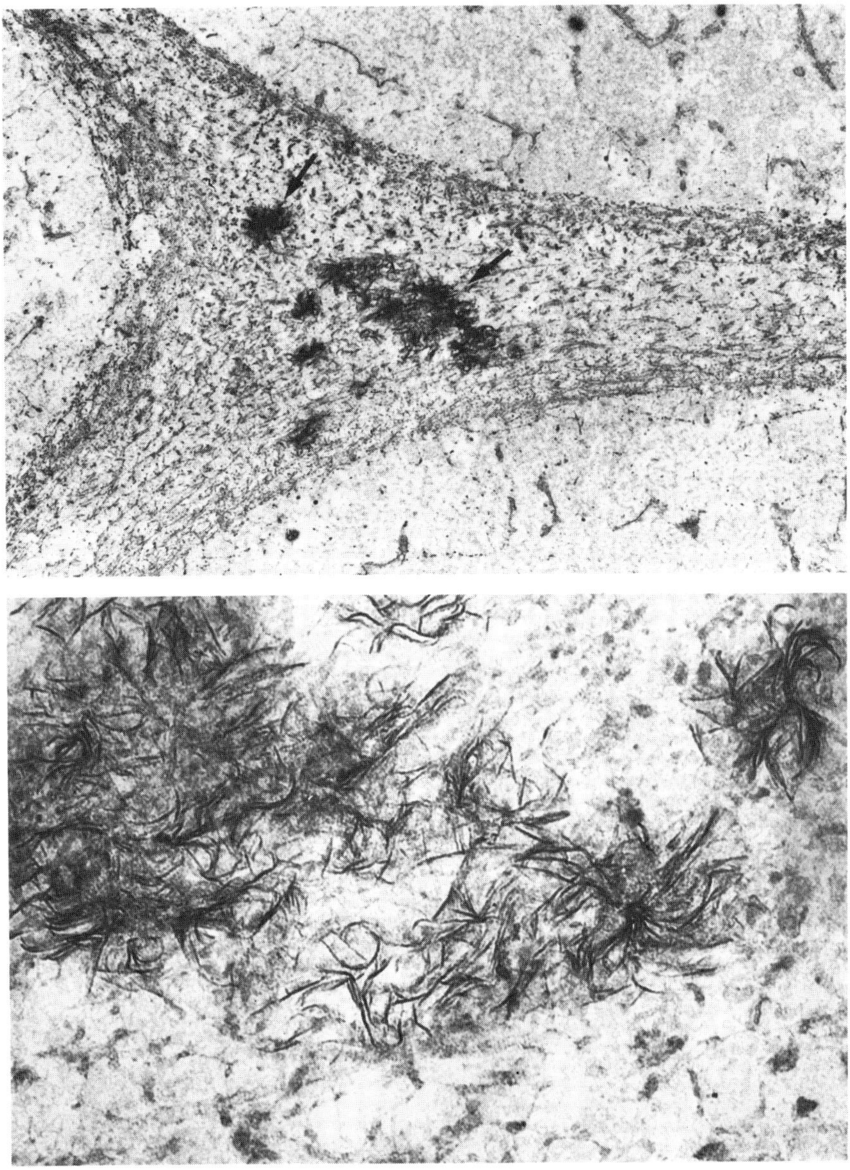

Fig. 2.7. (a) Electron micrograph showing calcification in the matrix septa of hypertrophic cartilage (arrowed); (b) at higher magnification the crystallites appear to emanate from electron-dense particles which may be proteoglycan.

the bone cells there appears to be a specific loading and unloading pattern for these elements. The intracellular material is deposited at the mineralizing front. Similarly it has been shown using staining techniques for calcium that chondrocytes and odontoblasts are involved in the transport of calcium during cartilage calcification and dentine formation (Fig. 2.8). Using $Ca^{45}$ it can be shown that mitochondria in the chondrocytes of calcifying cartilage have the ability to concentrate calcium which can be visualized in the form of intramitochondrial granules (Fig. 2.9). The mitochondria may also be involved in the transport of calcium and phosphate into the extracellular matrix.

Cells may also be directly involved in the initiation of calcification by the production of so-called "matrix vesicles". The vesicles are produced by the cells of calcifying systems by a process of budding from the cell membrane. Vesicles, it is suggested, are produced with the ability to form apatite crystallites internally which eventually rupture the enclosing membrane and are exposed to the tissues fluids with resulting further crystallite growth. These vesicles have been identified in all developing calcifying tissues except enamel, and have very specific features namely: (i) they are between 100 nM and 200 nM in diameter, (ii) they are surrounded by a distinct trilaminar membrane, (iii) they are electron-dense after osmium fixation due to the presence of lipid, (iv) they contain alkaline phosphatase and ATP actively (Fig. 2.10).

It is suggested that the alkaline phosphatase, probably hydrolysis organic phosphate, and together with calcium bound by the lipid or pumped across the vesicle membrane, forms an apatite crystallite within the vesicle. There is evidence to suggest that the vesicles can concentrate calcium against an unfavourable concentration gradient, since even in a rachitic animal, where the tissue fluids are low in calcium, crystallites form with the vesicles (Fig. 2.11).

### Intramembranous Ossification

Membrane bones are typically laid down in sheets at relatively high speed. Indeed it may be difficult to detect a layer of osteoid. The membrane bones of the skull are the first bones to develop, over the rapidly growing brain, at about 6 weeks of intrauterine life. Mesenchyme cells of the embryonic fibrous connective tissue enclosing the developing brain come together and differentiate into osteoblasts. At the same time fibres appear to form the primitive bone matrix or osteoid in which spicules of calcified tissue may be seen. These spicules by the addition of mineral increase in size to eventually become fine trabeculae (Fig. 5.2). The trabeculae may enclose spaces containing blood vessels. As the trabeculae enlarge, osteoblasts gradually become enclosed within the calcified matrix to form osteocytes. The outermost layers of differentiated cells take on the characteristics of a cellular layer of the periosteum. Experiments using radioisotopes have confirmed that this type of bone is fast growing.

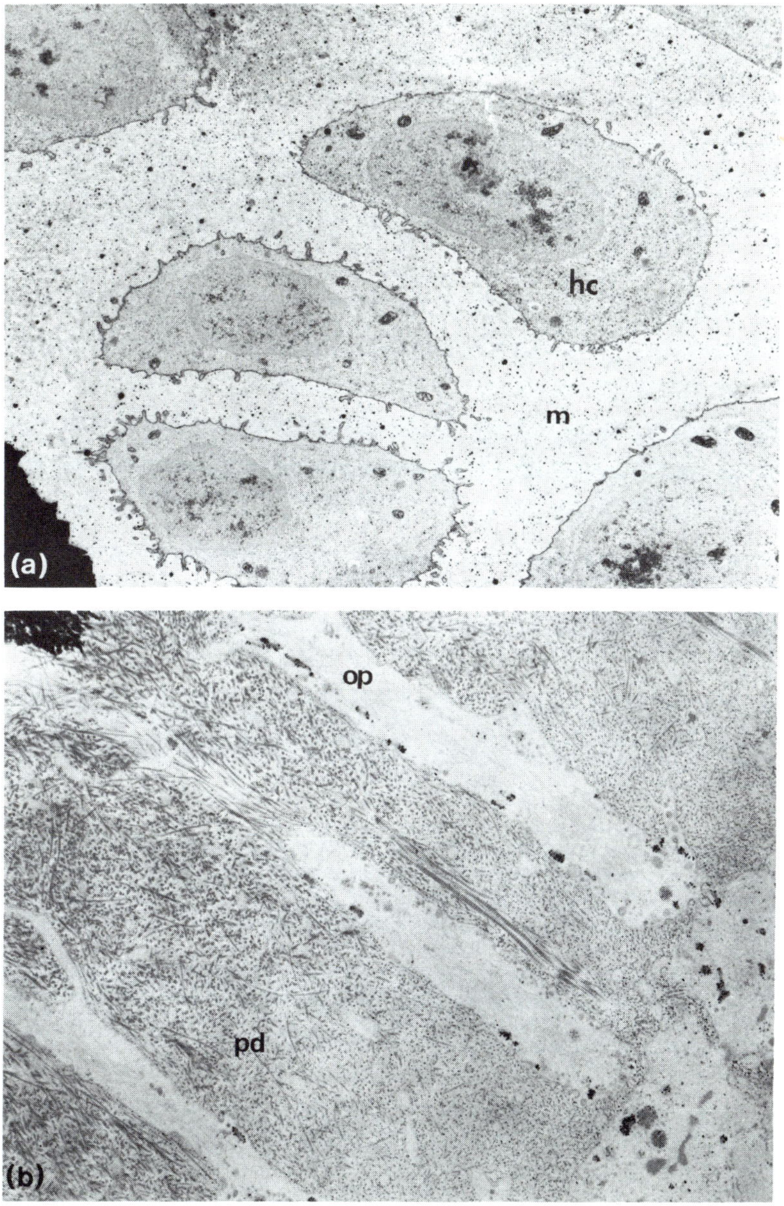


Fig. 2.8. Electron micrographs of (a) cartilage, (b) dentine, showing the intra and extracellular localization of calcium ions which form part of the electron-dense precipitates. hc, hypertrophic chondrocyte; m, matrix; op, odontoblast process; pd, pre-dentine.

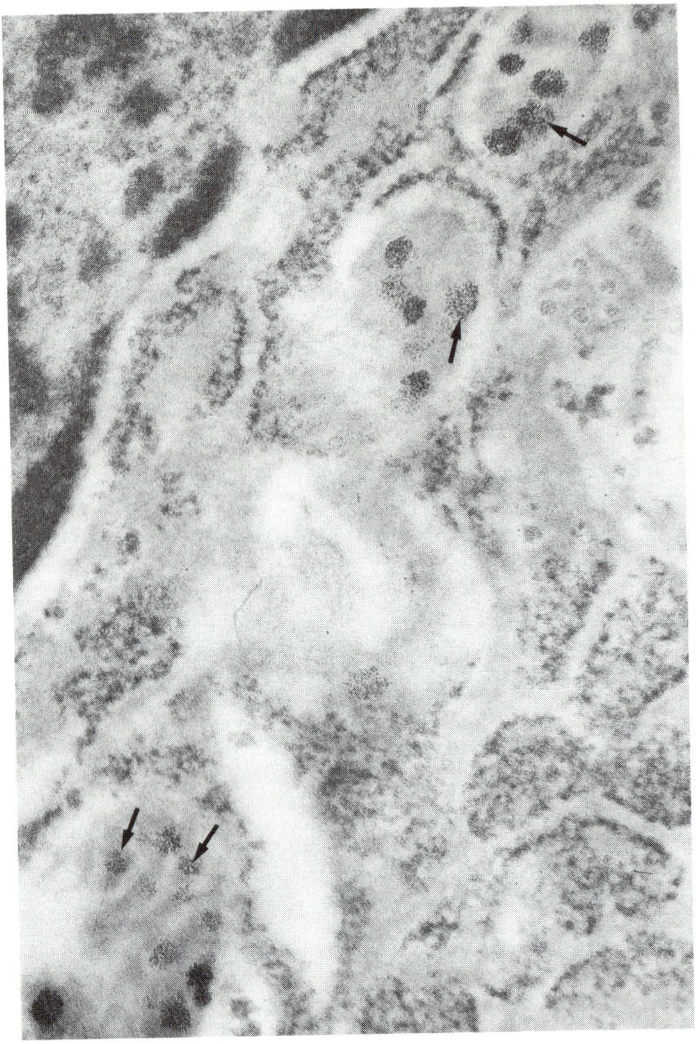

Fig. 2.9. Electron micrograph of bone cells processed anhydrously in which the mitrochondria contain electron-dense granules (arrowed) known to consist of calcium and phosphorus.

**Endochondral Ossification**

Endochondral ossification is the replacement of hyaline cartilage by bone. The detailed sequence of events during this process, as seen histologically, may differ from site to site within the developing skeleton, but the basic mechanism of cartilage replacement is the same. Endochondral ossification is usually described in relation to the development and growth of a long bone,

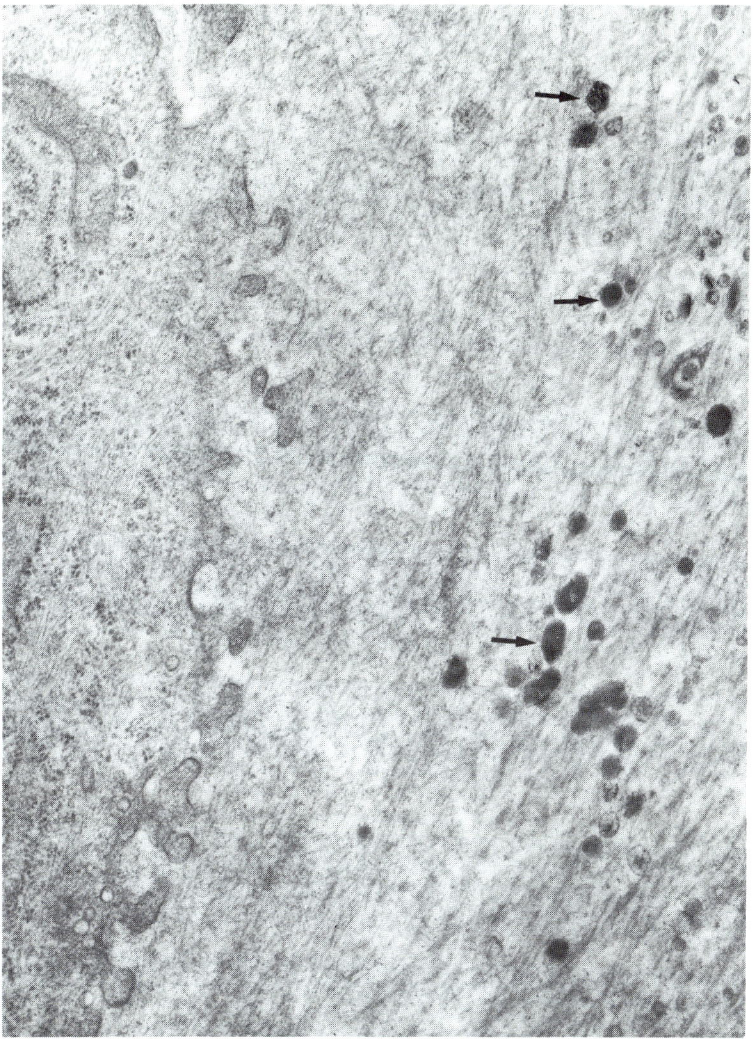

Fig. 2.10. Electron micrograph of cartilage in which numerous extra-cellular matrix vesicles may be seen (arrowed). Many are electron dense and some contain crystallites.

but the development and growth of the condylar process of the mandible serves the purpose equally well (Fig. 6.6).

The shape of the mandibular condylar process is mapped out by the development of the secondary mandibular condylar cartilage (see later chapter). This cartilage model, which appears at about 12 weeks of intrauterine life, develops from a condensation of mesenchyme cells or blastema. It is carrot shaped, with its narrower anterior end enclosed by the

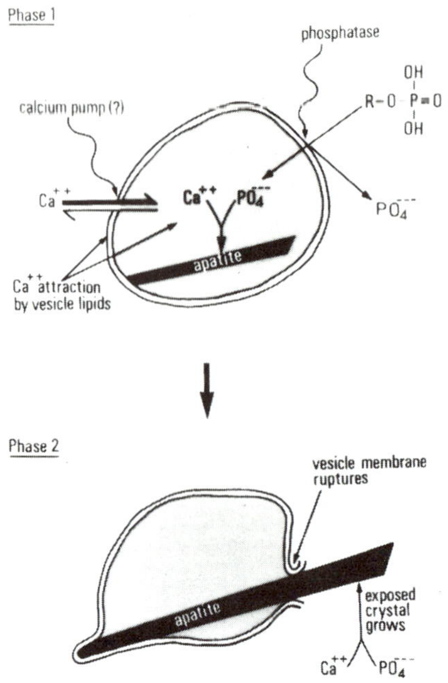


Fig. 2.11 *Phase 1.* During phase 1, intravesicular calcium concentration is increased by the affinity for lipids of the vesicle membrane and the interior. The possibility of an inwardly directed calcium pump is indicated in the diagram, but has not been proven to exist. Phosphatase (either alkaline phosphatase, pyrophosphatase or ATPase) at the vesicle membrane hydrolyses ester phosphate of the matrix fluid to produce a local increase in phosphate concentration. The intravesicular ionic product $(Ca^{2+}) \times (PO_4^{3-})$ is thereby raised, resulting in the initial deposition of calcium and phosphate as hydroxyapatite (and probably also an amorphous calcium phosphate).

*Phase 2.* With accumulation and growth, the intravesicular crystals are exposed to the extravesicular environment. Phase 2 begins with the exposure of preformed apatite crystals to the extravesicular fluid which in a normal animal is supersaturated with respect to apatite enabling further crystal growth. (by kind permission of Professor H. C. Anderson, University of Kansas Medical Centre, Kansas City and *Elsevier/ North-Holland Biomedical Press, Amsterdam.*

developing membrane bone of the body of the mandible. The cartilage grows upwards, backwards and outwards by appositional and interstitial growth at its posterior end, thereby giving rise to the condylar process of the mandible. At the anterior end the cartilage is gradually replaced by bone in the process of endochondral ossification.

The hypertrophic cartilage cells become increasingly separated by the formation of organic matrix. The organic matrix septa gradually calcify so that the hypertrophic chondrocytes become almost completely surrounded by the calcified matrix. This is followed by a vascular invasion of the calcified cartilage. Giant resorbing cells (chondroclasts) with several nuclei and a distinct brush border remove most of the calcified cartilage matrix. The precise origin of these giant resorbing cells is unknown, but similar cells are involved in the resorption of other hard tissues. Fine bone trabeculae are formed to replace the resorbed calcified cartilage matrix. The bone-forming cells, osteoblasts, probably differentiate from the undifferentiated mesenchyme cells which accompany the blood vessels invading the cartilage. When the condylar process of the mandible is fully developed, at the end of the second decade, only a thin layer or cap of cartilage remains. The condylar growth cartilage, therefore, after having mapped out the shape of the condylar process, is almost completely replaced by bone by the process of endochondral ossification.

## Bone Cells

Bone formation takes place in association with a layer of bone-forming cells or osteoblasts which cover the bone surface where active bone formation is taking place. As this proceeds, some of the osteoblasts may eventually become completely enclosed by bone to form osteocytes. Since bone is a dynamic tissue responding rapidly to the functional and physiological demands placed upon it, bone formation is often accompanied by bone resorption. This resorption is normally associated with giant multinucleated cells or osteoclasts.

*The osteoblast.* These cells are confined to the surface of bone where they form a monolayer (Fig. 2.12). The cells which immediately overlie the osteoblast are preosteoblast or osteoprogenitor cells which will replace the osteoblasts as they become involved in the forming bone. New bone matrix formation only occurs between the osteoblast and existing bone, so that there is always a zone of mineral-free matrix between the osteoblast and the calcification front (Fig. 2.12). Histologically the osteoblast has an eccentrically placed nucleus, highly basophilic cytoplasm and a large negatively stained Golgi region. In the electron microscope this is visualized as an extensive granular endoplasmic reticulum, a large and complex Golgi region consisting of several groups of lamellae and vesicles of varying types, sizes and electron density (Fig. 2.12).

The osteoblast is a cell, therefore, well differentiated to produce an organic matrix which under normal physiological conditions becomes calcified. Evidence of this function has been obtained from autoradiographic studies using tritiated glycine and other collagen precursors. However, the precise mechanism by which the collagen precursors leave the cell remain obscure. Since numerous cell processes extend through the unmineralized matrix to within a fraction of a micron of the mineral front, it has been suggested that the osteoblast may be directly involved in the process of matrix calcification. Indeed evidence now exists that these cells are directly involved in the transport of calcium and phosphorus during calcification.

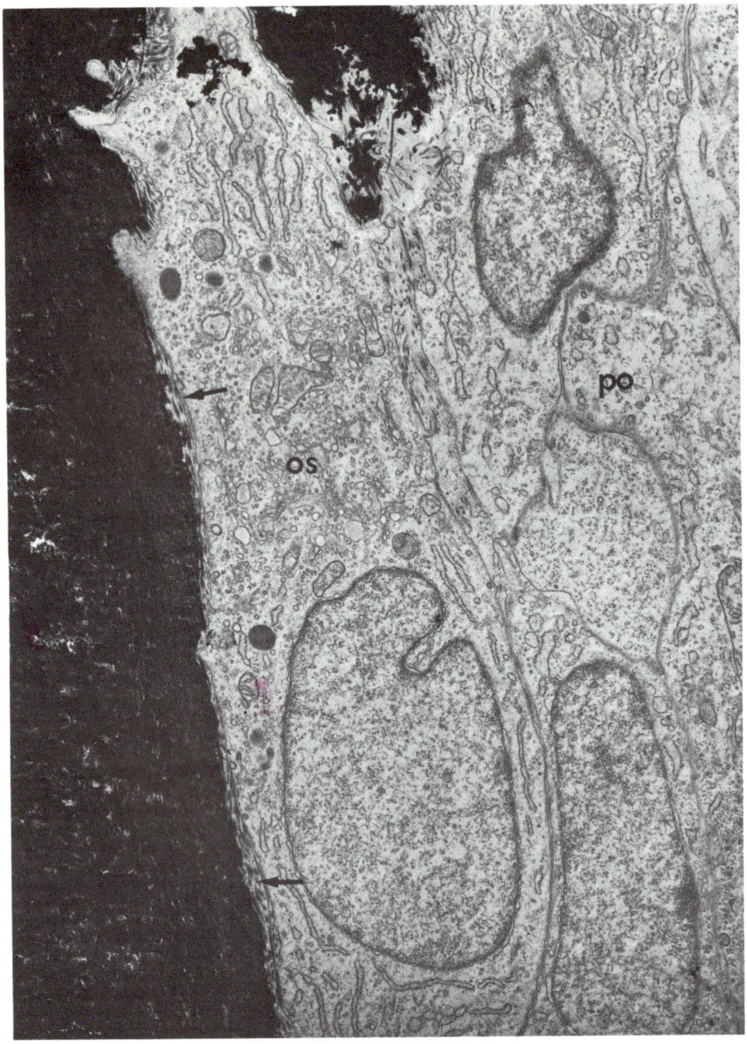


Fig. 2.12. Electron micrograph of preosteoblasts (po) and an osteoblast (os). The osteoblast is separated from the calcified bone matrix by a thin layer of osteoid (arrowed) in which collagen fibres may be seen.

Osteoblasts are clearly derived from the mesenchyme cells or preosteoblasts which overlie them. However, in cartilage undergoing endochondral ossification, some of the chondrocytes may survive to become osteoblasts.

*The osteocyte.* When the osteoblast becomes surrounded by newly formed bone it becomes an osteocyte. As it does so the morphology of the cell and its relationship with the bone gradually changes also (Fig. 2.13). It forms short cytoplasmic processes at points where the cell membrane is in contact with the bone matrix. The development of cell processes is one of the characteristics signifying the differentiation of the osteoblast to the osteocyte.

The cell processes of the osteocyte lie centrally in the canaliculi, occupying about 50 per cent of their volume, and are circular in transverse section. The plasma membrane is separated from the bone by a distance of about 30 nM and this area is translucent and devoid of structure. The cytoplasm of the process contains no organelles and is densely floccular in appearance.

The bone matrix lining the lacuna is frequently referred to as the osteocyte capsule, but consists of distinct layers. The inner layer in contact with the osteocyte consists of granular amorphous material outside which is a layer of banded collagen fibrils. The third outer layer is composed of loosely arranged apatite crystals which have been termed coastal crystals.

Not everyone would agree with the above description of the osteocyte capsule. However, inconsistencies in observation may be explained by the different ages and species of animals that have been used together with different methods of tissue preparation.

The osteocyte is similar in structure to the osteoblast, except that it is isolated in a lacuna and completely surrounded by bone matrix. In the young, where there is very active remodelling, the osteocytes probably do not remain in their lacunae long, but are released. It has been shown that the osteocyte has a life cycle and can be demonstrated in three phases, the formation phase, the resorption phase and the degeneration phase. In the resorptive phase the osteocyte resorbs the surrounding calcified matrix and is thereby released by osteocytic osteolysis.

The osteocyte lacuna stains with basic stains and gives a positive PAS reaction, suggesting that the amorphous granular material may represent protein polysaccharide. This material is similar, therefore, to any other connective tissue matrix and may be involved in the exchange of materials between cells and matrix. The coastal crystals may be a source of labile calcium and phosphate controlled by the metabolic activity of the cells. This would support the postulate that the osteocyte may be involved in calcium homeostasis by regulating their own environment.

*The osteoclast.* This is a large multinucleated cell up to 200,000 $\mu m^3$ and with up to 100 nuclei. Generally the osteoclast has an irregular shape, probably due to its motility, and it may be attached to the bone surface or lying free within the medullary spaces. Where resorption is taking place the plasma membrane is thrown into folds which constitute the "brush border" characteristic of these cells (Fig. 2.14). The folds or processes are finger-like, and the spaces between them extend into the cytoplasm of the cell where they may be dilated to form an area from which the large smooth vesicles of the

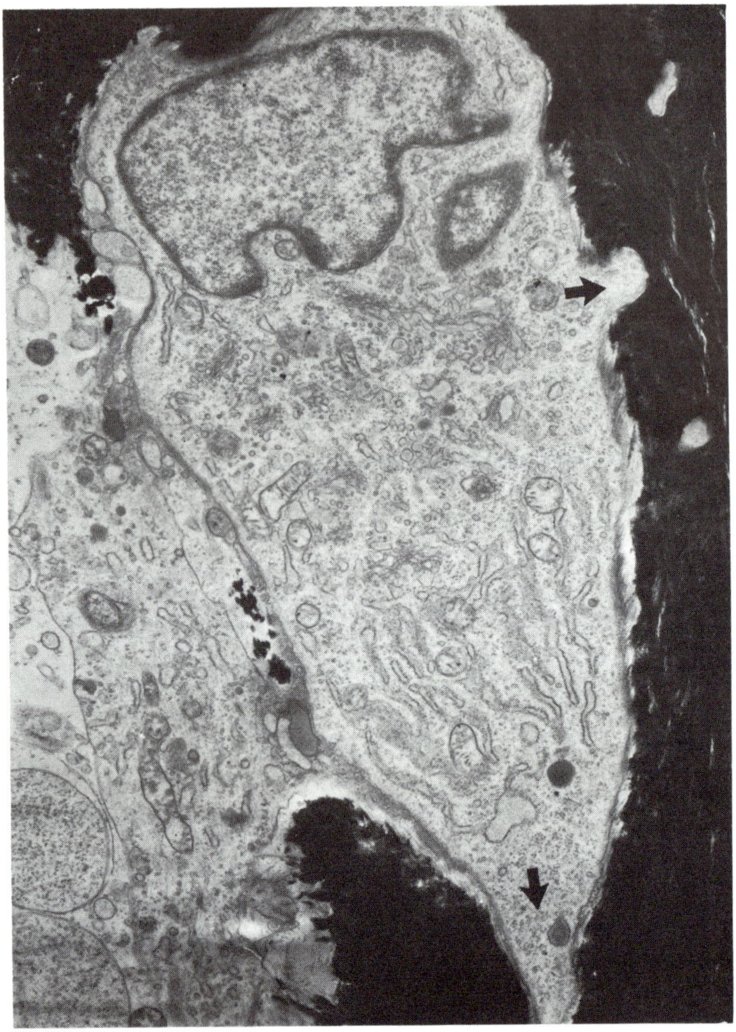

Fig. 2.13. Electron micrograph of an osteoblast becoming an osteocyte and forming the typical osteocyte processes (arrowed) as it becomes enclosed by bone matrix.

cytoplasm originate by micropinocytosis. The area of the brush border can become quite complex with the processes folding and interwining to form a system of tubules. Each cell may have several areas of brush border associated with different sites of absorption. Where the osteoclast is not associated with absorption, the plasma membrane is smooth apart from occasional blunt projections.

Beneath the brush border for a depth of 3 μm the cytoplasm is free of organelles apart from the polyribosome or small smooth vesicle. One of the

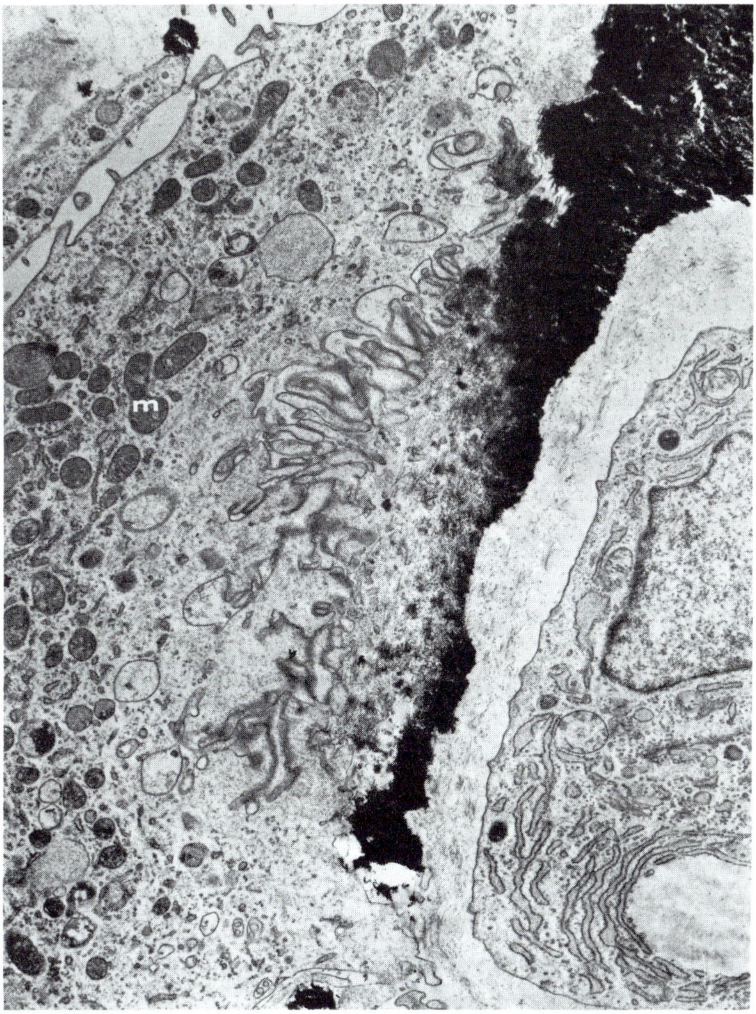


Fig. 2.14. Electron micrograph showing an osteoblast and an osteoclast separated by a spicule of bone. The osteoclast is clearly identified by a distinctly convuluted cell membrane associated with resorption of the bone. There are also numerous mitochondria (m).

most conspicuous features is the large numbers of mitochondria which are predominantly large and tubular. There are also large numbers of vacuoles of varying sizes throughout the cytoplasm. The larger vesicles are found more frequently in the region of the brush border and often seem to contain single crystals or groups of crystals. These vacuoles result from an invagination of the plasma membrane between the finger-like projections of the brush border and are most numerous beneath it. Smaller vesicles are often closely associated with the Golgi region, which consists of several discrete areas of lamellae forming a network around the nuclei. Also in the Golgi region are various types of multivesicular and lysosome-like bodies.

There is a distinct lack of granular endoplasmic reticulum which consists of a few dilated cisternae randomly distributed in the cytoplasm. Where the brush border comes in contact with the bone it is disrupted for a depth of about 1-2 μm. The collagen fibres lose their orientation and become separated from each other. Crystals become dissociated from the fibres and lie freely in the spaces between the folds of the brush border and in the large vacuoles beneath. From electron micrographs it is not possible to determine the exact sequence of events during resorption, that is whether the collagen fibres are first separated, resulting in the removal of crystallites, or whether the removal of the crystals precedes the separation of the collagen.

Osteoclasts are sensitive to parathydroid hormone and there is a significant increase in the numbers of osteoclasts and of intramitochondrial granules after the administration of parathyroid extract. The increase in the number of intramitochondrial granules may indicate increased mineral resorption, since these granules are involved in the movement of calcium and phosphate ions.

The osteoclast contains numerous lysosomes associated with the Golgi apparatus. Acid phosphate, which is used as a histochemical marker for lysosomes, has been demonstrated in osteoclasts. Collagenolytic enzymes have been found in bone cells, so it is possible that lysosomal enzymes of a collagenolytic character are involved in the dissolution of mineralized tissues.

## THE STRUCTURE OF BONE

Two types of bone may be seen by simple macroscopic examination of the skeleton. These are compact bone and spongy or cancellous bone. As the terms imply, compact bone contains little soft connective tissue, whereas spongy bone consists of a network of bone struts or trabeculae enclosing either red or fatty marrow. Compact bone is commonly found forming the cortical plates which enclose the trabecular spongy bone.

### Woven Bone

The first formed bone, which results from either intramembranous or endochrondral ossification, is referred to as embryonic, foetal or woven bone (Fig. 5.2). This type of bone is found chiefly in the embryo and foetus and has an organic matrix in which coarse collagen fibres are woven into a complex network. The fine trabeculae enclose vascular connective tissues and the trabecular surfaces are covered by a layer of osteoblasts. By producing further bone lamellae, the osteoblasts eventually become completely enclosed to form osteocytes. Consequently, the amount of intertrabecular connective tissue is progressively reduced. This type of bone is normally completely replaced, but some may persist near the insertion of tendons and attachment of ligaments.

### Immature Bone

Further layers of bone are successively produced so that lamellae containing osteocytes surround a central Haversian canal enclosing blood vessels and connective tissue. Thus a unit of bone described as a primary osteon or Haversian system develops (Fig. 2.15). The osteocytes within an osteon communicate with each other through canaliculi, but these do not extend across the cement line which forms a boundary to the osteon. Lamellae may also be produced by osteoblasts which differentiate from the periosteum to produce so-called circumferential lamellae. However, where rapid growth is taking place the periosteal surface does not have a layer of lamellar bone, but instead osteones are formed directly beneath the periosteal surface.

The immature bone thus formed consists of a mixture of woven bone and primary osteons. This bone may be in the form of trabeculae or in a more compact form where soft connective tissue is largely excluded.

### Mature Bone

The dynamic nature of bone as a tissue and its ability to respond to functional demands is well illustrated by the formation of mature bone. Existing or primary osteons are resorbed by osteoclasts which differentiate from cells within the vascular canals. Osteoblasts then lay down bone lamellae with an organic matrix which contains fine collagen fibres in contrast to that of the immature bone. The distinct junction that can be seen between the resorbing front and the newly deposited bone is known as a reversal line. Further generations of osteoblasts produce lamellae until the space created by resorption is filled with a secondary osteon. The secondary osteones have a more regular arrangement of lamellae and osteocytes around the central Haversian canal. This remodelling process may continue so that further generations of osteones may be found. The remnants of the earlier osteon are known as interstial lamellae.

The size of the osteones, the Haversian canals and the level of calcification within them varies within an individual bone. However, in young individuals and the elderly, the Haversian canals are larger and the mineral density lower.

## METHODS OF BONE GROWTH

The arrangement of the tissues where two or more individual bones meet is termed a joint or articulation. It is not necessary that movement be a function of such a meeting in order for these terms to be employed. In the skull the joints between the bones play an important role in growth and development and it is necessary, therefore, to understand the structure of such joints.

Joints may be classified according to their mode of development, structure or physiology. For the purposes of this text they will be classified according to structure, that is:

(1) syndesmoses — where bones are held together by bands of fibrous tissue.
(2) synchondroses — where two bones are joined by cartilage.
(3) synostoses — where bones are joined by bone.
(4) symphyses — where bones are capped by cartilage and held together by fibrous tissue.
(5) synovial joints — where a lubricating fluid, the synovial fluid, is present in a closed cavity or capsule where two bones capped by cartilage come together to form a joint.

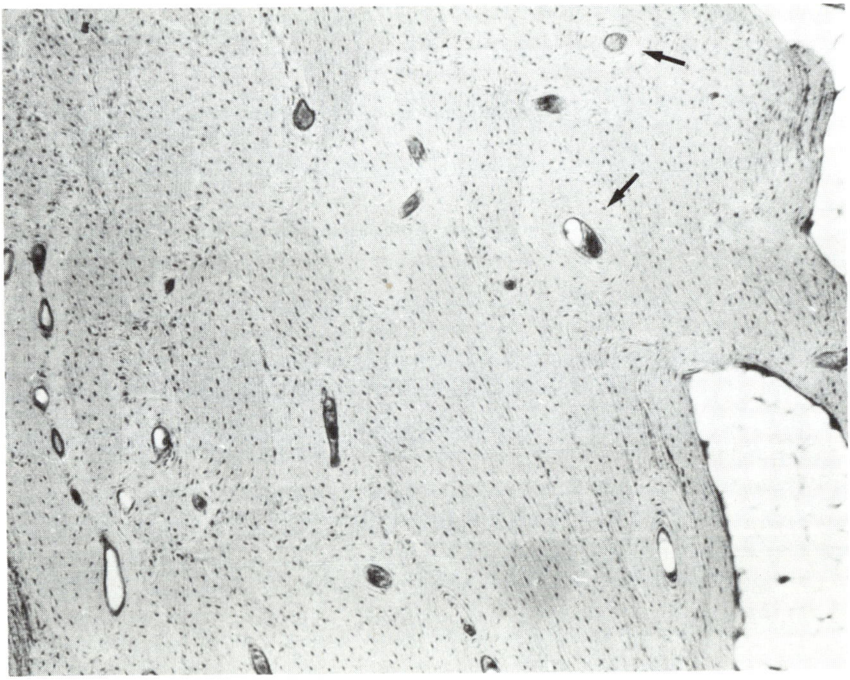

Fig. 2.15. Immature bone consisting of a mixture of woven bone and primary osteone (arrowed).

The primitive human skull contains elements which are formed both from primary and secondary cartilages and membranous connective tissue (see later chapters). In both primary cartilage and connective tissue growth is at first generalized, but with the onset of calcification and bone formation, growth becomes restricted to specific sites within the fibrous tissue and cartilage of the developing skull. In membrane bone these sites of localized growth are syndesmoses and in cartilagenous bone synchondroses. Where bone is formed by either of these methods further growth only takes place by the deposition of bone onto an existing bone surface. Surface deposition is a more important factor during the later periods of skull growth and in determining the final form of a bone is often accompanied by bone resorption. A balance between bone deposition and bone resorption is important for normal development and growth.

### Syndesmoses

The junction of syndesmoses that form between the membrane bones of the skull as known as sutures. These structures are a remarkably constant anatomical feature of the craniofacial skeleton. A growing suture has a characteristic structure (Fig. 2.16). During an active phase of growth new bone is added to the bony end surfaces bounding the suture. Since bone formation is a response to tensional forces, the stimulus for bone formation is probably the separation of bones bounding the suture by an increase in volume of the enclosed soft tissues. Tension is transmitted by the collagen fibres of the middle layer. Older views suggested that the proliferation of soft tissues within the suture itself provided the stimulus for bone formation.

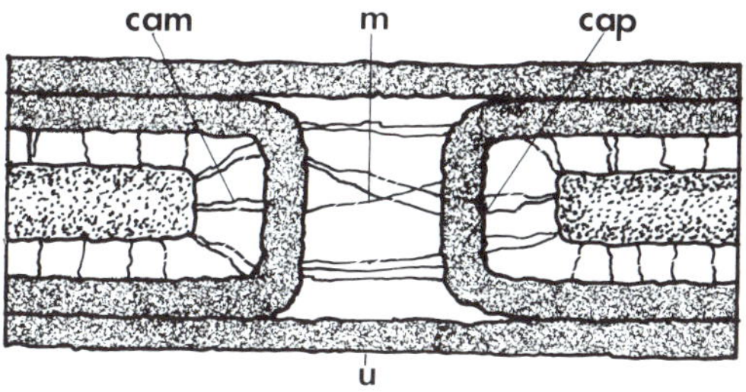


Fig. 2.16. Diagram illustrating the structure of a growing suture. u, uniting layer; m, middle layer; cam, cambial layer; cap, capsular layer.

However, it is clear that sutures are not structurally adapted to respond to pressure to produce bone, but to tension. When growth within a suture has ceased, the well-defined layers previously recognized disappear and complete bony fusion or synostoses occurs.

### Synchondroses

NB ↓

Synchondroses are what remains of the primary cartilagenous skeleton of the cranial base. Unlike a suture, this remaining area of growth cartilage is theoretically capable of growth under pressure. The structure of a synchondroses is basically that of a double epiphyseal plate and, therefore, has two major directions of linear growth (Fig. 2.17). Cells of the middle layers divide and produce an organic matrix which calcifies and is replaced by bone in endochondral ossification. The question arises as to whether the cartilage of the synchondroses intrinsically causes displacement or is the growth in response to changes in the soft tissues such as the enlarging brain.

The cartilages of the cranial base have been regarded as independent growth units developing in conjunction with the soft tissues it supports. Although the capacity for independent growth does not appear to be equal to that of epiphyseal growth cartilage, the cranial base will develop even where there is incomplete development or agenesis of the brain.

### Surface Deposition

This involves the formation of new bone laid down by osteoblasts beneath the surface periosteum or endosteum. All the bones of the skull enlarge by this method of growth whether they originated in membrane or hyaline cartilage. The complex process of bone growth often involves remodelling of existing bone and, therefore, surface deposition is accompanied by surface resorption. Surface deposition, however, may be restricted to specific growth sites or areas and is not necessarily a generalized phenomena.

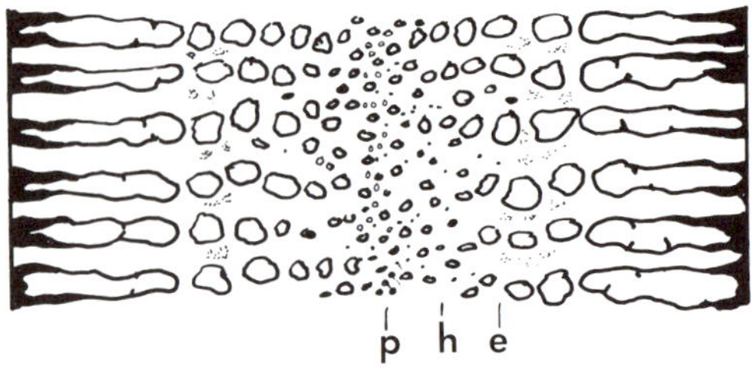


Fig. 2.17. Diagram illustrating the structure of a synchondrosis. p, proliferative zone; h, hypertrophic zone; e, endochondral bone formation.

## BIBLIOGRAPHY

AARON, J. E. and F. G. E. PAUTARD (1973) A cell cycle in bone mineralisation, in *The Cell Cycle in Development and Differentiation*, ed. M. Balls and F. S. Billet, Camb. Univ. Press, England.

ALI, S. Y., A. WISBY and J. CRAIG-GRAY (1978) Electron probe analysis of cryosections of epiphyseal cartilage, *Metab. Bone Dis. & Rel. Res.* **1**, 97.

ANDERSON, C. H. (1969) Vesicles associated with calcification in the matrix of epiphyseal cartilage, *J. Cell Biol.* **41**, 59.

ANDERSON, C. H. (1978) Introduction to the second conference on matrix vesicle calcification, *Metab. Bone Dis. & Rel. Res.* **1**, 83.

APPLETON, J. and D. C. MORRIS (1979) The use of the potassium pyroantimonate method as a means of identifying and localizing calcium at the ultrastructural level in the cells of calcifying system, *J. Histochem. Cytochem.* **27**, 676.

ARNOTT, H. J. and F. G. E. PAUTARD (1967) Osteoblast function and fine structure, *Israel J. med. Sci.* **3**, 657.

ASCENZI, A., E. BONUCCI and S. BOCCIARELLI (1967) An electron microscope study of primary periosteal bone, *J. Ultrastruct. Res.* **18,** 605.

BAUD, C. A. (1962) Morphology and inframicroscopic structure of osteocytes, *Acta Anat.* **51,** 209.

BAUD, C. A. and P. W. MORGENTHALER (1963) Structure submicroscopique du rebord lacuno canaliculaire orseux, *Morph. Jb.* **104,** 476.

BELANGER, L. F. (1969) Osteocytic osteolysis, *Calc. Tiss. Res.* **4,** 1.

BERNARD, G. W. and D. C. PEASE (1969) An electron microscopic study of initial intramembranous osteogenesis, *Am. J. Anat.* **125,** 271.

BONUCCI, E. (1967) Fine structure of early cartilage calcification, *J. Ultrastruct. Res.* **20,** 33.

BONUCCI, E. (1974) The organic-inorganic relationships in bone matrix undergoing osteoclastic resorption, *Calc. Tiss. Res.* **16,** 13.

CAMERON, D. A. and R. A. ROBINSON (1958) Electron microscopy of epiphyseal and articular cartilage matrix in the femur of the newborn infant, *J. Bone Jt. Surg.* **40A,** 163.

CAMERON, D. A. (1963) The fine structure of bone and calcified cartilage, *Clin. Orthop.* **26,** 199.

CAMERON, D. A., H. A. PASCHALL and R. A. ROBINSON (1967) Changes in the fine structure of bone cells after the administration of parathyroid extract, *J. Cell Biol.* **31,** 1.

CHAMBERS, T. J. (1980) The cellular basis of bone resorption, *Clin. Orthop. Rel. Res.* **151,** 283.

COOPER, R. R., J. W. MILGRAM and R. A. ROBINSON (1966) Morphology of the osteon. An electron microscope study, *J. Bone Jt. Surg.* **48A,** 1239.

DUDLEY, H. R. and D. SPIRO (1961) The fine structure of bone cells, *J. biophys. biochem. Cytol.* **11,** 627.

EASTOE, J. E. (1968) Chemical aspects of the matrix concept in calcified tissue organisation, *Calc. Tiss. Res.* **2,** 1.

FLEISCH, H. (1964) Role of nucleation and inhibition of calcification, *Clin. Orthop.* **32,** 170.

FURSETH, R. (1973) Tight junctions between osteocyte processes, *Scand. J. dent. Res.* **81,** 339.

GREENSPAN, J. S. and H. J. J. BLACKWOOD (1966) Histochemical studies of chondrocyte function in the cartilage of the mandibuler condyle of the rat, *J. Anat.* **100,** 615.

HANCOX, N. M. and B. BOOTHROYD (1963) Structure-function relationships in the osteoclast, in *Mechanisms of Hard Tissue Destruction,* ed. R. F. Sognnaes, Am. Ass. Advanc. Sci., Washington D.C.

HARTLES, R. L. (1964) Calcification, in *Modern Trends in Orthopaedics—Science of Fractures,* ed. J. M. P. Clark, Butterworths, London.

HERRING, G. M. (1968) The chemical structure of tendon, cartilage dentin and bone matrix, *Clin. Orthop.* **60,** 261.

FITTON JACKSON, S. (1957) The fine structure of developing bone in the embryonic fowl, *Proc. R. Soc. B,* **146,** 270.

FITTON JACKSON, S. (1960) Fibrogenesis and the formation of matrix, in *Bone as a Tissue,* ed. K. Rodahl, J. T. Nicholson and E. M. Brown, McGraw Hill, New York.

JONES, S. J., A. BOYDE and J. B. PAWLEY (1975) Osteoblasts and collagen orientation, *Cell Tiss. Res.* **159,** 73.

JOWSEY, J. (1973) Autoradiographic and microradiographic studies of bone, in *Biological Mineralization,* ed. I. Zipkin, John Wiley & Sons, New York.

LANDIS, W. J., M. C. PAINE and M. J. GLIMCHER (1977) Electron microscopic observations of bone tissue prepared anhydrously in organic solvents, *J. Ultrastruct. Res.* **59,** 1.

MATTHEWS, J. L., J. H. MARTIN, J. A. LYNN and E. J. COLLINS (1968) Calcium incorporation into the developing cartilagenous epiphysis, *Calc. Tiss. Res.* **1,** 330.

MATTHEWS, J. L., J. H. MARTIN and E. J. COLLINS (1968) Metabolism and radioactive calcium by cartilage, *Clin. Orthop.* **58,** 213.

MATUKAS, V. J. and G. A. KRIKOS (1968) Evidence for changes in protein polysaccharide associated with the onset of calcification in cartilage, *J. Cell. Biol.* **39,** 43.

MORRIS, D. C. and J. APPLETON (1980) Ultrastructural localization of calcium in the mandibular condylar growth cartilage of the rat, *Calc. Tiss. Int.* **30,** 27.

NEUMAN, W. F. and M. W. NEUMAN (1958) *The Chemical Dynamics of Bone Mineral,* Chicago Univ. Press, Chicago.

NYLEN, M. U., D. B. SCOTT and V. M. MOSLEY (1960) Mineralization of turkey leg tendon II. Collagen mineral relations revealed by electron and X ray microscopy, in *Calcification in Biological Systems,* ed. R. F. Sognnaes, Am. Acad. Advanc. Sci., Washington D.C.

OWEN, M. (1980) Bone cells: a review, *Radiat. Environ. Biophys.* **17,** 372.

PAUTARD, F. G. E. (1966) A biomolecular survey of calcification, in *Calcified Tissues.* Proc. 3rd European Symp., ed. H. Fleisch. H. J. J. Blackwood and M. Owen, Springer Verlag, New York.

PAUTARD, F. G. E. (1970) The mineral phase in calcified cartilage, bone and baleen, *Calc. Tiss. Res., Suppl.* **4,** 34.

POSNER, A. S. and F. BETTS (1975) Synthetic amorphous calcium phosphate and its relation to bone mineral structure, *Accts. Chem. Res.* **8,** 273.

POSNER, A. S., F. BETTS and N. C. BLUMENTHAL (1978) Properties of nucleating systems, *Metab. Bone Dis. & Rel. Res.* **1,** 179.

PRITCHARD, J. J., J. H. SCOTT and F. G. GIRGIS (1956) The structure and development of cranial and facial sutures, *J. Anat.* **90,** 73.

REVEL, J. P. and E. HAY (1963) An autoradiographic and electron microscope study of collagen synthesis in differentiating cartilage, *Z. Zellforsch., Mikrosk. Anat.* **61,** 110.

ROBISON, R. (1923) The possible significance of hexosephosphoric esters in ossification, *Biochem. J.* **17,** 286.

ROBISON, R. and A. H. ROSENHEIM (1934) Calcification of hypertrophic cartilage *in vitro, Biochem. J.* **28,** 684.

ROBINSON, R. A. (1979) Bone tissue: composition and function, *John Hopkins Med. J.* **145,** 10.

ROBINSON, R. A. and M. L. WATSON (1952) Collagen crystal relationships in bone as seen in the electron microscope, *Anat. Rec.* **144,** 383.

SCHENK, R. K., D. SPIRO and J. WIENER (1967) Cartilage resorption in the tibial epiphyseal plate of growing rats, *J. Cell Biol.* **34,** 275.

SIMKISS, K. (1976) Intracellular and extracellular routes in biomineralisation, in *Calcium in Biological Systems,* Symp. Soc. Exp. Biol. **30,** 423. Camb. Univ. Press, Cambridge.

SLAVKIN, H. C., J. P. BRINGAS, R. BROISSANT and L. BAVETTA (1972) Epithelial mesenchymal interactions during odontogenesis. II. Intercellular matrix vesicles, *Mechanisms Aging and Develop.* **1,** 139.

SLAVKIN, H. C., R. C. CROISSANT, P. BRINGAS, P. MATOSIAN, P. WILSON, W. MINO and H. GUENTHER (1976) Matrix vesicle heterogeneity: possible morphogenetic functions for matrix vesicles, *Fed. Proc.* **35,** 127.

SCHRAER, H. and C. V. GAY (1977) Matrix vesicles in newly synthesising bone observed after ultracryotomy and ultramicroincineration, *Calc. Tiss. Res.* **23,** 185.

TAVES, D. R. (1965) Mechanism of calcification, *Clin. Orthop.* **42,** 207.

URIST, M. R. (1973) Biologic initiators of calcification, in *Biological Mineralization,* ed. I. Zipkin, John Wiley & Sons, New York.

VAANANEN, H. K. (1980) Calcium incorporation in matrix vesicles isolated from chick epiphyseal cartilage, *Calc. Tiss. Int.* **30,** 227.

VAUGHAN, J. M. (1970) *The Physiology of Bone,* Clarendon Press, Oxford.

WASSERMAN, F. and J. A. YAEGER (1965) Fine structure of the osteocyte capsule and of the wall of the lacunae in bone, *Z. Zellforsch., Mikrosk. Anat.* **67,** 636.

WEIDMAN, S. M. (1963) Calcification of skeletal tissues, *Int. Rev. Connect. Tiss. Res.* **1,** 339.

# CHAPTER 3

# *Growth of the Cranium*

Having considered growth as a general process and mineralization in particular, it is now possible to look at more detail regarding the craniofacial region. Although most of the available literature describes what happens to the bony parts of this region, it must not be thought that the bones are genetically programmed to grow to a predestined size uninfluenced by other factors. This used to be the established view in the past, and presumably arose from the extensive study of skeletal material which appears, superficially, hard and unchanging. In addition, bones are easy to measure, whereas soft tissues such as the brain are not, and thus it is difficult to produce appropriate growth curves for them.

In recent years, however, the soft tissues have been given more prominence, and this is particularly evident in the theory of functional matrices (Moss and Salentijn 1969). This idea has been developed over the years, but broadly speaking it envisages growth in the craniofacial region in terms of certain essential matrices, for example the brain and its related membranes. Thus the brain enlarges from birth rapidly for the first few years and then more slowly, almost completely its growth by about 7 years. The bones of the cranial vault do not grow first, but respond to the increasing size of the brain, and tension on the sutures causes them to lay down bone between, for example, the parietal bones at the sagittal suture. A similar process may be envisaged for the growing eye. The bony orbit expands by both sutural growth, and bone deposition in response to the primary growth of its contents.

Both brain and eye with their surrounds are regarded in this concept as capsular matrices. A similar hypothesis exists for spaces such as those of the pharynx and larynx, which being vital to the life of the growing child are presumed to be the active force in the development of the nasomaxillary complex. As a result of this, the nasal cartilage, in addition to the sutures, has been given a secondary role of merely following the growth initiated elsewhere, and of providing stability in the region. Not all investigators, however, agree with this and the matter will be further discussed in Chapter 4.

Periosteal matrices are also invoked. These are the bones, including the muscles attached to them, such as in the case of the mandible. Although this theory has been very successful in getting away from the idea of a preconceived genetic plan which cannot be altered, there are a number of difficulties in accepting it in its entirety, and these will be dealt with more fully under the specific regions in this and subsequent chapters.

In this chapter the cranial base and cranial vault will be dealt with rather briefly, since much of the complex detail is not essential for understanding facial growth. A consideration of the midface and mandible follow in subsequent chapters, but it must, however, be realized that this is an artificial division for ease of presentation and that, of course, all parts are closely interrelated.

## CRANIAL BASE

Before considering some of the findings on growth of the cranial base it is perhaps as well to consider how it may be investigated and the limitations of the methods used.

Although the embryology of this area is fairly well understood, actual foetal quantitative data are not numerous. For example, there has been a lot of interest in the magnitude of the cranial base angle during growth, and different investigators have given quite opposing views. Presumably this is partly due to the difficulty in measuring the rather small dimensions involved, the lack of easily reproducible measuring points, and the large variability between specimens of the same age.

After birth, things are somewhat easier, but only a few direct measurements are possible, and so cephalometric radiography has been used to supplement these, with consequent further sources of error which will be discussed in detail in Chapter 7.

More accurate data have been accumulated from analyses of human postmortem material in which direct measurement may be made and the natural sites of growth identified histologically. Nevertheless, this is very time-consuming technique and so numbers have not always been large, with the consequent difficulty in comparing findings at different ages. Dried specimens have also been used, but shrinkage may occur in such specimens, which could invalidate observations.

Many animal experiments have been carried out, but those on rodents, etc., may be difficult to interpret in relation to man. Those on monkeys may have more relevance to human studies, and in these, for example, it is possible to insert metal markers which can be regarded as fixed points and growth can be measured from them.

### The Chondrocranium

This starts to form about 7 weeks in utero and is confined to the future base of the skull area, the rest of the cranium at this stage being a connective tissue capsule (covered by ectoderm) around the brain in which the future membrane bones of the vault will appear. The first appearance of the cartilage of the chrondrocranium around the cephalic end of the notochord is known as the parachordal cartilage; soon afterward appear areas in the future occipital region. Later there is a spread laterally and into the nasal area, while the inner ears are invested in the cartilagenous otic capsules which eventually unite with the occipital and hypophyseal (later sphenoid) cartilages.

At about 10 weeks the chondrocranium looks pear-shaped from above, as in the model in Fig. 3.1. An anterior view showing particularly well the nasal capsule and Meckel's cartilage is shown in Fig. 3.2.

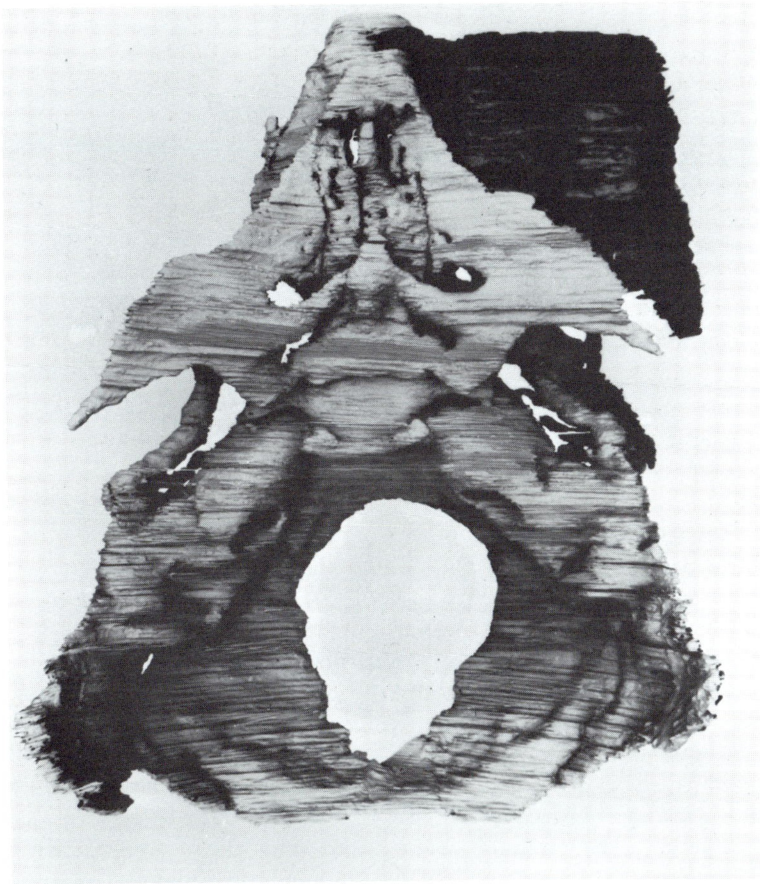

Fig. 3.1. The chondrocranium from above, from a model prepared by Dr T. H. M. Wynne, Liverpool A.H.A.(T). Note the recognizable aspects of the occipital and sphenoid areas. The frontal bone is shown darker, on the right-hand side only.

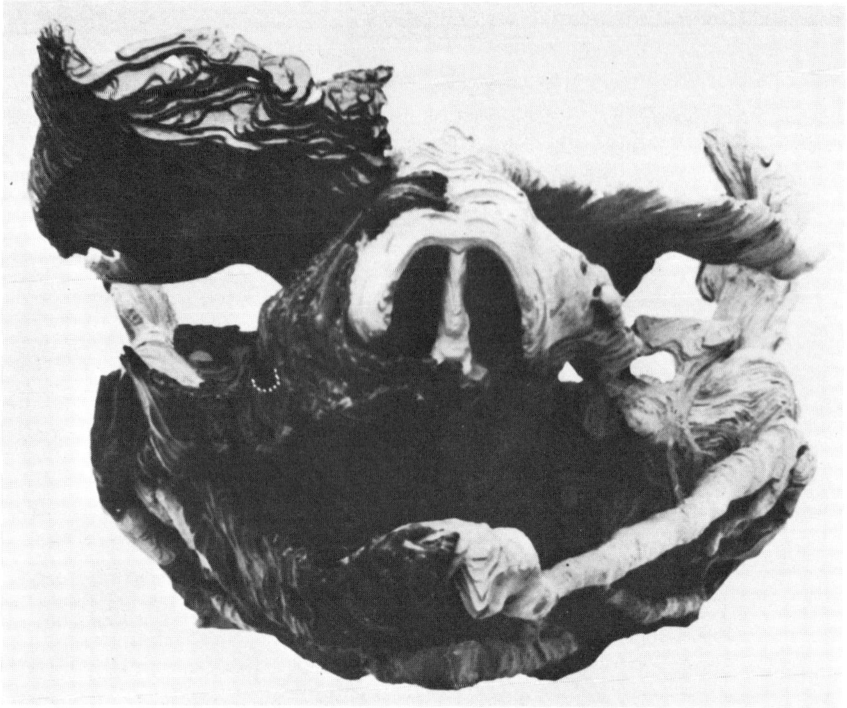

Fig. 3.2. The chondrocranium from the front from a model prepared by Dr T. H. M. Wynne, Liverpool A.H.A.(T). Note the nasal capsule in the middle and Meckel's cartilage and associated structures below on the right. The frontal bone has been shown above on the left-hand side only.

**Growth of the Cranial Base**

Ossification in the basilar part of the occipital bone occurs quite early at about 6 weeks and those for the lateral (condylar) parts about the 8th week. The interparietal part is later, and all parts are still united by cartilage at birth.

The sphenoid has several centres starting rather later, and at birth is in three parts, the greater wing and pterygoid process on each side with the body and lesser wings between. They fuse by the end of the first year.

The cribriform plate is not ossified until about the second year after birth, then uniting the perpendicular plate of the ethmoid and its lateral parts.

The cranial base appears to grow most rapidly from 14 to 32 weeks of foetal life, and then slows down before birth. It speeds up again after birth, slowing again at about 7 years. In foetal life the growth in the anterior part is faster than that of the posterior.

After birth, the main interest will be in the anteroposterior aspect of growth, and Fig. 3.3 shows the various parts of the cranial base in the

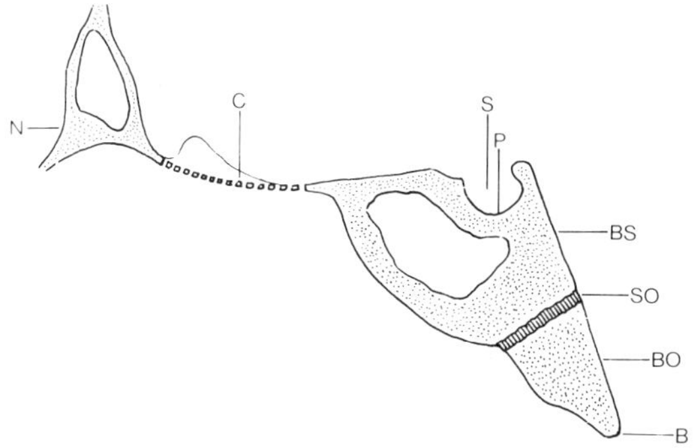


Fig. 3.3. Midline section of the cranial base. B, basion; BO, basiocciput; BS, basisphenoid; C, cribriform plate; N, nasion; P, pituitary point; S, sella point; SO, spheno-occipital synchondrosis. The crista galli is above the cribriform plate and the foramen caecum in front.

midline. It is important to realize that they do not all behave in the same way, some following a pattern of brain growth, others being more related to facial growth. Enlow (1975) points out that anatomically the anterior cranial fossa is specifically related to the nasomaxillary complex and that the pharynx is related to the middle cranial fossa.

The area from pituitary point to foramen caecum reaches adult proportions at about 7 years of age, and growth is thus related to that of the brain and will be mainly at the sphenoethmoidal and frontoethmoidal sutures.

The area from the foramen caecum to the nasion increases in length throughout childhood, and exhibits a pubertal spurt which, however, is seen primarily in males. The mechanism of growth is principally by bone deposition on the outer surface of the frontal bone and the increase in its thickness associated with the frontal sinus (Fig. 3.3).

These first two parts have often in the past been considered together in cephalometry, as the distance nasion to sella point (middle of the sella turcica), thus confusing two separate growth patterns. The nasion is, in any case, not a good reference point, as it is moving forward throughout growth and individuals may also show an upwards or downwards movement as well. There is in addition to forward growth some remodelling of bone on the cerebral surface in these areas both resorptive and appositional, which in general ceases by 4 years of age.

The sella turcica (Fig. 3.4) shows great variation in growth, apposition alternating with inactive periods. The anterior part appears to be stable at about 5 years, but elsewhere remodelling continues and posteriorly resorption is predominant even up to about 16 or 17 years of age. Thus the sella point cannot be regarded as stable during growth as a reference point. It is generally felt to move upwards and backwards, although some workers consider it more downwards and backwards.

Posteriorly the spheno-occipital synchrondrosis begins to close at about 12-13 years in girls and about 2 years later in boys, ossification starting in the cerebral surface first.

The area behind the sella turcica consists of the clivus, which is divided by the synchondrosis into sphenoidal and occipital parts, and the anterior margin of the foramen magnum (Fig. 3.3). The linear growth here is partly by the synchrondrosis already described, but also by apposition on the anterior margin of the foramen magnum (the posterior margin showing resorption). Thus the distance from the sella to the basion increases up to adulthood.

As mentioned earlier, the functional matrix theory assumes that the spheno-occipital synchrondrosis is not a growth centre in the active sense of

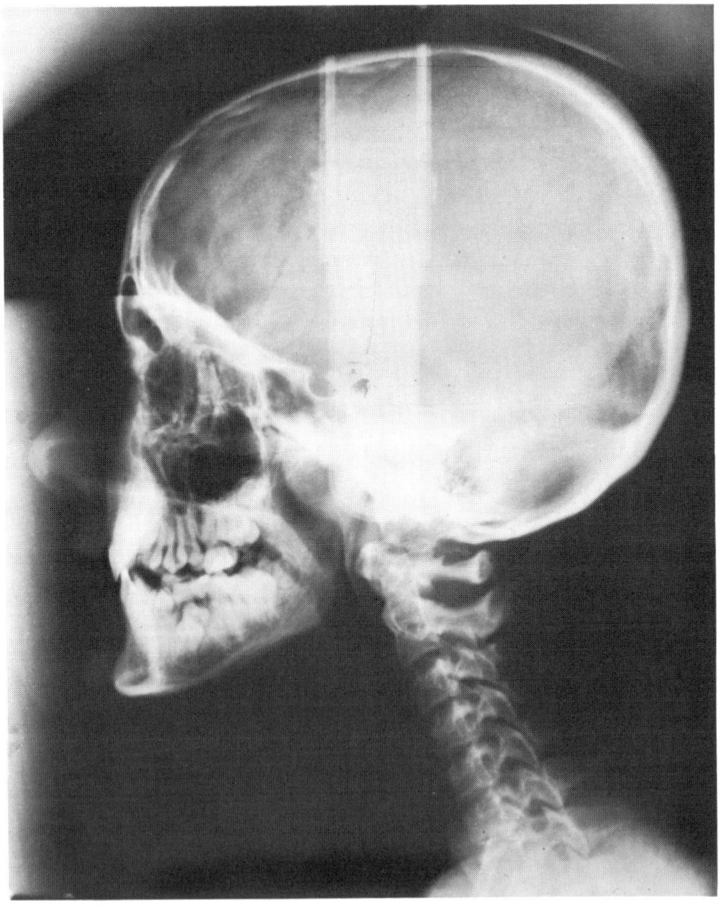

Fig. 3.4. Cephalometric radiograph showing a well-defined sella turcica. The basion is somewhat obscured.

the word. However, opinion is divided on this point as, for example, in organ culture where the cartilage shows a similar pattern of growth to epiphyseal cartilage. Also it continues growing after the brain has stopped.

There is also appositional growth on the cranial surface of the basisphenoid and resorption of the basiocciput and apposition on both their pharyngeal surfaces.

Whilst the midline region of the cranial base has been most studied, it is, of course, true that lateral parts also show growth. As the lobes of the brain grow, so does expansion occur via the sutures between the various skull bones. In addition, the endocranial surface shows resorption in general, but deposition occurs on structures such as the crista galli and the petrous elevations.

### Cranial Base Angle

Much work has been done on the question as to whether this angle changes in magnitude during growth. The angle is measured radiographically as nasion-sella point-basion (see Chapter 7), but in skeletal or postmortem material more often the pituitary point, the lowest part on the floor of the sella turcica, has been used rather than the sella. It is, of course, scarcely possible to measure this angle in embryonic life, and so consideration has usually been deferred to 10 weeks and over in foetal life. Ford (1956), in his investigation of 76 foetuses, found it "opened out" about 14-19° from 10 to 40 weeks. Most of the other investigators, however, have not found much change at different ages, and no more than could be explained by small sample variation. The angle varies in different studies, but appears to be around 130° (nasion-sella-basion) in general. Individual variations, however, are common due to different techniques and materials used. In certain pathological conditions, such as Down's syndrome or microcephaly, there may, however, be a flattening of the cranial base.

## CRANIAL VAULT

Whilst the cranial base is associated with both the growth of the brain and that of the face, the vault is entirely dependent at its inner surface on the brain. However, its external form is influenced by function in the shape of muscle attachments such as are found in the occipital and temporal regions. This is particularly evident in anthropoid apes with their large sagittal crests.

The pattern of development of the cranial vault is different from the rest of the body, as has already been indicated in Chapter 1. Half the increase in the circumference of the head is achieved by 9 months, about three-quarters by the end of the second year, the remainder of growth being very slow with a small but detectable spurt at adolescence. This latter phenomenon is probably due to thickening of the bones of the skull and the development of the sinuses.

In recent years it has proved possible to measure foetal heads by ultrasound, and therefore there are now available longitudinal studies. These suggest a peak velocity of head breadth about 13 weeks *in utero,* and a continuing fairly rapid rate until about 30 weeks.

At birth, bones of the cranial vault are not yet fully united and the cortices are thin and lacking diploë. Six fontanelles (spaces between the bones) exist at birth, the posterior one between the occipital and parietals closing soon after, the anterior one between the two halves of the frontal bone and the parietals closing at about one year, the anterolaterals rather earlier and posterolaterals rather later.

The expansion of the brain causes tension on the cranial sutures which stimulates bone formation there. In addition, deposition occurs on the surface of the cranial bones with resorption cranially. In order to allow for a relative flattening as the head gets larger, there are readjustments by resorption on the surface near the sutures and deposition cranially.

Adult cranial form can vary betwen individuals from longheaded or dolichocephalic to broadheaded or brachycephalic. The cephalic index (head breadth divided by length × 100) is the method of distinguishing between them and $<75$ is dolichocephalic and$> 80$ is brachycephalic. Between, the two individuals are regarded as mesocephalic.

What causes these differences is not entirely understood; for example, the medieval population in the United Kingdom tended towards brachycephaly, whereas populations both before and after tended towards dolichocephaly. Although it might be expected that in general the shape of the face would be related to that of cranium, in fact the correlations betwen facial breadth and cephalic index are very low (Goose 1981).

## BIBLIOGRAPHY


BJÖRK, A. (1955) Cranial base development, *Am. J. Ortho.* **41,** 198.

BURDI, A. R. (1969) Cephalometric growth analysis of the human upper face region during the last two trimesters of gestation, *Am. J. Anat.* **125,** 113.

ENLOW, D. H. (1975) *Handbook of Facial Growth,* Saunders, Philadelphia.

FORD, E. H. R. (1956) The growth of the foetal skull, *J. Anat.* **90,** 63.

FORD, E. H. R. (1958) Growth of the human cranial base, *Am. J. Ortho.* **44,** 498.

GILES, W. B., C. L. PHILLIPS and D. R. JOONDEPH (1981) Growth of the basicranial synchondrosis of adolescent *Macaca mulatta, Anat. Rec.* **199,** 259.

GOOSE, D. H. (1981) Changes in human face breadth since the Mediaeval period in Britain, *Arch. oral. Biol.* **26,** 757.

HARRISON, R. G. (1978) *Clinical Embryology,* Academic Press, London.

HRDLICKA, A. (1939) *Practical Anthropometry,* A.M.S. Press, New York.

LATHAM, R. A. (1972) Different relation of sella point to growth sites of cranial base in foetal life, *J. dent. Res.* **51,** 1646.

MARSHALL, W. A. (1977) *Human Growth and its Disorders,* Academic Press, London.

MELSON, B. (1974) The cranial base, *Acta Odont. Scand.* **32,** Suppl. 62.

MOSS, M. L. and L. SALENTIJN (1969) The capsular matrix, *Am. J. Ortho.* **56,** 474.

SCOTT, J. H. (1953) The cartilage of the nasal septum, *Brit. dent. J.* **95,** 37.

SCOTT, J. H. (1958) The cranial base, *Am. J. Phys. Anthrop.* **16,** 319.

STRAMRUD, L. (1959) External and internal cranial base, *Acta Odont. Scand.* **17,** 239.

STUTZMANN, J. J. and A. G. PETROVIC (1976) Experimental analysis of general and local extrinsic mechanisms controlling upper jaw growth, in *Factors Affecting the Growth of the Mid-face,* ed. J. A. McNamara, Jr., Center for Human Growth and Development, Univ. Michigan, Ann Arbor.

TANNER, J. M. (1978) *Foetus into Man: Physical Growth from Conception to Maturity,* Open Books, London.

THILANDER, B. and B. INGERVALL (1973) The human spheno-occipital synchondrosis II. A histological and microradiographic study of its growth, *Acta Odont. Scand.* **31,** 323.

WARWICK, R. and P. L. WILLIAMS (ed.) (1973) *Gray's Anatomy,* 35th ed., Longmans, London.

WYNNE, T. H. M. (1966) *Observations on the development of the human chondrocranium, Ph. D. Thesis, Univ. Liverpool.*

# CHAPTER 4

# *Midfacial Growth*

The position of the human face is different from that of other mammals in that the expansion of the cerebrum has caused increased flexion of the cranial base and the face has "rotated" downwards and backwards under the anterior part of the brain, making the maxilla rectangular rather than triangular. The orbits have also moved round towards each other and therefore the nasal region is reduced.

## PRENATAL DEVELOPMENT

At about 3 weeks in the early somite stage the basic features of what will become the face may be seen (Fig. 4.1). In the centre is the stomatodeum, which is to become the future mouth area. It is the site of the buccopharyngeal membrane, which is early differentiated in the embryo in front of the notochord. Outside it consists of ectoderm and inside endoderm, and at 4 weeks is already breaking down to leave a cavity. The eventual junction between ectoderm and endoderm is in the tonsillar region in the adult, showing how considerable has the growth been in this area.

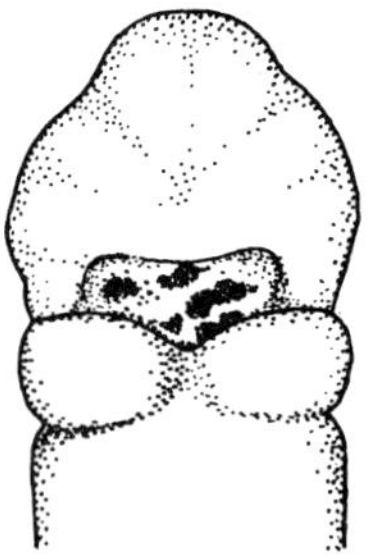

Fig. 4.1. Embryonic face at 3-4 weeks. Note stomatodeum with bucco-pharyngeal membrane breaking down in centre and mandibular processes below.

### The Face

Above is the forebrain covered with ectoderm and below is the mandibular arch, one of the six pharyngeal arches to develop in the future lower face and neck region.

Owing to the flexure of the head, the future face is rather crowded between the brain and the pericardial area containing the heart (Fig. 4.2). However, during development more room becomes available with the decrease in the flexure of the embryo, and by about 9-10 weeks the face looks more or less human (Fig. 4.3).

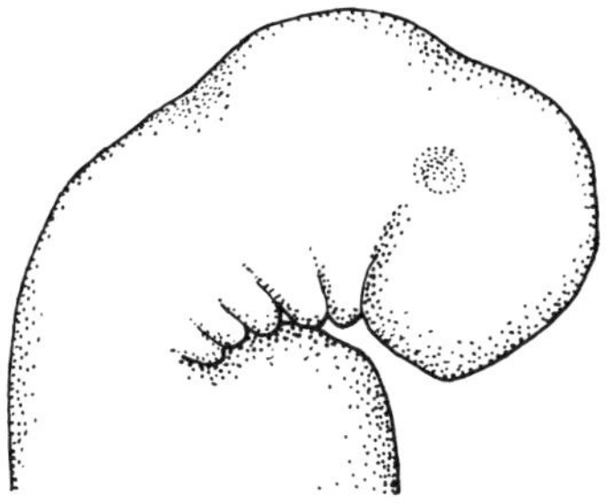

Fig. 4.2. Lateral view of 4-week embryo showing pharyngeal arches and lack of space between the brain and pericardial region.

At the earlier stage, however, the future facial area consists mainly of a framework of either ectoderm or endoderm, with a small amount of mesoderm. However, there is an invasion of neural crest cells which form adjacent to the neural tube and migrate into the future facial region and the pharyngeal arches. It is commonly called ectomesenchyme.

Before discussing the fusion of the various processes which will make up the future face, it may be as well to clarify the mechanisms probably involved. Proliferation of cells below the epithelium raise areas which are called processes and between them are often formed grooves or furrows. When adjacent processes "fuse", these furrows disappear. However, although in some cases there is true fusion (palatal shelves), whereby the epithelium disappears and the mesenchyme underlying actually joins together, often there is merely an increased cellular activity by the mesenchyme growing towards the surface which thereby makes the grooves disappear. This is better referred to as mergence.

### Nose and Nasal Cavities

At about 4 weeks (CR 5 mm) thickenings appear on each side of the surface ectoderm covering the forebrain called the nasal placodes. These are soon converted in the 5th week into pits by elevations of the underlying mesenchyme into a horseshoe shape on each side, termed the medial and lateral nasal processes. There may also be some growth inwards of the surface epithelium. The eventual result is in the formation of the anterior nares (Fig. 4.4).

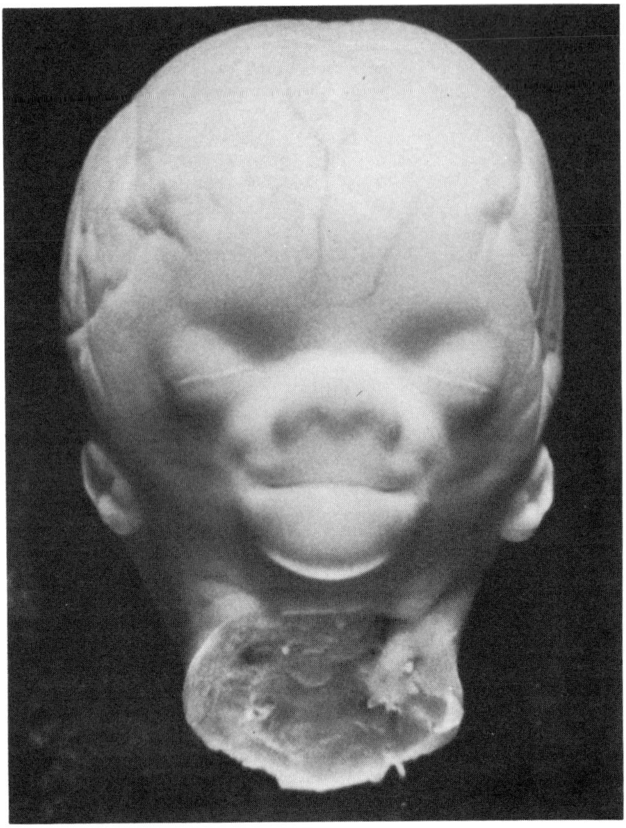

Fig. 4.3. Foetal head of about 10 weeks (by kind permission of Dr T. H. M. Wynne, Liverpool A.H.A.(T)).

Meanwhile, another process has arisen on each side from the mandibular arch, and this rapidly enlarges and comes into contact with the lateral nasal process which is separating the eye from the nasal pit along a line known as the nasolacrimal groove. As these processes merge, a rod of epithelium sinks into the underlying mesenchyme, establishing connections with the conjunctival sac and primitive nasal fossa, eventually forming the nasolacrimal duct.

The maxillary process grows further medially and eventually contacts the medial nasal process, and epithelial cells covering these processes become trapped between them and the mesenchyme fuses forming the nasal fin. The posterior aspect of this comes into contact with the bucconasal membrane, a horizontal epithelial structure which separates the early oral and nasal areas. This, however, ruptures near the end of the 5th week and disappears along with the nasal fin forming the choanae or posterior openings of the nasal sacs.

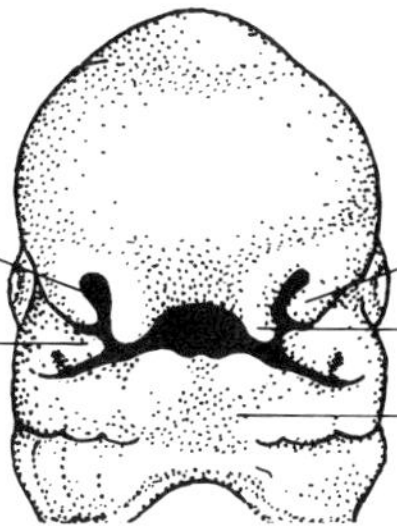


Fig. 4.4. Face at about 5 weeks, showing basic elements: LNP, lateral nasal process; MNP, medial nasal process.

As these enlarge, a nasal septum begins to form. Anteriorly the nasal pits will form the site of future nostrils and the alae of the nose will be formed by the lateral nasal processes. The medial nasal processes form the middle part of the nose and the philtrum of the upper lip, the lateral part of which being formed by the maxillary processes (Fig. 4.5).

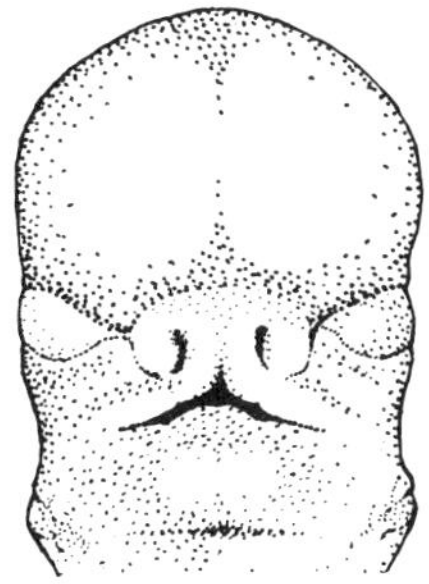

Fig. 4.5. Face with processes fused at about 7-8 weeks.

### The Palate

There is not entire agreement on the formation of the palate owing to the difficulty of studying all stages of early human development. However, the formation is certainly in two separate stages, the primary palate and the secondary palate. The former represents three components: a medial portion of the upper lip or prolabium, a premaxillary part of the upper jaw with incisor teeth and a palatal portion which is continuous with the future nasal septum and forms the hard palate in front of the secondary palate, the junction being at the region of the future incisive foramen.

The primary palate is formed by the merging of the two medial nasal processes and tissue between, although some investigators think that the rapid growth of the maxillary processes merging with the medial nasal processes makes some contribution. The primary palate thus partially closes off the oral and nasal cavities anteriorly (Fig. 4.6).

The secondary palate begins as ridges of tissue growing from the medial aspect of the maxillary processes about the 6th week, and at first they are directed downwards on either side of the tongue. During the 7th week they become reorientated horizontally above the tongue, and this may partly be due to the less cramped position of the facial area owing to the decreased flexure of the embryo referred to earlier and possibly to tongue movements in swallowing. The adjacent margins begin to fuse and the epithelium is broken up and may leave epithelial pearls in the line of fusion of the palate. Contact is made first near the anterior one-third of the processes, and progresses both forwards joining with the primary palate in the region of the future incisive foramen and backwards too. The process is normally complete by about the 10th week.

During the development of the face there is an effective movement of the eyes round to the front, but, of course, as there is growth all the time they are not nearer together than they were formerly. Sometimes there are disturbances which leave the eyes wider apart than normal (hypertelorism).

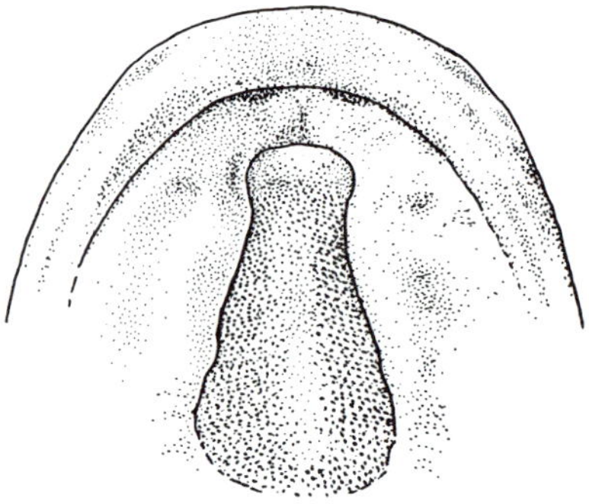

Fig. 4.6. View of palate from below at about 6-7 weeks. Note that the primary palate is complete anteriorly, but the secondary palate is still incomplete. The shelves at this stage will be facing downwards, but later will move upwards over the tongue to fuse together.

### Pharyngeal Arches

Proliferation of neural crest material and mesoderm in the wall of the primitive pharynx form processes which grow ventrally around the lateral aspects of the foregut, starting in the late somite period and eventually merging in the midline with their opposite number (Fig. 4.2). Originally there are six, but the fifth one disappears. The body of the arches is mesenchyme covered on the inside with endoderm and on the outside ectoderm. The parts between are termed clefts outside and pouches inside. Each arch has a cartilagenous rod, a primordial striated muscle element the branchiomere, a vascular component or aortic arch artery and a mixed motor and sensory nerve grows into each arch from the lateral aspect of the hindbrain.

Only the first two arches, the mandibular and hyoid, are of interest in connection with the face. The mandibular arch, as has been seen, produces laterally the maxillary processes and the lower jaw and face is derived from it too. The cartilagenous part forms Meckel's cartilage and its derivatives which will be described in more detail in the next chapter. The muscle element becomes the muscles of mastication, tensor tympani, tensor veli palatini, mylohyoid and anterior belly of digastric and they bring their nerve supply with them, the mandibular division of the fifth cranial nerve.

The second, or hyoid, arch is chiefly of interest in that its muscular element migrates some way to form the facial muscles, stylohyoid and posterior belly of digastric. With them comes their nerve, the facial or seventh cranial. The first ectodermal cleft between the mandibular and hyoid arches persists as the external auditory meatus and the dorsal part of the endodermal pouch develops into the Eustachian tube and the middle ear cavity. Mesenchyme from the adjacent first and second arches form the external ear.

Occasionally there are faults in development in the pharyngeal arches, and one well-known one is mandibulofacial dysostosis affecting the first arch. The malformations affect the eyes, giving antimongoloid obliquity of the palpebral fissures and coloboma of the lids, underdevelopment of the mandible and cheek bones as well as some ear defects.

### Cleft Lip and Palate

With the complexity of the development of the face it is not surprising things sometimes go wrong, and one of the relatively common results is cleft lip and palate, although there are occasionally other facial clefts.

The classification of these conditions is generally accepted as being:

1. Clefts of primary palate, that is cleft lip with or without cleft of the alveolar process (Fig. 4.7).
2. Clefts of the secondary palate, the so-called isolated cleft palate (Fig. 4.8).
3. Clefts of primary and secondary palates (Fig. 4.9).

Clearly factors affecting the primary and secondary palate are different, and so the frequencies with which the types occur are found to be different. For example, cleft lip with or without cleft palate is more common in boys and occurs in about 1 in 1000 births, varying with different races, being more common in Japanese and less common in Blacks. Cleft palate alone occurs more frequently in girls and is seen in about 1 in 2500 births.

The frequency of cleft lip and palate seems to vary in different years, and there may be some suggestion that it is increasing at present.

Although clefts may readily be produced experimentally in animals by various factors, for example cortisone, or folic acid deficiency, there seems to

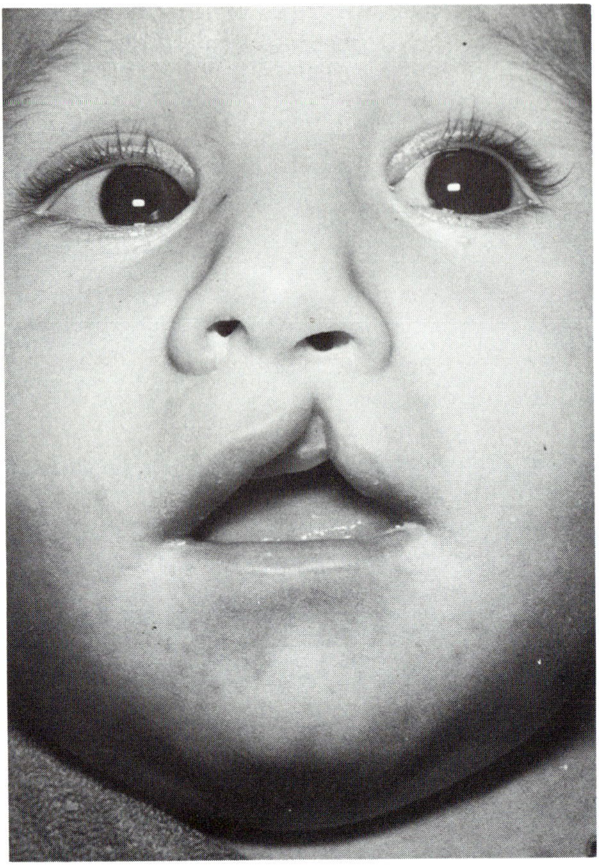

Fig. 4.7. Incomplete cleft on the left side of the primary palate only (by kind permission of Mr P. G. Bush, Liverpool A.H.A.(T)).

be no obvious causation of this type in man.

Three-fifths of cases of cleft lip (and palate) and four-fifths of cleft palate are found as solitary cases, and it is probable that usually there is a combined genetic and environmental causation, but that inheritance does not follow a simple Mendelian pattern. In studying the incidence among relatives it is found that recessive inheritance is unlikely, because of the close resemblance of the proportion of sibs and children affected, while dominant inheritance is also unlikely owing to the sharp fall in the proportion affected as one passes from monozygotic twins to first-degree and further relatives. The most likely mode of inheritance is multifactorial, with a threshold beyond which there is risk of malformation. That is to say there is an underlying liability to cleft lip or palate which may be distributed in a normal way. When sufficient genes are involved, the threshold is passed and the condition manifested. In this way

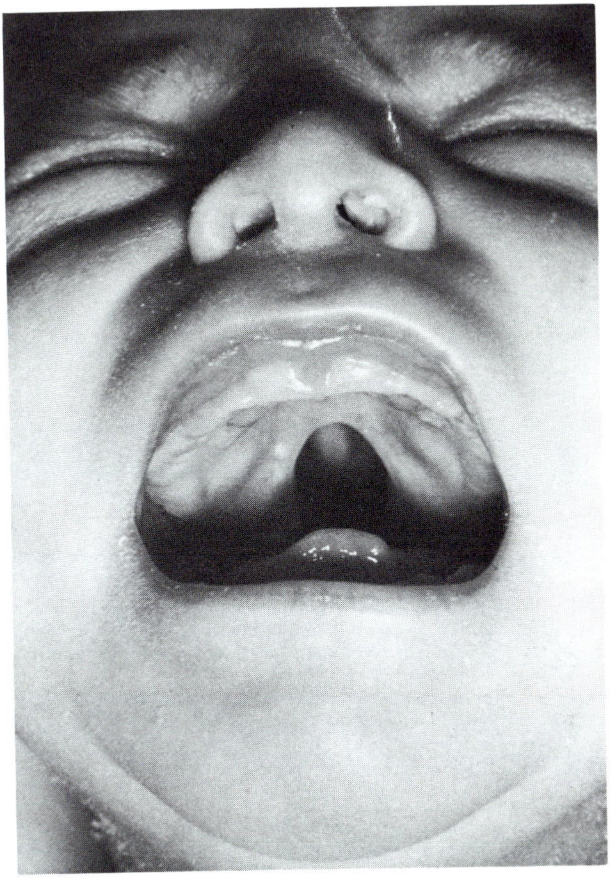

Fig. 4.8. Cleft of the secondary palate only (by kind permission of Mr P. G. Bush, Liverpool A.H.A.(T)).

it can be seen that families with existing cases of cleft will be more likely than others to have further cases, and the risk of parents having further children with clefts has been summarized by Blyth and Carter (1969) in the following terms.

*Cleft lip with/without cleft palate:* Both parents normal, risk to other sibs or children 4 per cent; if one parent and one child affected, 12 per cent risk to subsequent sibs.

*Cleft palate median, uncomplicated:* Risk to subsequent sibs when parents normal, 1 in 50; when parents normal but another relative affected, 1 in 10; when one parent affected, 1 in 6.

Cleft lip and palate, however, also occur in association with other abnormalities; in some cases chromosomal aberrations, in others a mutant gene may be responsible.

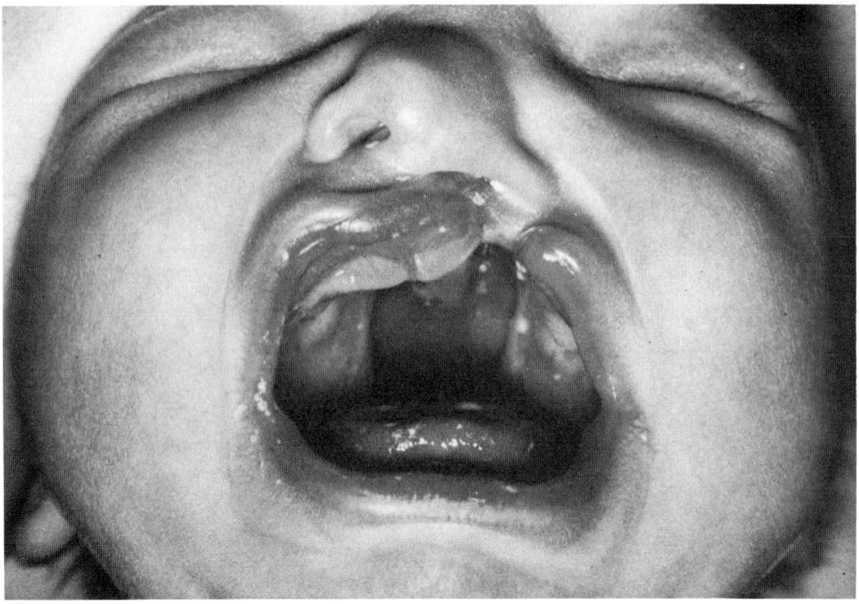

Fig. 4.9. Incomplete cleft of primary palate on left side and of secondary palate too (by kind permission of Mr P. G. Bush, Liverpool A.H.A.(T)).

## Ossification

At an early stage in the foetus the skeleton of the midfacial region is cartilagenous, as is the base of the skull to which it is connected. It develops in the maxillary and frontonasal processes and may be referred to as the nasal capsule.

Medially in the septal cartilage and laterally in the side walls of the nasal cavities above is where the lateral mass of the ethmoid will later ossify, and below the inferior turbinate process (Fig. 4.10). Later between these two areas the cartilage atrophies and the developing maxillary sinus appears.

Cartilage is important in early foetal life as a framework, since the ossification centres of bones related to it have not yet joined up and therefore provide no support for the structures developing in the facial area.

The maxilla appears early as a centre of membranous ossification on the outer side of the nasal capsule about the 6th week. The site is immediately lateral to and below the infraorbital nerve, where the anterior superior dental nerve branches off. Ossification extends backwards towards the zygomatic bone, and between these arise a mass of secondary cartilage which, however, only lasts for a short time, unlike that in the mandible. The zygomatic bone is also ossifying at this time and forming part of the cheek and the lateral floor of the orbit.

The ossification of the maxilla continues forward in front of the anterior

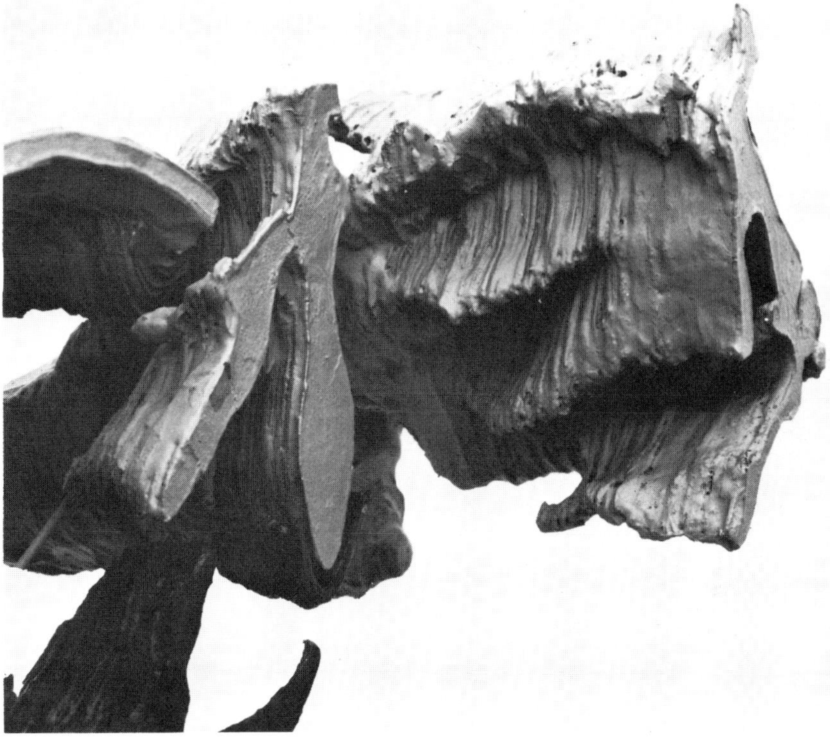

Fig. 4.10. Internal view of posterior part of lateral nasal wall from a model prepared by Dr T. H. M. Wynne, Liverpool A.H.A.(T). Note the nasal septum centrally and the superior, middle and inferior turbinates on the right-hand side.

superior dental nerve towards the developing premaxilla and provides an upward extension to form the frontal process of the maxilla. Also on the lateral aspect of the nasal capsule, the nasal and lacrimal bones arise in membrance at about 8 weeks (Fig. 4.11).

The premaxilla has arisen from the area of the primary palate at about 7 weeks, and shortly after fuses with the medially directed process of the maxilla to form the majority of the hard palate. A suggestion of their separate origins is provided by the remains of a suture at birth on the palate between the incisor foramen posteriorly and the alveolar process between the canine and lateral incisor. However, it should be noted that not all investigators consider there is a definitive premaxillary centre of ossification, as serial sectioning does not necessarily reveal it.

The palatine bone develops in membrane about the 7th to 8th week. The centre of ossification first appears on the inner side of the posterior part of the nasal capsule cartilage and is related to the palatal nerves. It continues inwards to form the back of the hard palate and upwards as a vertical plate

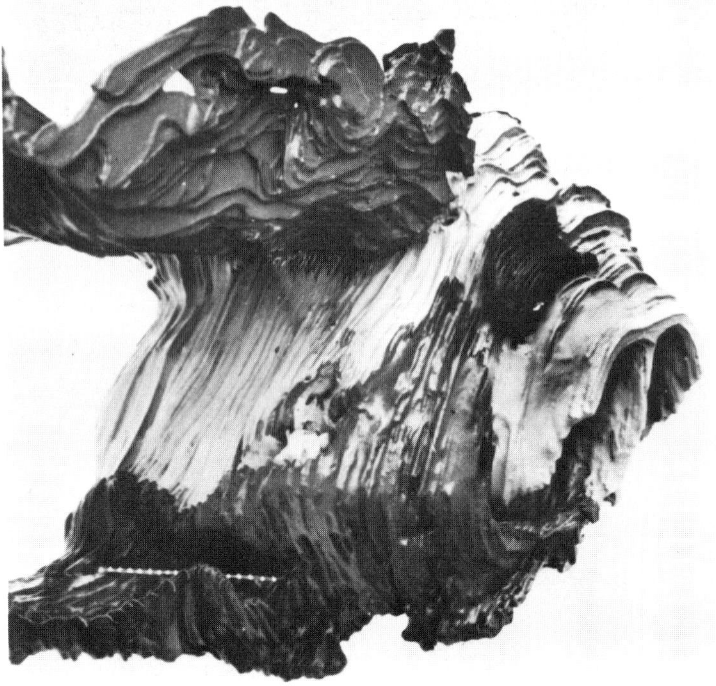

Fig. 4.11. Right side of nasal capsule from a model prepared by Dr T. H. M. Wynne, Liverpool A.H.A.(T). The membrane bones are shown darker, the frontal bone above, nasal bone in front and the maxilla below.

overlapping the back of the nasal surface of the maxilla and between the lower parts of the medial and lateral pterygoid plates.

The perpendicular plate of the ethmoid ossifies in due course within the nasal septum posteriorly and superiorly and, laterally, the lateral mass of the ethmoid also ossifies. They become united after birth, when the cribriform plate is ossified. The inferior turbinate bone develops laterally in the process mentioned earlier. Below the septal cartilage the vomer develops, about 12 weeks, forming a groove in which the cartilage is loosely attached, the nasovomerine groove (Fig. 4.12). There appears to be a structure attaching the anterior border of the nasal septum to the premaxilla, termed the septopremaxillary ligament.

It is important to realize that, even early in foetal life, growth as well as development is occurring in the face and the processes of remodelling of bone to be described later in connection with postnatal growth is already at work. However, investigation of prenatal growth in man is not easy because of the lack of availability of human foetuses of some ages and also due to the variability exhibited.

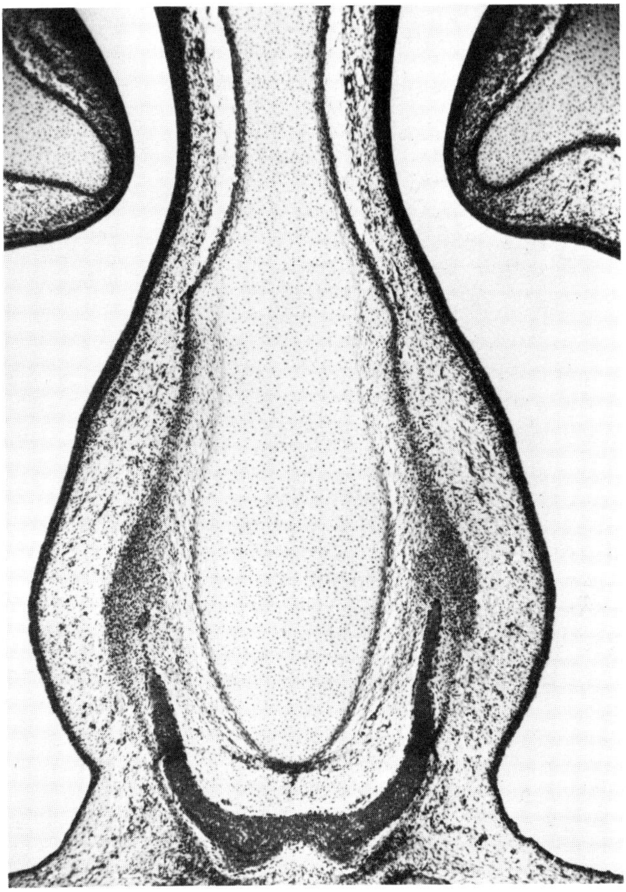

Fig. 4.12. Section through the nasal septum showing its relation to the vomer below (by kind permission of Dr. T. H. M. Wynne, Liverpool A.H.A.(T)).

Burdi (1969) investigated growth of the nasomaxillary complex between the 12th week and term. Using sixty-eight specimens of foetal heads which he sectioned parasagittally just lateral to the nasal septum, he obtained enlarged photographs in which standard cephalometric points could be identified.

The entire nasal septum as well as individual regions of it demonstrated significant correlations between increasing septal height and crown rump length (a measure of foetal age). Septal length was also significantly correlated with crown rump length, the largest relative increase in length being in the posterior region of the septum (measured, on a line parallel to the palatal plane, from perpendiculars through crista galli and through posterior nasal spine).

Both hard and soft palates increased in length at a rate which was significantly correlated with increasing crown rump length. The proportionality between soft and hard palate length remained approximately constant, soft palate being about one-third of total palate length.

No significant changes in regression coefficients were observed for the upper facial profile, and so the major finding was that growth of the upper face during this period followed a trend characterized by progressive enlargement of a relatively stable profile.

However, not all investigators agree that the regression with time is linear, and they suggest that more rapid growth occurs in the first part of foetal life with a slowing down later.

Part of the controversy about foetal facial growth arises from the variability shown by specimens and the difficulty in dating them exactly. Also the use of fixed cephalometric points, some of which are not accurately determinable at this age, gives rise to errors. In addition, in some cases the points themselves are not stable with age.

## POSTNATAL GROWTH

Growth of the midface is achieved by a number of mechanisms, and the apparent growth downwards and forwards shown by cephalometric studies oversimplifies the complex nature of growth in this region.

The midface is involved in a number of very important functions, for example respiration, mastication, swallowing and vision. The facial skeleton is naturally important for supporting the exercise of these functions, but it is now generally agreed that in growth the determining factors are often those of these functions rather than intrinsic predetermined growth of bones alone.

It is easy to see this in connection with the eyes, where it has been shown that orbit size is related to its contents and the absence of an eye will restrict growth in this area. There is also some evidence that normal turbinate morphogenesis requires an intact structural nasal frame which is loaded in both incisal and molar occlusal function by muscular activity. Further evidence relating to mastication and deglutition will be dealt with in later chapters.

Respiration is, of course, of paramount importance biologically, and the maintenance of an effective airway must be allowed for during growth. Moss (1964), in elaborating his theory of functional matrices, states that the form of the nasal or oral cavities must not be thought of as space merely left over by adjacent bone growth. On the contrary, they are the biologic prerequisite to normal function. It is, however, difficult to visualize what actual mechanism is involved.

**General Factors**

Before going into the details of midfacial growth it will be as well to discuss in general terms the following four factors: Sutures, cartilage, displacement growth and surface deposition and resorption.

*Sutures.* Although no longer considered an active means of growth, they are necessary to allow filling in of bone following growth mediated elsewhere. The sutural system in the midfacial region is partially indicated in Fig. 4.13, and superficially, anyway, seems to provide for a forward and downward direction of growth. However, they are not all simple sutures and, for example, the zygomaticomaxillary one would not, in fact, readily allow growth downwards and forwards as the articular surface of the maxilla faces outwards.

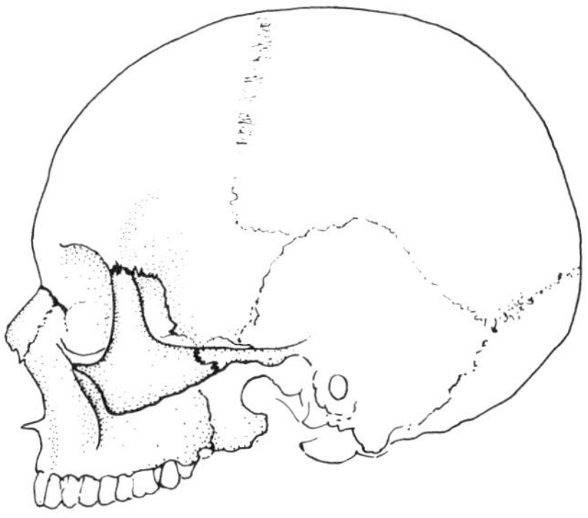

Fig. 4.13. Lateral view of skull of an adult showing the position of the sutures which seem to indicate a general downward and forward direction.

*Cartilage.* The importance of the nasal septum has been debated considerably over the years, some workers such as Scott (1967) considering it an active growth centre, others feeling it only follows behind growth already proceeding.

Many experiments have been carried out to investigate this problem. For example, Sarnat and Wexler (1966) removed areas of the cartilagenous nasal septum in developing animals and found a reduction of growth in the snout with a reversal of the incisal relationship and overeruption of the lower incisors. However, there has been some criticism of experimental work in general, saying that the trauma involved might cause fibrosis and therefore inhibit growth of the region anyway.

Other workers have grown nasal cartilage by transplantation to see how much growth continues in the new environment. In general the earlier experiments were disappointing, indicating little potential for growth of the cartilage. More recently, however, considerable proliferation activity has been found, indicating there is substantial potential for growth.

Success has also been achieved in tissue culture where definite growth of nasoseptal cartilage occurred which could be increased by various humoral agents such as somatomedins.

In any case, if the septal cartilage is an important growth centre it is probably mainly operative in the foetal and early postnatal period.

*Displacement.* As the midface is connected with the cranial base, growth there will also affect it. This growth has been dealt with in Chapter 3, so will not be repeated here except to say there results a passive downward and forward movement of the midface.

*Surface deposition and resorption.* In the course of growth, inevitably parts of the midface will be resorbed and at other times deposition will occur. In the maxilla, for example, the major deposition is backward in the tuberosity region but resorption occurs anteriorly.

The most detailed work on this subject has been carried out by Enlow and Bang (1965). They sectioned a number of human maxillae, and other areas of the midface, of children of various ages, and looked at the type of bone in the different regions. Thus areas of periosteal deposition or resorption were identified, the same also being charted for the endosteum.

Björk (1966 and 1968) has contributed to these findings by inserting small metal markers in various places in the maxilla during childhood. Subsequent radiographs can then monitor where deposition or resorption of bone has occurred as the markers remain as fixed points. Some points were inserted on either side of the median palatal suture and their movement apart indicated actual sutural growth.

## REGIONS OF GROWTH

Since all the face, cranial vault and base are developing simultaneously, it is somewhat artificial to deal with only one aspect at a time. However, for ease of comprehension it is helpful.

In addition to the cranial vault, base and auditory capsules which have been dealt with in Chapter 3, Scott (1955) enumerates the following regions descriptively:

The nasal region
The orbital cavities
The alveolopalatal region
The facial buttress system
The pharyngeal region

He also mentions the muscular processes, but, apart from the zygomatic arch and lateral pterygoid plates, which can be dealt with under the buttress system, these are mainly concerned with the mandible and occipital regions and therefore need no further description here.

*Nasal region.* The bones involved are:

*Roof:* nasal, frontal, cribriform plate of ethmoid, body of sphenoid.
*Lateral wall:* maxilla, vertical plate of palatine, lateral part of ethmoid, lacrimal and inferior turbinate.
*Medial wall:* perpendicular plate of ethmoid, septal cartilage and vomer.
*Floor:* palatal process of maxilla and palatal process of palatine bone.

A line drawn along the lower borders of the orbits divides the nasal cavities into an upper interorbital and a lower maxillary part. The proportions of these change with growth. At birth the upper part is about twice as high as the lower; however, in the adult the two are about equal in height. By the end of the first decade the upper part has reached its full dimensions, while the lower part continues to grow into adult life (Fig. 4.14).

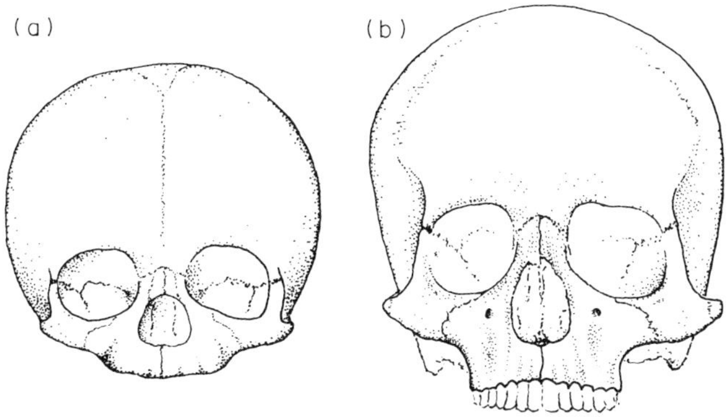


Fig. 4.14. Skulls showing the proportions of the midface in a child and an adult.

Apart from the uppermost part of the roof of the nasal chambers the surfaces of the walls and floor are primarily resorptive, including the nasal bone, and therefore there is a lateral and anterior expansion of the nasal chambers with a downwards movement of the palate.

The ethmoidal turbinates are depository laterally and inferiorly and resorptive superiorly and medially, and this moves them downward and laterally with the growth of the nasal region.

The expansion of the maxillary sinus is in a downwards forwards and outwards direction by resorption on all its walls except the medial one, on which there is deposition. By the 3rd year the sinus has extended above the deciduous molars and the unerupted 1st permanent molar and the developing permanent canine is close to its anterior wall. It continues to enlarge and in the adult the floor is related mainly to the premolars and molars.

During the 1st year the perpendicular plate of the ethmoid ossifies at the back of the septal cartilage and by the 3rd year has met the vomer with which it unites by about the 10th year. Irregular remodelling gives rise to variable amounts of septal deviation or possibly it may be partly due to cartilagenous growth after the bony skeleton is consolidated.

The nasal bones have resorption on their inner surfaces and deposition on the outer surfaces and, indeed, the position of the nasion is not as constant during growth as is sometimes assumed in cephalometry.

There is a displacement of the whole nasomaxillary complex in an inferior direction, and new bone is added at the frontomaxillary, ethmomaxillary, ethmofrontal, nasofrontal frontolacrimal and vomerine sutures. In addition, more laterally, bone is also added at the zygotemporal, zygosphenoidal and zygomaxillary sutures.

*The orbital cavities.* The growth of the orbit is related to the expanding contents of the orbit, that is the eye and its associated structures. As the eye is relatively mature at birth, growth is probably more or less complete by 7 years of age.

The medial wall of the orbit, which consists of the ethmoid, maxillary and lacrimal bones, expands in a lateral direction with the enlargement of the ethmoidal sinuses. The roof shows mainly deposition and so does the floor. This does not decrease the size of the orbit as it can be considered as a V facing anteriorly and the growth goes in the direction of the larger part of the V.

The whole orbit is also displaced downwards along with the rest of the mid-face in association with growth at the sutures within and outside the orbit.

The medial rim of the orbit in the child is only slightly in front of the lateral, but it grows forward together with the nasal wall and in the adult is in front of the lateral rim which has effectively moved backwards with the cheek.

*Alveolopalatal region.* As will be seen in Chapter 9, the gum pads are not closely related to each other at birth, but during growth the alveolar process moves downwards both as a result of general displacement of the maxilla downwards and forwards and also due to deposition on its inferior surface. This is related to the developing and erupting teeth, but it is important to realize that eruption is an additional mechanism going on as well independently. When the dentition is established, there is a tendency for mesial drift of teeth to occur, the cause of which is somewhat disputed. In earlier populations such as the Saxons, where much approximal attrition occurred, this allowed room for eruption of the posterior molar teeth.

The hard palate being composed of the palatal process of the maxilla in front and the horizontal plate of the palate bone posteriorly achieves downward growth by bone deposition on its oral surface and, as has been mentioned before, the nasal floor which is its upper side undergoes resorption. The palate also grows wider by this mechanism, on the V-principle with direction of growth towards the open part of the V, that is downwards. Laterally, growth is also achieved by growth at the mid-palatal suture early in life and later by deposition on the lateral aspect of the maxilla. The importance of the first method has been debated at length in the past, but implant studies have demonstrated actual separation of the markers which must indicate sutural growth.

*The facial buttress system.* The forces of mastication are transmitted to the cranium through the ramal element of the mandible and the buttress system of the face. This comprises the palatal vault, the zygomaticofrontal and zygomaticotemporal arches, the frontomaxillary and pterygopalatalmaxillary articulations.

The maxilla grows backwards by deposition on the posterior-facing maxillary tuberosity, allowing for the erupting molar teeth and maxillary sinus. There is also, laterally, growth by deposition on its buccal surface, thus widening the dental arch. In front of the malar protuberance, however, the surface is resorptive. Anteriorly, deposition occurs in relation to the anterior nasal spine above, but below there is resorption to allow downward movement of the spine, thus retaining its contour.

The overall effect of growth in the maxilla is to place it more forward and downwards, although there is some dispute as to how backward growth can do this. It may be that the nasal cartilage or the functional matrix is moving everything in this region forward or there may be a pushing against the connective tissue in the pterygomaxillary space by the newly forming bone posteriorly.

The zygomatic bone also shows deposition posteriorly and inferiorly. Resorption probably occurs anteriorly, so that it relocates posteriorly as it grows to keep in line with the maxilla. However, not all investigators agree about there being resorption anteriorly. The zygomatic arch moves outwards by resorption medially within the temporal fossa and by deposition laterally to keep the proportion of the cheek bone in relation to the face.

The sutures in this region allow adjustments in growth in different directions and are secondary to the other changes already described.

*The pharyngeal region.* This is at the back of the midface, bounded by the cervical vertebrae posteriorly and the posterior segment of the cranial base above (Fig. 4.15). Its growth is, of course, associated with the respiratory and alimentary systems partially mediated presumably by growth of the cervical vertebrae in height. The anterior posterior depth is associated with the cranial base growth at the spheno-occipital synchondrosis.

In addition, however, cervicofacial posture plays an important part. This is

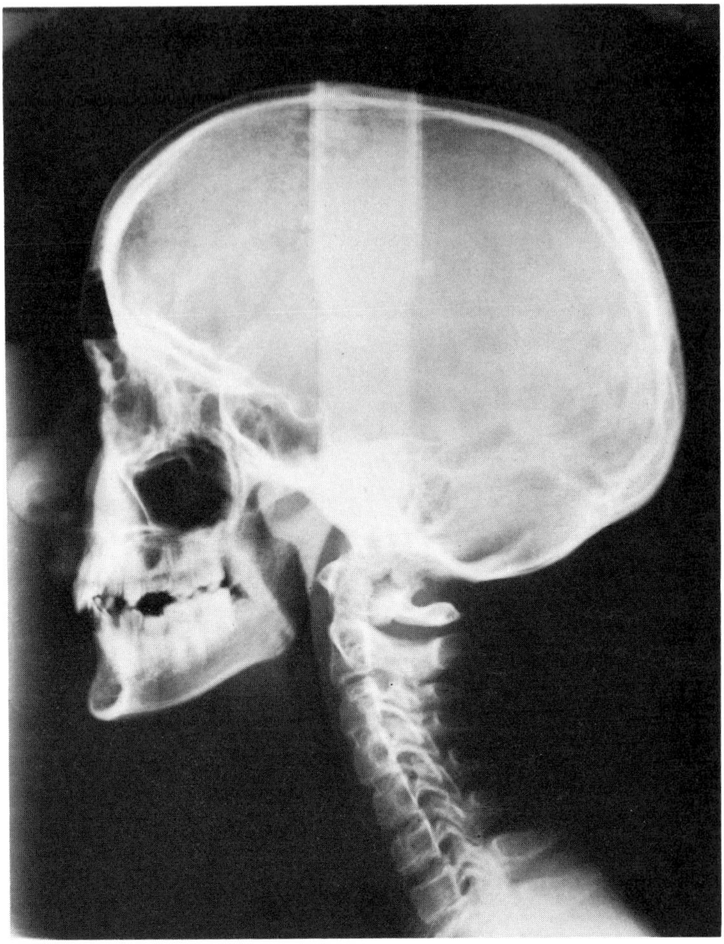

Fig. 4.15. Cephalometric radiograph showing position of nasopharynx (dark shadow) with relation to the cervical vertebrae, midface and cranial base. (A filter has been put on the radiograph anteriorly to show up the soft tissues.)

noticeable, particularly in cases where adenoids are enlarged, thus reducing the airway. There is a tendency for the lips to be kept open, a degree of actual mouthbreathing may result and the child will extend his head backwards somewhat to allow a better airway.

The overall effects of adenoids on facial growth has been studied extensively over the years, but the original concept that it produced a long face with pinched nose and open mouth with proclined maxillary incisors has been disproved. However, there are facial changes, the main ones being a larger lower facial height, open lips with the tongue more inferiorly placed and also

Narrow upper arch.

often an open bite. The incisors are usually retroclined, however. After removal of the adenoids there is a tendency to revert to a more normal growth pattern.

## MAGNITUDE OF GROWTH

There are very many investigations aimed at quantifying the amount of growth going on in the facial region, and some of the radiological ones will be discussed in the chapter on cephalometrics.

It is important to realize that individuals show great variability in facial growth both in pattern and magnitude, so that a series of mean values of size at different ages, even if accompanied by standard deviations, is of little value to the clinician interested in a particular patient. Also standards obtained, for example, in the United States, will not necessarily be applicable to children in the United Kingdom or elsewhere.

Some of the general features of growth in this connection have already been discussed in Chapter 1. It is, however, useful to have some idea of the magnitude of various dimensions of the face and their behaviour during growth, so a few illustrations are given herewith.

Savara and Singh (1968) examined 52 boys radiologically from 3 to 16 years in a mixed longitudinal study and found that measurements involving facial height such as from nasomaxillary suture to prosthion showed more growth than those of length (anterior nasal spine—pterygomaxillary fissure). Facial width as measured between zygomaticomaxillary sutures or pterygomaxillary fissures showed even less.

Although there were variations, the general pattern was a slowing of growth from 3 years to about 10 years of age and a pubertal spurt round about 13-14 years.

The actual figures were height 4.99 cm at 3 years and 7.08 cm at 16 years, length 4.83 cm at 3 years and 6.08 cm at 16 years. Width between zygomaticomaxillary sutures was 7.62 cm at 3 years and 9.53 cm at 16 years.

In comparison with boys, another study of girls in the same region showed the adolescent spurt of growth 2 or 3 years earlier and dimensions overall smaller. Other investigators have also found this, and also that boys show greater forward growth in the lower face at puberty, making their faces straighter, squarer and more angular. Individual variation is, again, wide both in the age of pubertal changes and their magnitude.

It should be noted that facial dimensions are increasing after cranial ones have slowed down, and, for example, between 4 and 20 years of age the increase of upper face width is twice that for head width. The size of a child's face at an early age gives very little predictive value regarding the rate at which he will grow in the ensuing years of childhood.

## BIBLIOGRAPHY


BJÖRK, A. (1966) Sutural growth of the upper face studied by the implant method, *Acta Odont. Scand.* **24**, 109.

BJÖRK, A. (1968) The use of metallic implants in the study of facial growth in children: method and application, *Am. J. phys. Anthrop.* **29**, 243.

BJÖRK, A. and V. SKIELLER (1976) Postnatal growth and development of the maxillary complex, in *Factors Affecting the Growth of the Midface,* ed. J. A. McNamara, Jr., Center for Human Growth and Development, Univ. Michigan, Ann Arbor.

BLYTH, H. and C. CARTER (1969) *A Guide to Genetic Prognosis in Paediatrics,* Heinemann, London.

BURDI, A. R. (1969) Cephalometric growth analysis of the human upper face region during the last two trimesters of gestation, *Am. J. Anat.* **125**, 113.

ENLOW, D. H. (1975) *Handbook of Facial Growth,* Saunders, Philadelphia.

ENLOW, D. H. and S. BANG (1965) Growth and remodelling of the human maxilla, *Am. J. Ortho.* **51**, 446.

HARRISON, R. G. (1978) *Clinical Embryology,* Academic Press, London.

HARVOLD, E. P., B. S. TOMER and G. CHIERICI (1981) Primate experiments in oral respiration, *Am. J. Ortho.* **79**, 359.

LATHAM, R. A. (1976) An appraisal of the early maxillary growth mechanism, in *Factors Affecting the Growth of the Midface,* ed. J. A. McNamara, Jr., Center for Human Growth and Development, Univ. Michigan, Ann Arbor.

LATHAM, R. A. and W. R. BURSTON (1966) The postnatal pattern of growth at the sutures of the human skull, *Dent. Practit.* **17**, 61.

LEVIHN, W. C. (1967) A cephalometric roentgenographic cross-sectional study of the craniofacial complex in fetuses from 12 weeks to birth, *Am. J. Ortho.* **53**, 822.

LINDER-ARONSON, S. (1979) Naso-respiratory function and craniofacial growth, in *Naso-Respiratory Function and Craniofacial Growth,* ed. J. A. McNamara, Jr., Center for Human Growth and Development, Univ. Michigan, Ann Arbor.

LINDER-ARONSON, S. and D. G. WOODSIDE (1979) The growth of the sagittal depth of the bony nasopharynx in relation to some other facial variables, in *Naso-Respiratory Function and Craniofacial Growth,* ed. J. A. McNamara, Jr., Center for Human Growth and Development, Univ. Michigan, Ann Arbor.

MEREDITH, H. V. (1959) Recent studies on growth of the body and face, *Am. J. Ortho.* **45**,110.

MOSS, M. L. (1964) Vertical growth of the human face, *Am. J. Ortho.* **50**, 359.

MOSS, M. L. (1976) The role of nasal septal cartilage in midfacial growth, in *Factors Affecting the Growth of the Midface,* ed. J. A. McNamara, Jr., Center for Human Growth and Development, Univ. Michigan, Ann Arbor.

MOSS, M. L. and L. SALENTIJN (1969) The capsular matrix, *Am. J. Ortho.* **56**, 474.

SARNAT, B. G. and M. R. WEXLER (1966) Growth of the face and jaws after resection of the septal cartilage in the rabbit, *Am. J. Anat.* **118**, 755.

SAVARA, B. S. and I. J. SINGH (1968) Norms of size and annual increment of seven anatomical measures of maxillae in boys from three to sixteen years of age, *Angl. Ortho.* **38**, 104.

SCOTT, J. H. (1955) Craniofacial regions, *Dent. Practit.* **5**, 208.

SCOTT, J. H. (1967) *Dentofacial Development and Growth,* Pergamon Press, Oxford.

SOLOW, B. and E. GREVE (1979) Craniocervical angulation and nasal respiratory resistance, in *Naso-Respiratory Function and Craniofacial Growth,* ed. J. A. McNamara, Jr., Center for Human Growth and Development, Univ. Michigan, Ann Arbor.

STUTZMANN, J. J. and A. G. PETROVIC (1976) Experimental analysis of general and local extrinsic mechanisms controlling upper jaw growth, in *Factors Affecting the Growth of the Midface,* ed. J. A. Mcnamara, Jr., Center for Human Growth and Development, Univ. Michigan, Ann Arbor.

WYNNE, T. H. M. (1966) *Observation on the development of the human chondrocranium,* Ph.D. thesis, Univ. Liverpool.

# CHAPTER 5

# *Growth of the Mandible*

The skeleton of the lower part of the face is formed by a single bone, the mandible, which in addition to providing attachment for the facial soft tissues and masticatory muscles, encloses the muscles used in speech, supports the teeth and forms part of the temporomandibular articulation (Chapter 6). The structural changes in development and growth of the mandible are well documented, but the detailed mechanisms by which these changes take place are still the subject of debate. In particular, the role of the secondary condylar cartilage in mandibular growth is questioned.

Since the growth of the mandible, following cephalometric analysis, is described in Chapter 7, this chapter should be read in conjunction with the relevant section on the mandible.

## DEVELOPMENT

The mandible develops in relation to the first pharyngeal arch where it is preceded by the cartilage of the primary cartilagenous skeleton, Meckel's cartilage. This bar of hyaline cartilage surrounded by a distinct fibrous perichondrium extends from the midline upwards, backwards and outwards towards the otic capsule. It attains its fullest form by 6 weeks of intrauterine life and has a close relationship with the mandibular nerve (Fig. 5.1). Meckel's cartilage takes no direct part in the formation of the corpus of the mandible, but acts as a support not only for the mandibular nerve but for the membrane bone which will develop later. Part of the fibrous perichondrium, however, remains to form the sphenomalleolar and sphenomandibular ligaments. The most dorsal part of Meckel's cartilage will later ossify and form the malleus of the middle ear.

Intramembranous ossification commences during the 7th week of intrauterine life as a mass of fibrous tissue lateral to the bifurcation of the incisive and mental nerves (Fig. 5.1). The rapid spread of membrane bone encloses the mental nerve in a groove and forms a plate extending laterally to the inferior dental nerve. From below the groove containing the nerve, bone formation extends beneath the incisive nerve and upwards between the incisive nerve and Meckel's cartilage. The groove containing the mental nerve becomes the mental foramen by the extension of bone over the nerve. With

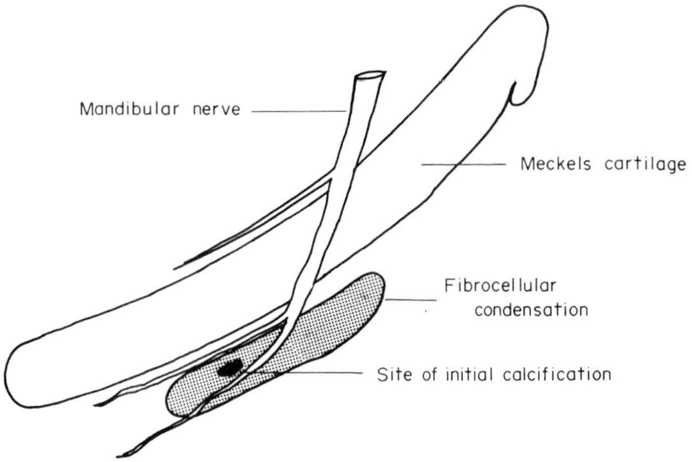


Fig. 5.1. Diagram showing the relationship of Meckel's cartilage to the mandibular nerve and the site where membrane bone formation is initiated.

the formation of bone over the incisive nerve, the incisive canal is formed. The bone of the two halves of the mandible comes into close relationship in the midline where they are separated by fibrous tissue to form a symphysis in which nodules of the remnants of Meckel's cartilage may be seen until birth. Complete bony union to form a synostosis is not complete until the end of the first year after birth (Chapter 2).

Bone formation also spreads backwards, resulting in a plate lateral to the inferior dental nerve. At this stage the developing dental lamina is remote from the bone of the mandible (Fig. 5.2). Later, as the tooth germs differentiate, they will become enclosed by the lateral and medial plates of the mandibular bone. These plates will extend above the level of the roof of the canals for the incisive and inferior dental nerves to form the alveolar plates. As a result, the tooth germs become enclosed in a trough which is later divided by septa extending mediolaterally to form crypts or alveoli.

Between 12 and 14 weeks, secondary or accessory cartilages appear in relation to the developing foetal mandible. These are the symphysial, coronoid and condylar cartilages. The symphysial and coronoid cartilages disappear before birth, but the most important in relation to the development and growth of the mandible is the condylar cartilage. This attains its fullest form at about 12 weeks of intrauterine life and is a carrot-shaped structure enclosed by a fibrous perichondrium extending upwards, backwards and outwards. Its narrow proximal end is related to the membrane bone of the mandibular corpus. It grows rapidly at its distal end both appositionally and interstitially (Chapter 2). By 14 weeks endochondral ossification is taking place and the bone thus formed is indistinguishable from the membrane bone of the

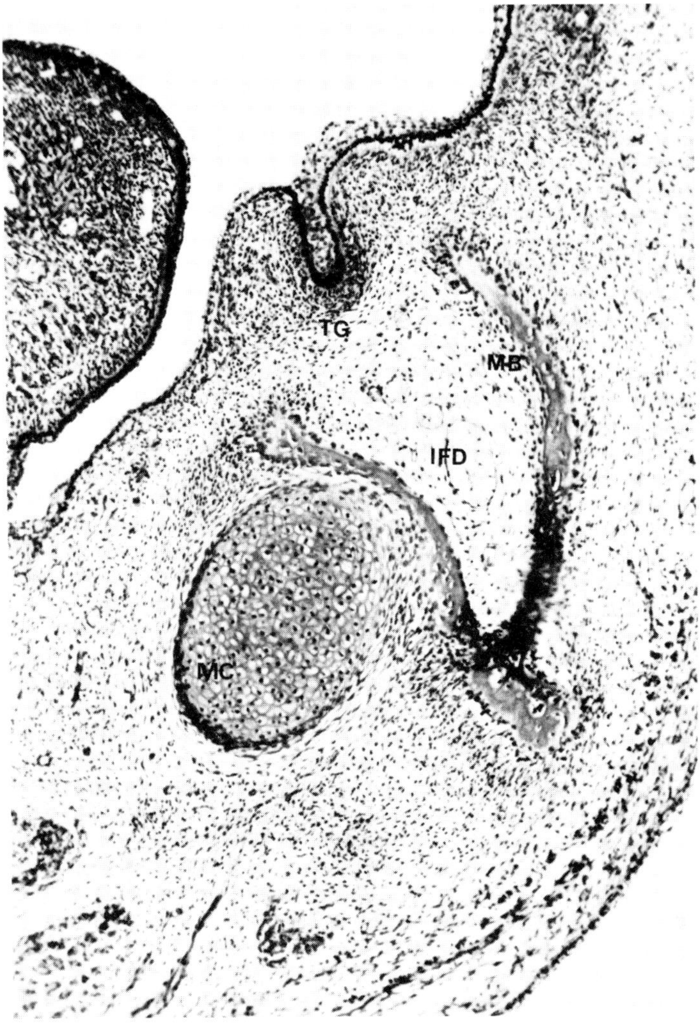


Fig. 5.2. Photomicrograph of a coronal section through the developing mandible. MC, Meckel's cartilage; MB, membrane bone of mandible; IFD, inferior dental nerve; TG, tooth germ.

mandibular corpus. The role of this cartilage in mandibular growth will be discussed later in this chapter.

## GROWTH

In the earliest stages of mandibular development growth takes place by surface deposition with resorption beginning at about 10 weeks around the expanding tooth germs. At 13 weeks, however, resorption fields appear on the buccal surface of the coronoid process and the lingual surface of the posterior part of the corpus. The anterior border of the ramus is resorptive, the posterior border depository and the anterior tip of the coronoid process is also depository. By 26 weeks the future postnatal growth pattern is well established, except in the incisor region (Fig. 5.3).

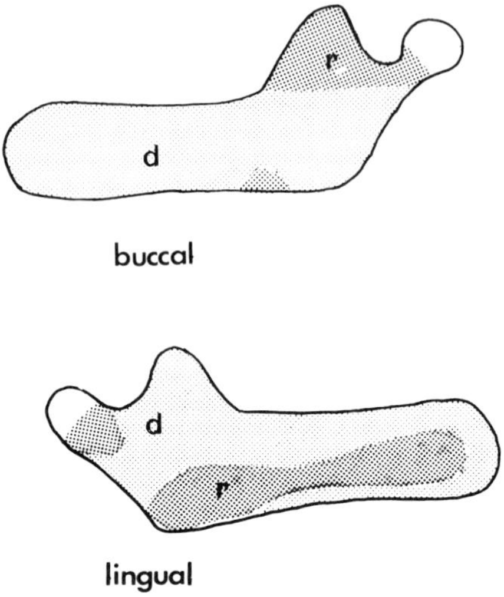


Fig. 5.3. Foetal mandible showing the resorptive (r) and depository (d) fields.

At birth the mandible has the essential structures of the adult, but differs in that the mandibular angle is obtuse, the ramus is small compared with the corpus and there is no dense cortical bone. The body has both neural and alveolar elements and constructed around the bony core developed by the condylar cartilage are the coronoid and angular muscular processes (Fig. 5.4).

In the early postnatal mandible, after about 15 weeks, the labial surface of the anterior part of the corpus is depository and the lingual side resorptive. This produces a forward growth movement of the incisor region, thereby lengthening the mandible to accommodate the deciduous dentition. By the age of 5-6 years, however, the labial surface becomes resorptive, so that further lengthening of the arch is accomplished posteriorly where ramus is remodelled to form corpus. This posterior growth is sufficient to accommodate the developing permanent molar teeth. The mandible, therefore, may be divided into two parts, the corpus and the ramus. During further development and growth their relative proportions are altered by bone resorption and deposition so that the ramus becomes relocated posteriorly with consequential lengthening of the corpus (Fig. 5.5). The ramus increases in its dimensions anteroposteriorly to allow for the growth of the middle cranial fossa and pharynx. Increase in the vertical height of the ramus accommodates for the vertical growth of the nasomaxillary complex and tooth eruption. Remodelling changes, therefore, position the mandibular corpus correctly in relation to the maxilla.

### Corpus

Enlow (1975) suggests that the mandible has a growth field which is a direct anatomical equivalent to the maxillary tuberosity, the lingual tuberosity. The presence of the lingual tuberosity is emphasized by a resorptive field immediately beneath. This area, aligned vertically beneath the maxillary tuberosity, grows by deposition on its posterior facing surface at an equal rate to that of the maxillary tuberosity (Fig. 5.6). Growth is in a posterior direction by surface deposition on the posterior facing surface of the tuberosity. The dental arch is brought into alignment by a growth field immediately behind the tuberosity. This produces growth medially, so that this part of the ramus will become corpus, since at the same time the ramus is being transformed into corpus. There is little increase in bicondylar width since the lateral growth of the cranial base is complete by 3 years (Fig. 5.6).

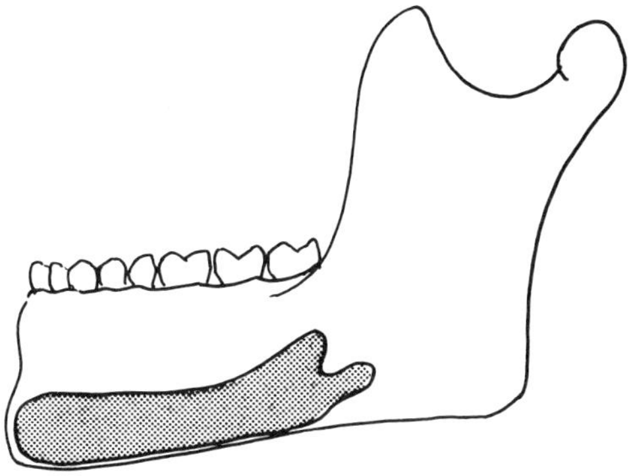

Fig. 5.4. Diagram illustrating the differences between the mandible at birth and in the adult.

Since any individual maintains the same distance between his teeth throughout life, the mandible has to increase its vertical height. This compensates for the eruption movement of teeth, the increase in height of the alveolar process and the forward growth of the mandible.

### Ramus, Coronoid and Condylar Processes

As we have seen during the growth of the mandible, the whole of the mandibular ramus is relocated, bone resorption taking place on the anterior border and deposition on the posterior border. This is somewhat of an oversimplification since at the same time there is enlargement of both the coronoid

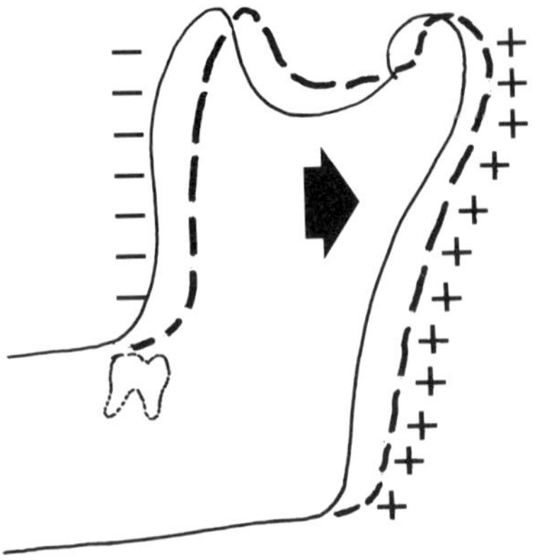

Fig. 5.5. The ramus of the mandible is relocated by resorption on its anterior border and deposition on its posterior border.

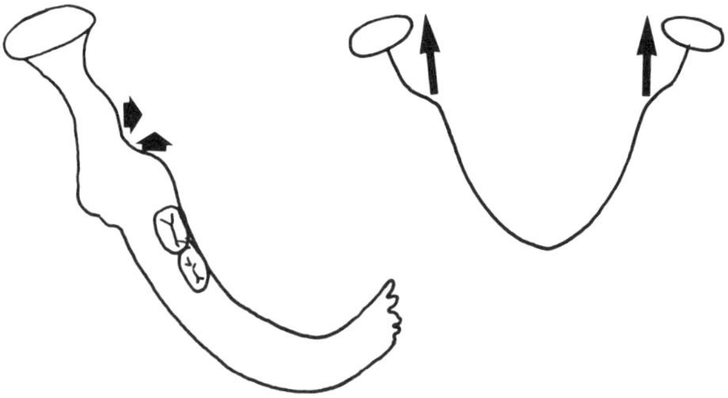

Fig. 5.6. Growth by surface deposition at the lingual tuberosity is accompanied by surface deposition in a growth field immediately behind the tuberosity. This produces growth medially, so that the dental arch is brought into alignment as this part of the ramus becomes corpus.

and condylar processes. The coronoid process has a lingual surface that faces superiorly, posteriorly and medially. The deposition of bone onto this surface will, therefore, increase the vertical height of the coronoid process, produce posterior growth and move the base of the coronoid process medially (Fig. 5.7). The buccal side of the coronoid process has a resorptive surface with the inside surface undergoing apposition. In each case growth is an example of the expanding V principle propounded by Enlow. The ramus beneath the coronoid process also has a twist, so that the buccal side faces posteriorly and is depository while the lingual side is resorptive.

The posterior border of the ramus is a major growth site which keeps pace with the growth of the mandibular condyle. Although the two sites are physically close they, according to Enlow, are independent and localized

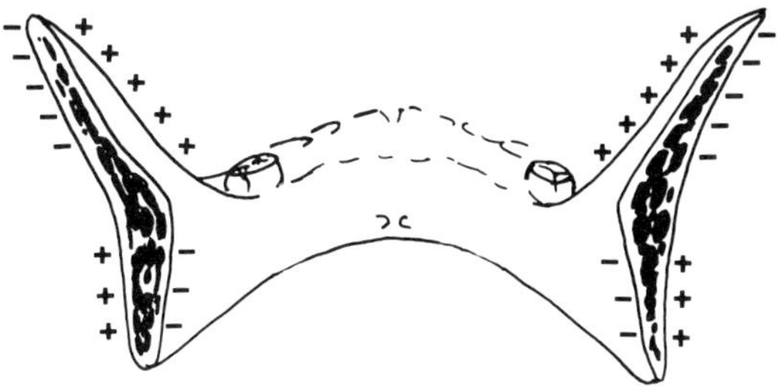

Fig. 5.7. A transverse section through the coronoid processes of the mandibular ramus indicating how growth takes place according to the expanding V principle.

areas of growth. Together they represent the most active areas in mandibular growth in terms of the amount of bone deposited.

The mandibular foramen throughout maintains a fairly constant position halfway between the anterior and posterior borders of the mandibular ramus.

### The Mandibular Condyle

The secondary cartilage of the mandibular condyle provides both a major growth centre and an articular surface for the ramus of the mandible. Its detailed structure will be described in Chapter 6. It functions as a growth centre up to the end of the second decade, during which it is replaced by bone in endochondral ossification. The endochondral bone forms the core of the condylar process around which the bone is produced periosteally or endosteally in a fibrous membrane. It is clear that cartilage is the ideal tissue to form the rapidly growing articular mandibular condyle, since it is a pressure-adapted tissue.

Beneath the condylar head the lingual and buccal surfaces of the condylar process are resorptive. As the broad condyle grows backwards, upwards and outwards, the neck is formed from the condyle by remodelling (Fig. 5.8). This is yet another example of the expanding V principle.

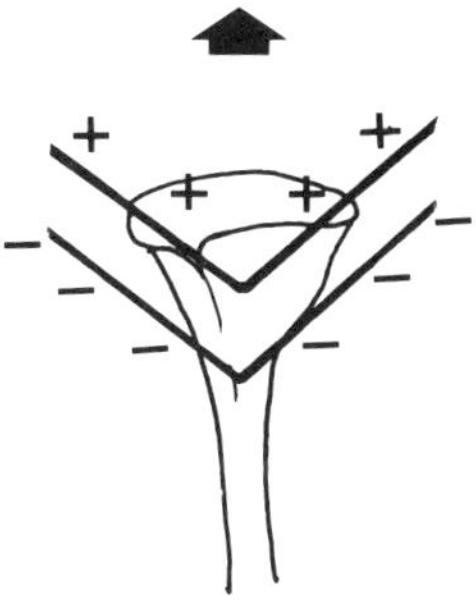

Fig. 5.8. As the condyle grows, the neck is formed from the condyle by remodelling and provides further illustration of the expanding V principle.

*The role of the mandibular condylar cartilage.* While agreeing that the condylar cartilage is an important growth centre, there are two basic concepts concerning its role in mandibular development and growth. The earlier suggestion embodied the idea that the condyle was the master control centre for mandibular growth and that this capacity was genetically determined. Accordingly, the growing pressure-adapted cartilage pushed against the articular surface of the glenoid fossa thereby creating a force which displaced the mandible downwards and forwards (Fig. 5.9A). It was suggested, furthermore, that the cartilage, therefore, controlled by direction of its growth, the relationship between the corpus and ramus. Also, since the growth of the ramus controlled the distance between the upper and lower jaws, this in turn determined the amount of alveolar bone required to maintain interocclusal vertical dimensions. The above, if true, would indicate an overall control of mandibular growth by the condylar cartilage. However, it must be acknowledged that mandibles lacking condyles develop normally, which would tend to invalidate the concept outlined above.

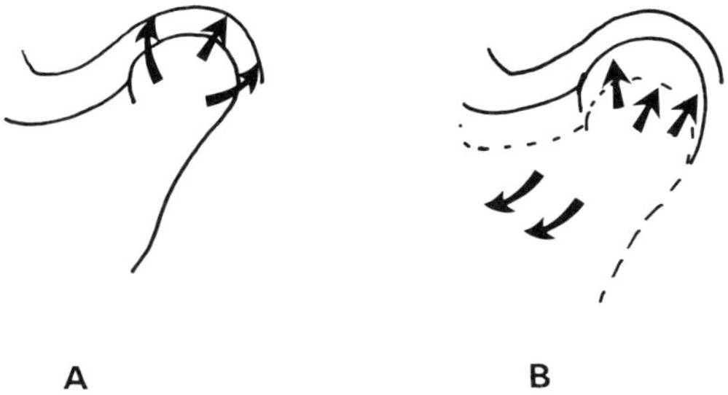


Fig. 5.9. The mandibular condyle may (A) push against the cranial base to propel the mandible downwards and forwards, (B) grow to fill in the space created by the forward displacement of the mandible by the surrounding soft tissues.

Alternatively, the mandible may be simply carried downwards and forwards by the growth of all the enclosing soft tissues, that is the soft tissue matrix. Therefore, the mandible is displaced downwards and forwards and the condylar cartilage grows to fill in the space created (Fig. 5.9B). Although the cartilage of the condyle is genetically programmed to produce bone, the organization of the tissue is not determined by the condylar cartilage but by external agencies, that is the soft tissues. The mechanism may be more complex than simple physical stimulation, however, and probably involves nerve muscle control mechanisms reacting to sensory input from the orofacial soft tissues. The total sum of these soft tissue influences has been termed by Moss (1969) the "functional matrix".

### Function and Mandibular Size

The fact that the size of the mandible is influenced by function has been indicated in both animals and man, and thus lends credence to the importance of soft tissues in growth. Watt and Williams (1951) showed that weanling rats fed on a soft diet developed significantly narrower dental arches than their litter mates. More recently, Beecher and Corruccini (1981) showed a similar effect in a small sample of Rhesus macaques.

In man, comparisons between British medieval and 17th-19th-century populations indicate a reduction in size of the mandible has occurred during this period, and is more marked in those parts of the mandible which are muscle bearing (Moore *et al.* 1968, Goose and Frake 1977). Since there were no appreciable incursions of different racial groups at this time and it is too short for evolutionary changes, the effect would seem to be environmental. The only clear factor to be isolated was the change to softer diet which occurred in the 17th century.

## BIBLIOGRAPHY


BEECHER, R. M. and R. S. CORRUCCINI (1981) Effects of dietary consistency on maxillary arch breadth in Macaques, *J. dent. Res.* **60,** 68.

BJÖRK, A. (1955) Facial growth in man studied with the aid of metallic implants, *Acta Odonto. Scand.* **13,** 9.

BJÖRK, A. (1963) Variations in the growth pattern of the human mandible; longitudinal radiographic studies by the implant method, *J. dent. Res.* **42,** 400.

BJÖRK, A. (1969) Prediction of mandibular growth rotation, *Am. J. Ortho.* **55,** 585.

ENLOW, D. H. (1975) *Handbook of Facial Growth,* Saunders, Philadelphia.

ENLOW, D. H. and D. B. HARRIS (1964) A study of the postnatal growth of the human mandible, *Am. J. Ortho.* **50,** 25.

GOOSE, D. H. and S. E. FRAKE (1977) A comparison between medieval and modern British mandibles, *Arch. oral Biol.* **22,** 55.

MANSON, J. D. (1968) *A Comparative Study of the Mandible,* Kimpton, London.

MAUSER, C., D. H. ENLOW, D. O. OVERMAN and R. E. McCAFFERTY (1975) A study of the prenatal growth of the human face and cranium, in *Determinants of Mandibular Form and Growth,* ed. J. A. McNamara, Jr., Center for Human Growth and Development, Univ. Michigan, Ann Arbor.

MOORE, W. J., C. L. B. LAVELLE and T. F. SPENCE (1968) Changes in the size and shape of the human mandible in Britain, *Brit. dent. J.* **125,** 163.

MOSS, M. L. (1960) Functional analysis of human mandibular growth, *J. Prosth. Dent.* **10,** 1149.

MOSS, M. L. (1969) The primary role of functional matrices in facial growth, *Am. J. Ortho.* **55,** 566.

MOSS, M. L. and R. RANKOW (1968) The role of the functional matrix in mandibular growth, *Angl. Ortho.* **38,** 95.

MOSS, M. L. and L. SALENTIJN (1970) The logarithmic growth of the human mandible, *Acta Anal.* **77,** 341.

SCOTT, J. H. (1954) The growth of the human face, *Proc. Roy. Soc. Med.* **47,** 1.

SCOTT, J. H. (1967) *Dentofacial Development and Growth,* Pergamon Press, Oxford.

SCOTT, J. H. (1969) The doctrine of functional matrices, *Am. J. Ortho.* **56,** 38.

SICHER, H. (1947) The growth of the mandible, *Am. J. Ortho.* **33,** 30.

WATT, D. G. and C. H. M. WILLIAMS (1951) The effects of the physical consistency of food on the growth and development of the mandible and maxilla of the rat, *Am. J. Ortho.* **37,** 895.

CHAPTER 6

# *The Temporomandibular Joint*

The temporomandibular joint is the joint between the condylar process of the mandible and the squamous temporal bone of the cranium (Fig. 6.1). Because of its anatomical and histological characteristics, this joint is unique to and diagnostic of all mammals including man. Although the temporomandibular joint may be classified as a synovial joint, unlike almost all other synovial joints, the articular surfaces do not consist of hyaline cartilage but are formed of a dense avascular mixture of connective tissue fibres and fibroblasts. Also unlike most other synovial joints, apart from the sternoclavicular, acromioclavicular, wrist and knee joints, the joint cavity is divided into an upper and lower joint compartment by a fibrous intra-articular disc. It is also highly significant in understanding joint function to realize that the joint consists of two physically separate articulations, one on either side of the face, whose movements are completely interdependent. A given movement in one joint results in a certain and predeterminable movement in the other.

Because of its importance in relation to the development and growth of the mandible and the phylogeny of the mammals, the temporomandibular joint has been the subject of considerable basic biological investigation. Clinical interest has been stimulated by the common problem of temporomandibular joint dysfunction syndrome and the problems relating to growth and functional adaptation. However, there are numerous questions waiting to be resolved. Not least concerns the role of the secondary mandibular condylar cartilage in the development and growth of the temporomandibular joint (Chapter 5). Earlier ideas suggested that the mandibular condylar cartilage was a primary growth centre in much the same way as an epiphyseal growth plate. More recent views have concluded that the condylar cartilage is highly adaptive and responds to a wide variety of chemical and physical stimuli. Therefore, during growth changes in orofacial function can result in adaptive changes within the temporomandibular joint. However, the adult joint appears to be more stable and resistant to change.

### Phylogeny

During the evolution of the mammals from reptiles, the lower jaw underwent radical modifications and in the process an entirely new jaw joint evolved.

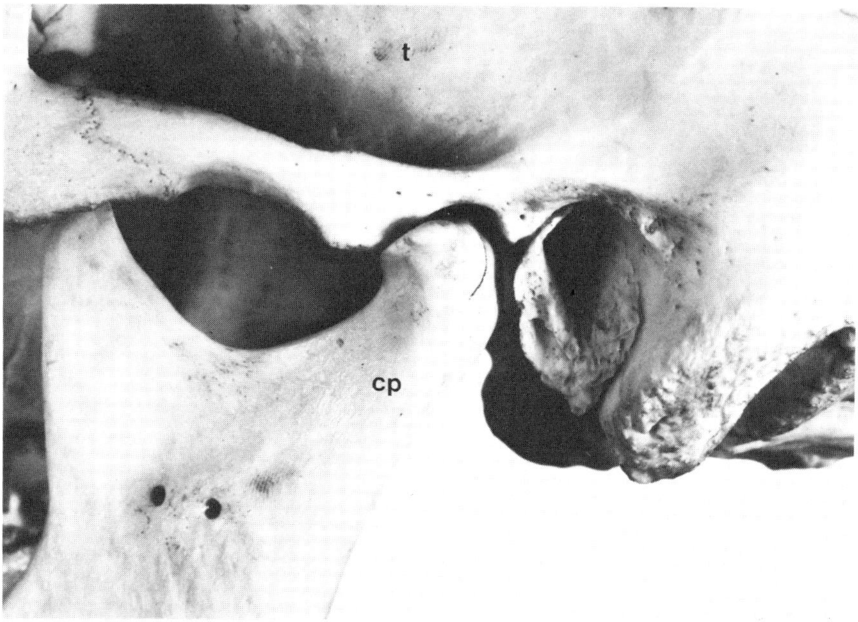


Fig. 6.1. Skeletal preparation showing the bony components of the temporomandibular joint that is the condylar process of the mandible and squamous temporal bone of the cranium.

In reptiles the lower jaw consists of several membrane bones which ensheath a rod of cartilage, Meckel's cartilage. The posterior end of Meckel's cartilage ossifies to become the articular which articulates with the quadrate to form the jaw joint. The largest and tooth-bearing bone of the lower jaw is the dentary. The fossil record suggests that during evolution of mammals the dentary gradually increased in size lateral to Meckel's cartilage and eventually came to form part of the articulating surface of the lower jaw. At the same time the temporal bone (squamosal) developed a flange for articulation with the dentary and gradually displaced the quadrate as the bone with which the lower jaw articulated. A number of fossils of mammal-like reptiles show the intermediate stage in which the articular surface is formed partly of Meckel's cartilage and partly by the dentary, with the opposing surface formed by the quadrate and the temporal. Therefore, the joint is one in which both the reptilian type of jaw joint and mammalian type coexist. In these mammal-like reptiles the quadrate was loosely attached to or had an articulation with the temporal bone and so was already becoming free to assume its later function as an ear ossicle.

With the emergence of the mammals proper, the reptilian jaw joint underwent further changes and moved back to become incorporated in the ear, thereby contributing to a more efficient hearing mechanism. The proximal end of Meckel's cartilage, the articular, detached from the lower jaw to become the malleus, and another bone of the reptilian lower jaw, the angular, becoming the tympanic bone. The lower jaw became a single bone, the dentary or mandible, which articulated with the squamous part of the temporal bone to form the temporomandibular joint.

The transition from reptiles to mammals, as described above, is in evolutionary terms a relatively recent phenomenon. However, rapid functional and behavioural adaptation of the masticatory apparatus throughout mammalian evolution has produced a wide range of structural modification. This would further suggest that this region is functionally and structurally susceptible to modification, as suggested earlier.

### Development

The temporomandibular joint develops at about 12 weeks, which is late in embryonic life when compared with the major synovial joints, and is closely associated with the development of the mandible and middle ear.

A bar of cartilage, Meckel's cartilage, appears in the mandibular arch and extends from the developing cartilagenous otic capsule to the middle line (Chapter 5). Posteriorly it ends in a thickened articular process. In the area between the posterior end of Meckel's cartilage and the otic capsule two other pieces of cartilage differentiate which will become the incus and stapes of the middle ear. Posteriorly Meckel's cartilage and the incus cartilage grow and become adapted in shape to each other forming a joint, the malleoincal joint.

At about 6 weeks of intrauterine life, several pieces of membrane bone appear; one, the mandible, arises from a condensation of mesenchyme tissue at the bifurcation of the inferior alveolar nerve. Another, the squamous part of the temporal bone, appears lateral to the brain as part of the cranium. A further piece of membrane bone is formed close to the posterior end of Meckel's cartilage. This piece of membrane bone develops to become the tympanic bone which, growing extensively in association with an extension of the temporal bone, helps to shut off the developing malleus and the other ear bones into the middle ear.

The membrane bones grow and gradually assume their definitive form. The developing mandible acquires two secondary cartilages between 10-14 weeks of intrauterine life, which will form the coronoid and condylar process respectively. The anterior coronoid process gives attachment to the temporal muscle. The more posterior condylar process grows towards the base of the zygomatic process of the temporal bone with which the condylar process forms the jaw joint (see Chapter 5).

In man, the first sign of the developing jaw joint is about 12 weeks, when two clefts appear amongst the mesenchymal cells separating the secondary cartilage of the condylar process and the temporal bone. These clefts enlarge to become the upper and lower joint cavities. The lateral part of the disc develops from a condensation of mesenchyme extending between the masseter and lateral pterygoid muscles and passing posteriorly over the condyle. The medial part of the disc appears to be derived from an extension of the lateral pterygoid tendon which also runs over the condyle and inserts with the lateral part onto the posterior end of Meckel's cartilage. It does not transfer to its definitive attachment on the posterior part of the joint capsule until the Glasserian fissure closes at 21 weeks. When this happens the portion of the perichondrium of Meckel's cartilage running from the mandible to the cranium differentiates into the sphenomandibular ligament.

## The Functional Anatomy of the Temporomandibular Joint

*The mandibular condyle.* The mandibular component of the temporomandibular joint is formed by the mandibular condyle, which can be defined as the expanded superior part of the condylar process enclosed within the articular capsule. There is considerable variation in size and shape of the mandibular condyle, but some broad generalizations may be made.

The long axis of the condyle is orientated posteriomedially and if extended would pass through the anterior border of the foramen magnum. The mature condyle measures about 20-25 mm posteriomedially and 8-10 mm anteroposteriorly. Anteriorly and superiorly, the articulating surfaces of the condyle are rounded, with the anterior-facing slope about half as long as the posterior-facing slope (Fig. 6.1).

Medially and laterally, the surfaces of the condyle are granular in appearance, where the collagen fibre bundles of the capsule and meniscus are inserted. The anterior surface of the neck dips towards the ramus and bears an area to which the external pterygoid muscle attaches. Below the articular surface at the back of the condyle is a triangular-shaped area to which the articular disc and capsule are attached. Also closely related to the area are the auriculotemporal nerve and the glenoid process of the parotid gland.

*The glenoid fossa and articular eminence.* Like the mandibular condyle, the various parts of the articular surface of the squamous temporal show considerable structural variation. The temporal articulation is situated anteriorly to the tympanic bone on the squamous temporal and comprises the concave glenoid or articular fossa and the convex articular eminence or tubercule (Fig. 6.2). The glenoid fossa measures about 20 mm anteroposteriorly and 25 mm mediolaterally. Posteriorly, the articular fossa is elevated to form a ridge, the posterior articular lip, and is separated from the tympanic plate by the squamotympanic fissure. Laterally, the posterior articular lip is to form a cone-shaped prominence, the postglenoid process. The lateral border of the glenoid fossa is frequently elevated to form a narrow low ridge. Medially, the fossa is bounded by a bony lip which leans up against the angular spine of the

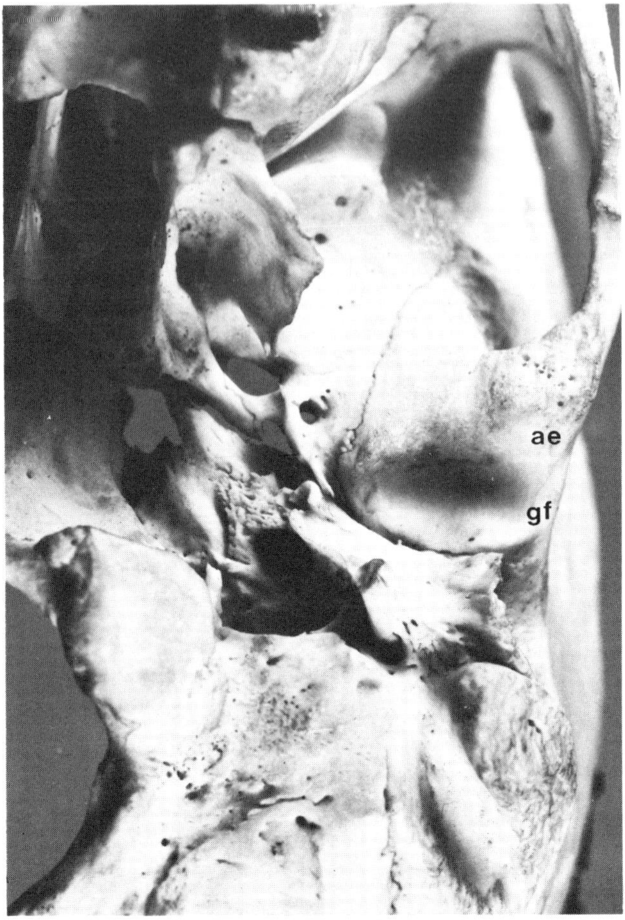


Fig. 6.2. Skeletal preparation showing the concave glenoid fossa and anteriorly the convex articular eminence.

sphenoid bone. The cortical bone separating the glenoid fossa from the middle cranial fossa is always thin.

Anteriorly, the articular surface of the glenoid fossa is continuous with the convex articular eminence, which is structurally the root of the zygomatic arch. At this point the bone becomes thicker and denser.

*The intra-articular disc or meniscus.* An intra-articular disc is always present in eutherian mammals, but is absent in monotremes and marsupials. The monotremes and marsupials retain more of the primitive mammalian characteristics than the eutherian. Therefore, it seems likely that the intra-articular disc is a refinement of the temporomandibular joint that evolved later. However, it is possible that the absence of the disc in non-eutherian mammals is due to secondary loss.

The meniscus sits characteristically like a close-fitting cap on the head of the condyle (Fig. 6.3). The inferior surface is concave and oval in shape with the long axis orientated mediolaterally. The superior surface is convex posteriorly, but anteriorly it is said to be "saddle-shaped", being convex from side to side but concave from before backwards. Viewed from above, the disc is pear-shaped with the apex situated anteriorly. According to Rees (1954), the disc is not of uniform thickness, but has four well-defined ellipsoidal bands or zones (Fig. 6.3):

(i) the anterior band
(ii) the intermediate band
(iii) the posterior band
(iv) the bilaminar region

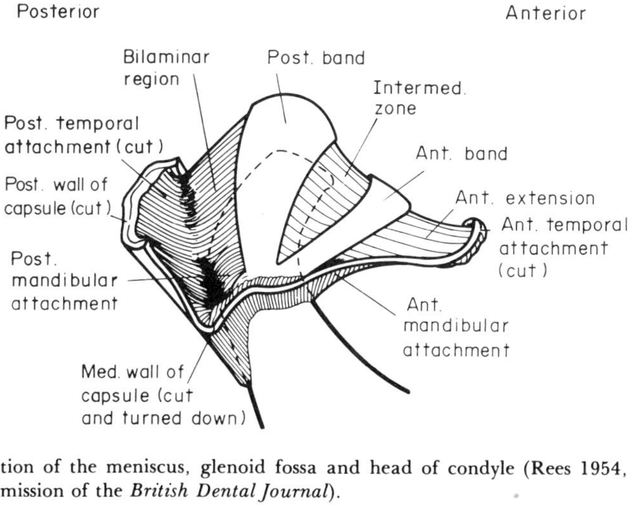


Fig. 6.3. Section of the meniscus, glenoid fossa and head of condyle (Rees 1954, with kind permission of the *British Dental Journal*).

The anterior band is moderately thick, but narrow anteroposteriorly, the intermediate band is thinnest and narrowest. The posterior band is the thickest of the bands and is widest anteroposteriorly. Continuous with the posterior band is the bilaminar region, which consists of an upper stratum attached to the posterior wall of the glenoid fossa and squamotympanic fissure and a lower stratum which is attached to the back of the condyle beneath the articular surface.

Medially and laterally, the articular disc blends with the capsule and both are attached to the medial and lateral poles of the condyle. Anteriorly, the

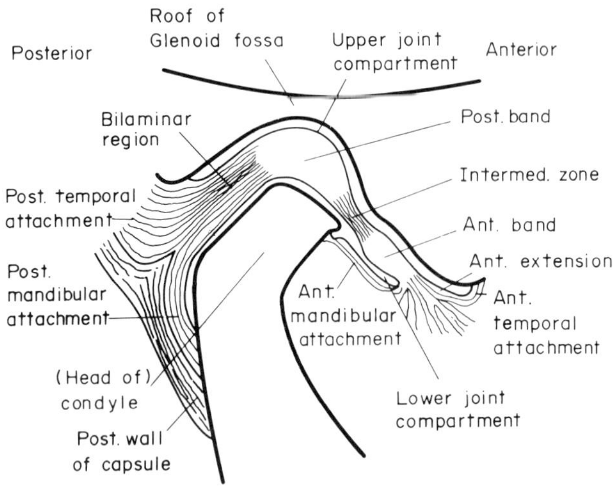


Fig. 6.4. Diagram showing the parts of the meniscus in relation to the head of the condyle (Rees 1954, with kind permission of the *British Dental Journal*).

disc is attached to the anterior margin of the articular eminence and below to the anterior margins of the condyles (Fig. 6.4). The disc also has an attachment to muscles and in the case of the lateral pterygoid tendonous fibres merge with the disc anteriorly to form a true insertion. There are also connections with the masseter and temporalis muscles and the anterior part of the disc. These consist of fibrous bands at right angles to the direction of the muscle fibres.

*The articular capsule.* This consists of an outer fibrous layer and an inner synovial layer of connective tissue and numerous blood vessels and is blended with the articular disc posteriorly. Medially, the articular capsule is loose and weak and is separated from the disc by a deep extension of the joint compartment, except below where the capsule and disc are jointly attached to the medial pole of the condyle. Anteriorly, where the disc is attached to the tendon of the lateral pterygoid, the capsule is deficient.

Laterally and posteriorly, the capsule is loose and thin, but more anteriorly it is strengthened by the triangular-shaped temporomandibular ligament. The broad base of the ligament passes downwards and forwards from its attachment to the root of the zygoma to the neck of the condyle below the lateral pole (Fig. 6.5).

*Synovial membrane.* A true synovial membrane, that is a thin vascular layer of connective tissue covered with flattened polygonal cells, is not present. Traces of a synovial membrane are found only in the fornices of the joint cavities and commonly in the posterior part of the upper joint cavity where

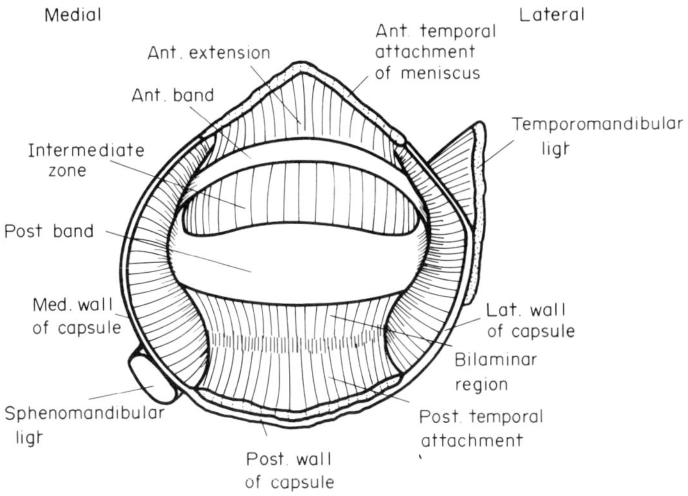


Fig. 6.5. The surface of the meniscus as seen from above, showing the menisco-capsular sulcus (Rees 1954, with kind permission of the *British Dental Journal*).

there may be a few folds of synovial tissue which appear to form part of the bilaminar "retrodiscal pad".

## The Histology and Ultrastructure of the Articular Tissues and Intra-articular Disc

The articular surfaces within the mandibular joint consist of avascular fibrous connective tissue consisting of bundles of collagen fibres and some elastic fibres (Fig. 6.6). Over most of the surface of the mandibular condyle the fibrous articular tissue is uniform in thickness, but becomes thinner at the periphery where it is continuous with the periosteum of the condylar process. Covering the glenoid fossa there is a comparatively thin layer of fibrous tissue which is continuous with a thicker layer over the slope of the articular eminence.

Beneath the fibrous articular surfaces, when growth of the mandibular condyle is occurring, are tightly packed cells with a high nucleocytoplasmic ratio. These cells form the so-called transitional or intermediate zone. This zone is continuous with a layer of cartilage in which the cells hypertrophy and become increasingly separated by organic matrix. Deep within the hypertrophic zone the matrix calcifies irregularly and is gradually resorbed and replaced by bone in endochondral ossification (Fig. 6.6) (Chapter 2).

In the adult, where the growth has ceased, the cell zones described above can be recognized, except that the intermediate zone is reduced in width and cellularity. Hypertrophic cartilage is absent and is represented by a zone of fibrous cartilage which is continuous with cortical bone. Calcification may spread for a varying distance into the hypertrophic cartilage and consistently reaches a higher mineral density than the adjacent cortical bone.

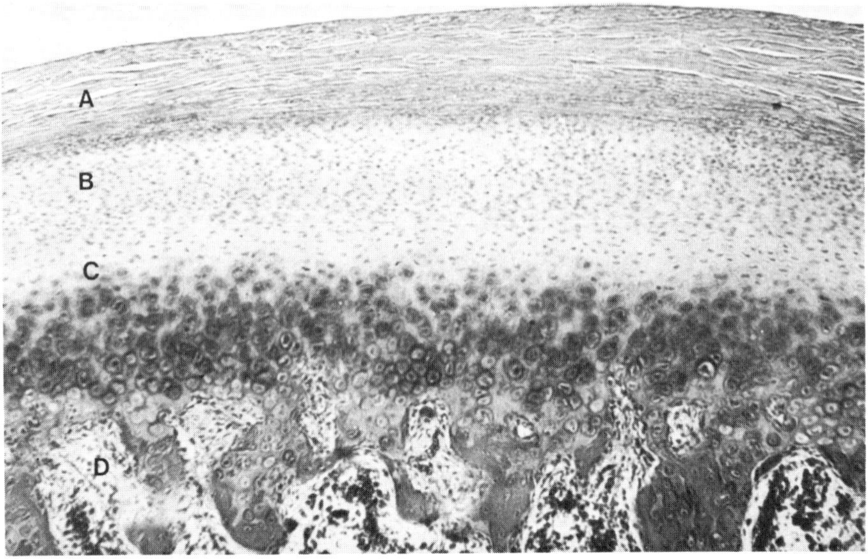


Fig. 6.6. Section through the growing condylar cartilage of a 13-year-old child showing A, fibrous articular zone, B, intermediate or proliferative zone, C, hypertrophic cartilage, D, endochondral bone formation.

In the transmission electron microscope the collagen fibres forming the articular tissue can be seen in bundles orientated parallel to the articulating surface, but at the articulating surface individual collagen fibres are present (Fig. 6.7). Throughout the fibrous articular tissue are fibroblasts, which do not approach the articulating surface and decrease in numbers with age. Randomly orientated elastic fibres are also present, some of which are close to the articulating surface (Fig. 6.7). In the transmission electron microscope the articulating surfaces appear smooth, but only a relatively small area is sampled. In the scanning electron microscope, where a larger area can be examined, the surfaces are irregular and have fine ridges and grooves passing in an anteroposterior direction (Fig. 6.8). The ridges probably represent the bundles of collagen fibres near the articulating surface. Shallow oval-shaped depressions probably represent the subsurface location of fibroblasts which have shrunk as a result of dehydration during tissue preparation.

The meniscus is composed chiefly of anteroposteriorly orientated bundles of collagen fibres together with some randomly orientated elastic fibres. Elastic fibres in large numbers extend from the disc into the squamotympanic fissure (Fig. 6.3). Anteriorly, elastic fibres are also present at the attachment of the lateral pterygoid muscle. The fine randomly orientated fibres dispersed

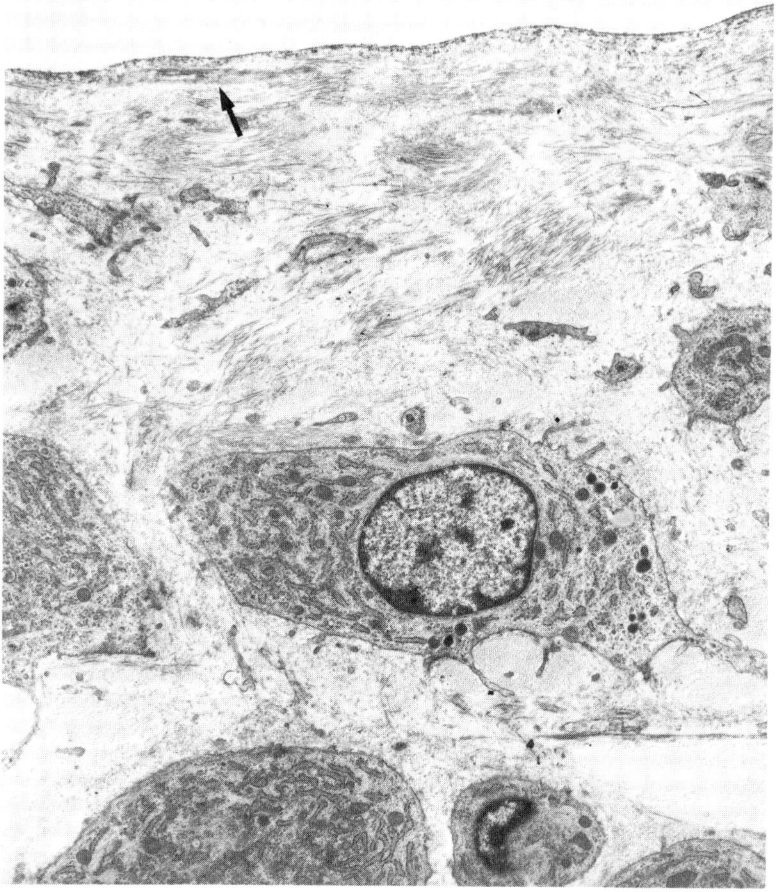

Fig. 6.7. Transmission electron micrograph (T.E.M.) showing the fibrous articular tissue of the mandibular condyle in the rat with an elastic fibre close to the articulating surface (arrowed).

throughout the disc have all disappeared by the end of the 3rd decade.

There are large vascular spaces in the bilaminar region which are predominantly venous and appear to be extensions of the pterygoid venous plexus. Small blood vessels may penetrate about two-thirds towards the centre of the disc, but nerve endings are confined to the posterior part of the disc.

## Joint Movements

It is only in man that an articular eminence and the complexities of movement associated with it are a dominant feature. In man, the first fraction of mouth opening is a simple hinge movement (Fig. 6.9). Further opening of the

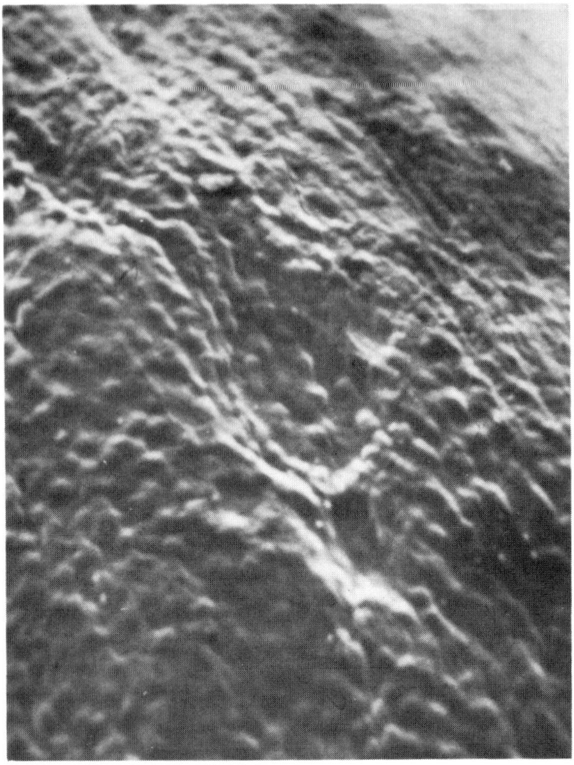

Fig. 6.8. Scanning electron micrograph (S.E.M.) of the articulating surface of the mandibular condyle in the monkey, which shows that it is not as smooth as indicated in the T.E.M.

mouth is associated with translocation forwards and downwards of the mandible with the condyle and the intra-articular disc sliding forwards on the posterior slope of the articular eminence. This adaptation is probably associated with the evolution of the upright posture in man which, by flexing the head forward on the trunk, tends to restrict the amount of space available for the angle of the mandible to move back in simple hinge movements.

Most of the lateral pterygoid muscle is inserted into the anterior surface of the neck of the condyle. Its function is to draw the mandible forward and when only the muscle on one side contracts to rotate the mandible laterally upon the condyle. By drawing the condyle forwards and downwards on the posterior slope of the articular eminence it also plays a significant part in mouth opening. Some of the fibres of the tendon of the lateral pterygoid muscle are inserted into the anterior border of the disc, mostly into its medial aspect. This muscle insertion into the disc has an important function in ensuring that the disc is pulled forward at the same time as the condyle moves forward. The tension put upon the disc by the lateral pterygoid in opening

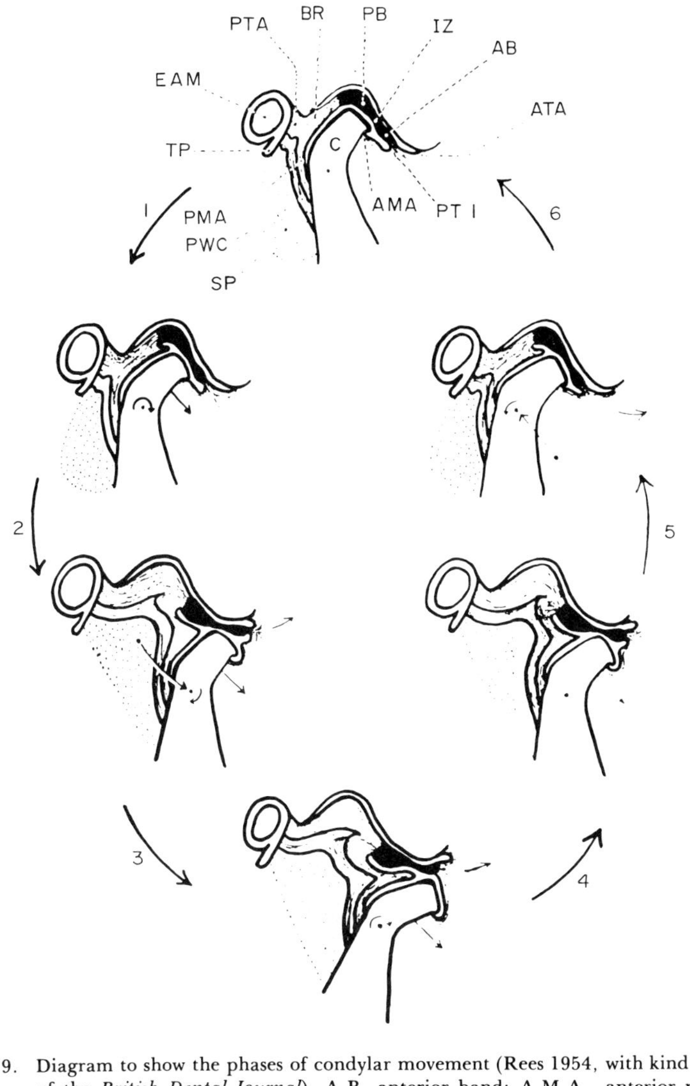


Fig. 6.9. Diagram to show the phases of condylar movement (Rees 1954, with kind permission of the *British Dental Journal*). A.B, anterior band; A.M.A., anterior mandibular attachment; A.T.A., anterior temporal attachment; B.R., bilaminar region; E.A.M., external auditory meatus; I.Z., intermediate zone; P.B., posterior band; P.M.A., posterior mandibular attachment; P.T.A., posterior temporal attachment; P.T.I., lateral pterygoid insertion; P.W.C., posterior wall of capsule; S.P., soft tissue pad; T.P., tympanic plate.

must tend to flatten the disc a little, though it would appear to be too closely applied to the convex surface of the condyle for this to occur. It has also been suggested that there are slender fibrous attachments between the disc and parts of the masseter and temporalis muscles that are in relation to the joint.

The function of the disc is not completely resolved, though it helps in more complex joints as found in the human to establish congruity between the bony articular surfaces. In addition, the disc also reduces the space between the articular surfaces so that fluid film lubrication can take place. Being attached to tissues behind the joint, it would seem to provide a means of drawing tissue into the interarticular space that would otherwise tend to remain when the condyle moved forward.

Posterior to the densely fibrous part of the disc, there is the bilaminar area. There is a relatively thin extension of the inferior layer of the fibrous tissue of the disc over the rounded posterior surface of the condyle head. This is the inferior lamina, above which the fibrous part of the disc ends abruptly and is attached to a loosely textured highly vascular tissue which contains many elastic fibres, the superior lamina. The superior lamina appears to be an important element in the joint mechanism. By virtue of its attachment to the disc as the condyle and disc move forwards in opening or lateral movement, the tissue is drawn forward to replace it. Therefore, at the same time blood is drawn into it by negative pressure so that its size and shape is modified to fit the glenoid cavity. As the condyle moves backwards in closure, blood is displaced from the vessels and the tissue returns to its original position by virtue of its elastic fibres which have been put under tension by its translation forwards.

## BIBLIOGRAPHY


APPLETON, J. (1975) The ultrastructure of the articular tissue of the mandibular condyle in the rat, *Arch. oral Biol.* **20,** 823.

APPLETON, J. (1978) The fine structure of a surface layer over the fibrous articular tissue of the rat mandibular condyle, *Arch. oral Biol.* **23,** 719.

BARNETT, C. H., D. V. DAVIES and M. A. MACCONAILL (1961) *Synovial Joints. Their Structure and Mechanics,* Longmans, London.

BAUME, L. J. and J. HOLZ (1970) Ontogenesis of the human temporomandibular joint: development of the temporal components, *J. dent. Res.* **49,** 864.

BLACKWOOD, H. J. J. (1965) Cell differentiation in the mandibular condyle of rat and man, *Les Congrés et colloques de L'Universite de Liege,* **31,** 23.

BLACKWOOD, H. J. J. (1965) Vascularization of the condylar cartilage of the human mandible, *J. Anat.* **99,** 551.

BLACKWOOD, H. J. J. (1966) Growth of the mandibular condyle of the rat studied with tritiated thymidine, *Arch. oral Biol.* **11,** 493.

BLACKWOOD, H. J. J. (1976) The mandibular joint development, structure and function, *in Scientific Foundations of Dentistry,* ed. B. Cohen and I. R. H. Kramer, Heinemann, London.

CARLSON, D. S., J. A. McNAMARA, Jr., L. W. GRABER and D. L. HOFFMAN (1980) Experimental studies of growth and adaptation of TMJ, in *Current Advances in Oral Surgery,* Vol. III, ed. W. B. Irby, Mosby, St. Louis.

CARLSSON, G. E. and T. OBERG (1974) Remodelling of the temporomandibular joints, *Oral Sci. Rev.* **6,** 53.

DIXON, A. D. (1962) Structure and functional significance of the intra-articular disc of the human temporomandibular joint, *Oral Med., Oral Surg., Oral Pth.* **15,** 48.

DURKIN, J. F., J. T. IRVING and J. D. HEELEY (1969) A comparison of the circulatory and calcification patterns in the mandibular condyle in the guinea pig with those found in the tibial epiphyseal and articular cartilage, *Arch. oral Biol.* **14,** 1365.

DURKIN, J. F., J. D. HEELEY and J. T. IRVING (1973) The cartilage of the mandibular condyle in temporomandibular joints, function and dysfunction I, *Oral Sci. Rev.* **2,** 29.

ENLOW, D. H. (1975) *Handbook of Facial Growth,* Saunders, Philadelphia.

FAHRENBACH, W. H., L. B. SANDBERG and E. G. CLEARY (1966) Ultrastructural studies on early elastogenesis, *Anat. Rec.* **155,** 563.

FURSTMAN, L. (1963) The early development of the human temporomandibular joint, *Am. J. Ortho.* **49,** 672.

GARDNER, D. L. (1972) The influence of microscopic technique on knowledge of cartilage surface structure, *Ann. rheum. Dis.* **31,** 235-258.

GREENLEE, T. K., R. ROSS and J. L. HARTMAN (1966) The fine structure of elastic fibres, *J. Cell Biol.* **30,** 59.

GREENSPAN, J. S. and H. J. J. BLACKWOOD (1966) Histochemical studies of chondrocyte function in the cartilage of the mandibular condyle of the rat, *J. Anat.* **100,** 615.

GRIFFIN, C. J. and C. J. SHARPE (1962) Distribution of elastic tissues in the human temporomandibular meniscus especially in respect to compression areas, *Austral. dent. J.* **7,** 72.

GRIFFIN, C. J., R. HAWTHORN and R. HARRIS (1975) Anatomy and histology of the human temporomandibular joint, *Monogr. Oral Sci.* **4,** 1.

LEVY, B. M. (1964) Embryological development of the temporomandibular joint, in *The Temporomandibular Joint,* 2nd ed., ed. B. G. Sarnat, Charles C. Thomas, Springfield, Illinois.

MILES, A. E. W. and J. A. DAWSON (1962) Elastic fibres in the elastic fibrous tissues of some joints, *Arch. oral Biol.* **7,** 249.

MOFFETT, B. C. (1957) The prenatal development of the human temporomandibular joint. *Contributions to Embryology,* Publication No. 243, **36,** 21.

MOFFETT, B. C. (1966) The morphogenesis of the temporomandibular joint, *Am. J. Ortho.* **52,** 401.

NOBLE, H. W. (1973) Comparative functional anatomy of temporomandibular joint, *Oral Sci. Rev.* **2,** 3.

REES, L. A. (1954) The structure and function of the mandibular joint, *Brit. dent. J.* **96,** 126.

SYMONS, N. B. B. (1952) The development of the human mandibular joint, *J. Anat.* **86,** 326.

THILANDER, B. (1964) Innervation of the temporomandibular joint, *Acta Odont. Scand.* **22,** 151.

WRIGHT, W., D. DOWSON and J. KERR (1973) The structure of joints, *Rev. Connective Tissue Res.* **6,** 105.

YUODELIS, R. A. (1966) Ossification of the human temporomandibular joint, *J. dent. Res.* **45,** 192.

YUODELIS, R. A. (1966) The morphogenesis of the human temporomandibular joint and its associated structures, *J. dent. Res.* **45,** 182.

## CHAPTER 7

# *Cephalometrics and Facial Growth*

A cephalometric radiograph is a view of the skull to show primarily the facial area taken with a standard degree of magnification and with the head in a standard reproducible position. The view studied is usually a lateral view with the left side of the face closest to the film, but postero-anterior or frontal cephalograms are also taken.

A cephalometer or cephalostat consists of the head-holder and radiographic equipment used to produce a cephalometric radiograph.

Cephalometrics is the expression used to describe the analysis of cephalometric radiographs.

### CEPHALOMETRIC TECHNIQUES AND ITS USES

Anthropologists had used the craniostat to measure dried skulls since the 19th century. It was a natural progression to wish to look at the bony structures within the living skull, and radiographs became used for this purpose. Later there was developed a technique for the examination of the skull fixed in a standardized position, primarily as a research tool to study the growth of the skull and jaws (Broadbent 1931 and Hofraff 1931).

Subsequently, cephalometrics have been used in orthodontic assessment and treatment planning, in monitoring treatment progress and as a method of describing treatment changes. The study of cross-sectional and more particularly longitudinal data has added substantially to the clinician's knowledge of facial growth. Attempts have been made to predict facial growth and to plan orthodontic treatment in conjunction with the predicted growth.

Cephalometrics have supplied data for a vast orthodontic literature. There has been a temptation to compare the individual patient with population norms in the belief that arithmetical formulae would simplify treatment planning, playing what has been described as "the numbers game". However, there has been an increasing awareness of the shortcomings of cephalometrics, and before examining its contribution to the study of facial growth it is necessary to make a critical appraisal of cephalometric techniques and principles.

**Radiographic Principles**

The patient's head is held in the cephalostat which has two graduated ear rods enabling the head to be placed in a central and consistent position within the cephalostat (Fig. 7.1). Head position in the sagittal plane of space is controlled variably by a nose rest, infra-orbital pointer, or simply by asking the patient to look straight ahead into a mirror on the wall. The X-ray tube is ideally fixed and placed exactly 5ft away from the mid-point of the cephalostat, which lies between the two ear rods. Thus the central ray passes along the central axis of both ear rods. The X-ray film contained in a cassette is also at a fixed distance from the X-ray tube and the patient's head. In this way, an orientated or standardized head position can be obtained upon each occasion that a lateral cephalogram is taken. A frontal cephalogram can be taken by turning the head-holder through 90°.

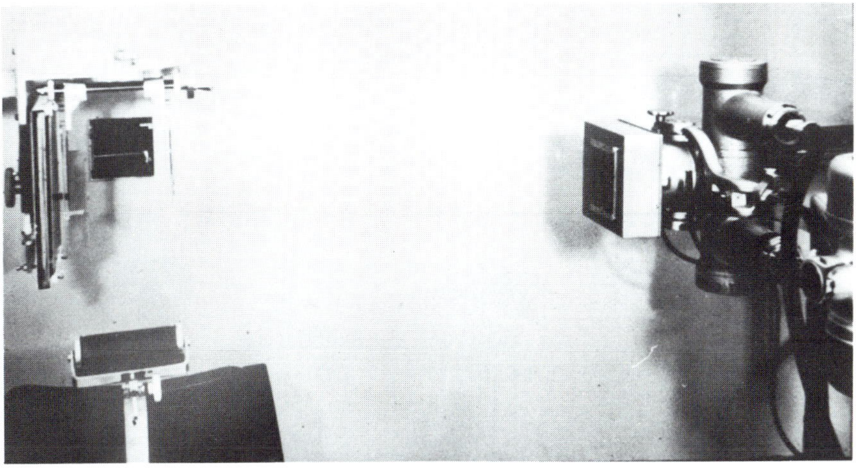

Fig. 7.1. Cephalometer and X-ray source.

The technical problems of producing consistent cephalograms are well reviewed by Horowitz and Hixon (1966), and the interested student is recommended to read their work. The problem of enlargement of the image, however, will be briefly discussed (Fig. 7.2). The enlargement of an image is inversely proportional to the ratio between the distances from the focal spot of the tube to the centre of the target and to the film in the cassette holder. Thus, enlargement is minimized by placing the film as close to and the X-ray tube as far away from the subject's head as is practicable. The normal tube distance of 5 ft and a film placed less than 1 in from the head gives a 6-7 per cent enlargement of structures in the mid-sagittal plane. In fact, this enlargement factor is increased slightly, but made more consistent, by placing the film cassette approximately 5 in from the centre of the target or head.

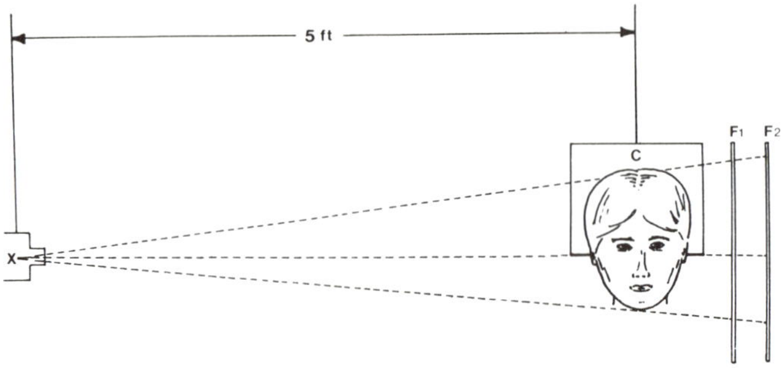


Fig. 7.2. Representation of cephalometer and X-ray source. X, X-ray; C, Cephalostat; F, Film (in cassette). Enlargement is illustrated by images F1 and F2.

Thus, the cephalometric radiograph produced is of consistent enlargement, with the head in an orientated or standardized position. Unfortunately, head positioning is not always completely accurate. Shaw (1977), discussing posing error in the infant cephalometer, describes head rotation, tilting and nodding. Encouragingly on lateral films, he found sagittal measurements were consistently reproducible with quite small posing errors, provided the structure examined was in the midline. On the other hand, on frontal films small variations in head position produced large errors in measurement from the sagittal plane.

**Cephalograms in Use**

An impression of the spatial relationships of teeth, jaws and soft tissues may be obtained by direct visualization. However, detailed examination is usually carried out by placing the lateral cephalogram upon a lighted tracing box; acetate tracing paper is placed upon the radiograph and both are secured with Sellotape. A sharp hard pencil is used to trace in selected anatomical landmarks. Points are chosen and joined to create planes whence angular measurements between intersecting planes are obtained. Electronic measurement using an XY digitizer has made the analysis of cephalometric radiographs simpler and faster, and has enabled large quantities of data to be handled by direct access to the computer.

The technical problems of faulty radiographic technique, magnification and posing error have been briefly discussed. These problems can be overcome by an awareness of their presence and careful technique. However, there are further sources of error less easily controlled. The cephalogram is a two-dimensional shadow of a three-dimensional object. Thus, structures are superimposed upon one another. Not only may desired landmarks be obscured in this way, but the true spatial relationship of structures cannot be ascertained and assumptions have to be made. For instance, articulare and posterior nasal spine (Fig. 7.3) are just two points formed by the intersection

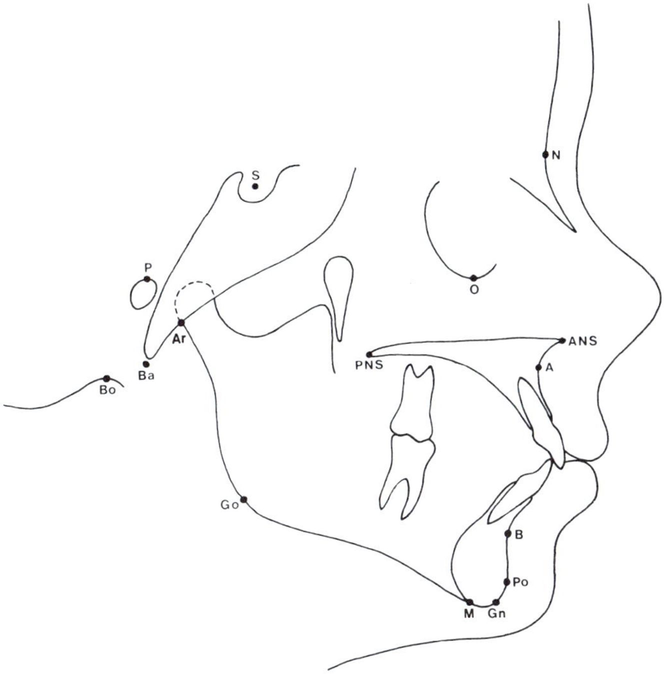


Fig. 7.3. Lateral tracing to show standard cephalometric points. S, Sella point; N, Nasion; P, Porion; O, Orbitale; Ar, Articulare; PNS, Posterior nasal spine; ANS, Anterior nasal spine; A, 'A' point; B, 'B' point; Go, Gonion; Po, Pogonion; Gn, Gnathion; M, Menton; Bo, Bolton point; Ba, Basion.

of two shadows, one superimposed upon the other. Anatomically the structures which make the shadows are spatially separated, no such anatomic points exist.

Many of the landmarks used are sites of bone resorption or deposition and are therefore constantly changing. Moreover, in the growing individual, landmarks will be altering their relationship to one another. Hence, one of the greatest problems of analysis has been to find horizontal or vertical reference planes in the skull that permit serial analysis of cephalograms to be carried out.

Tracing technique itself is a further source of error. Errors of measurement are well documented and vary from point to point. For example, the identification of the centre of Sella Turcica, point S, is consistently good, whereas Gonion or point A are more difficult to identify and therefore the error is higher.

Thus, there exist many conceptual problems regarding the analysis of cephalometric radiographs. The identification of landmarks can be difficult and errors occur during tracing. When examining serial cephalograms of the same patient, the clinician is often faced with the problem of knowing how much change is real change and how much is due to one of the many sources of error.

### Cephalometric Points, Planes and Angles

The more commonly employed cephalometric points, planes and angles are displayed in Figs. 7.3, 7.4 and 7.5 and are defined in the text.

DEFINITIONS

| | |
|---|---|
| *Points* | |
| Sella point ('S') | The mid-point of the sella turcica estimated by eye. |
| Nasion | The anterior point of the suture at the junction of the frontal and nasal bones in lateral view. |
| Porion | The uppermost contour of the bony external auditory meatus (usually taken as the upper point on the ear rod on the cephalostat, as it is not a clearly distinguishable bony landmark). |
| Tragion | The uppermost point of the supratragal notch. The soft-tissue equivalent of the porion. |
| Orbitale | The lowest point on the lower margin of the bony orbit. |
| Articulare | The point of intersection of the dorsal contours of the articular process of the mandible and the temporal bone. |
| Posterior nasal spine | The most posterior projection of the hard palate seen in lateral view. |
| Anterior nasal spine | The most anterior projection of the pre-maxilla below the nasal cavity seen in lateral view. |
| 'A' point (subspinale) | The most posterior point of the concavity on the anterior surface of the premaxilla in the midline, below the anterior nasal spine. |
| 'B' point (supramentale) | The most posterior point of the concavity on the anterior surface of the mandible in the midline, above the pogonion. |
| Gonion | A point midway between the anterior and posterior points on the angle of the jaw, obtained by bisecting the angle formed by a tangent to the mandibular base and the posterior margin of the ascending ramus. |
| Pogonion | The most anterior point on the bony chin. |
| Gnathion | The point on the chin determined by bisecting the angle formed by the facial and mandibular planes. |
| Menton | The lowest point on the symphyseal shadow. |
| Bolton Point | The highest point on the notch immediately posterior to the occipital condyle. |
| Basion | The lowest point on the anterior margin of the foramen magnum. |

## DEFINITIONS

| | |
|---|---|
| *Planes* | |
| Sella-nasion plane | The line drawn through sella point and nasion. |
| Frankfurt horizontal plane | The line connecting the lower border of the orbit and the porion. |
| Maxillary plane | The line drawn through the anterior and posterior nasal spines. |
| Occlusal plane | The line from the mid-point between the tips of the upper and lower incisors to the anterior contact between the upper and lower first molars in occlusion. |
| Mandibular plane | The line drawn from menton to gonion. |
| Bolton plane | The line joining the Bolton point and the nasion. |
| Pterygoid vertical plane | The line drawn perpendicular to the Frankfurt plane, passing through the distal of the pterygopalatine fossa. |
| 'APo' line | The line joining 'A' point to the pogonion. |
| 'E' plane (aesthetic plane) | The line drawn from the tip of the nose to the most anterior point of the soft-tissue chin. |
| Facial plane | The line joining nasion to pogonion. |
| De Coster's line | The outline of the internal surface of the anterior cranial base. |
| *Angles* | |
| SNA | The angle formed between the lines drawn from sella to nasion and from nasion to 'A' point. |
| SNB | The angle formed between the lines drawn from sella to nasion and from nasion to 'B' point. |
| Maxillary mandibular plane angle | The angle formed between the maxillary and the mandibular planes. |
| Maxillary incisor angle | The angle formed between the maxillary plane and the long axis of the most proclined maxillary incisor. |
| Mandibular incisor angle | The angle formed between the mandibular plane and the long axis of the most proclined mandibular incisor. |
| Inter-incisal angle | The angle formed between the long axis of the most proclined maxillary and mandibular incisors. |
| Y-Axis | Is the line drawn from the sella point to gnathion and related angularly to the Frankfurt plane. |
| Cranial base angle | The angle formed between the lines drawn from nasion to sella and from sella to basion. |
| Facial angle | The angle formed between the Frankfurt plane and the Facial plane. |

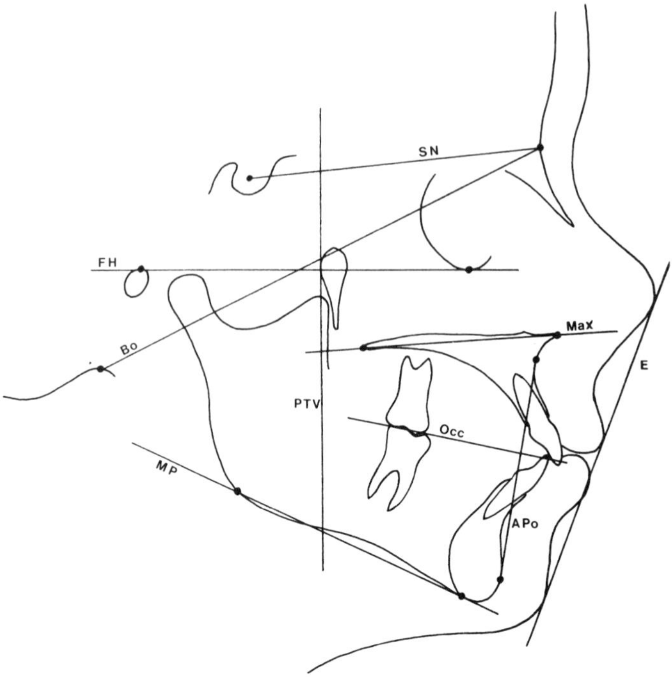


Fig. 7.4. Lateral tracing to show standard cephalometric planes. SN, Sella-nasion plane; FH, Frankfurt horizontal plane; Max, Maxillary plane; Occ, Occlusal plane; MP, Mandibular plane; Bo, Bolton plane; PTV, Pterygoid vertical plane; APo, 'APo' line; E, Aesthetic plane.

**Cephalometric Analyses**

A large number of cephalometric analyses have been reported. This partly reflects the purpose, that is whether the analysis is to be used for diagnostic purposes, treatment planning, treatment change analysis, growth analysis or prediction, or for research into particular areas of facial growth. However, it also reflects the search for non-growing stable horizontal and vertical planes to which may be related the points, planes and angles to be analysed.

The advent of the X-Y digitizer and computer has greatly increased the complexity of analyses undertaken, without unfortunately necessarily reducing the main defects of cephalometric analysis, radiographic technique, posing and tracing errors, or the problems of analysing three-dimensional growing subjects by means of a two-dimensional shadow.

**Diagnostic and Treatment Planning Analyses**

In most diagnostic analyses the main purpose is to examine the variation of the patient from population norms (mean values). The reference planes may

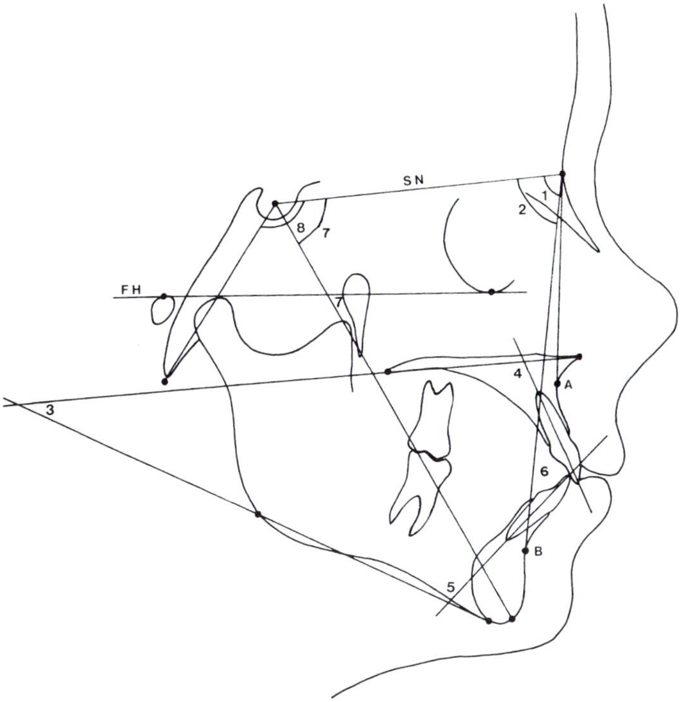


Fig. 7.5. Lateral tracing to show standard cephalometric angles. 1, SNA; 2, SNB; 3, Maxillary-mandibular planes angle; 4, Maxillary incisor angle; 5, Mandibular incisor angle; 6, Inter-incisal angle; 7, Y-axis; 8, Cranial base angle.

vary, but are often common to a number of analyses. Variation exists in the manner in which the dentoalveolar structures are analysed in relation to the skeletofacial structures. The orthodontist today knows that the individual patient cannot be made to fit precisely population norms. Individual variability is large, but fortunately dentobasal adaptations readily occur (Solow 1980). Treatment analyses may be used to indicate areas of variation and as wide guidelines to treatment objectives.

Though many cephalometric analyses are common to both diagnostic and research procedures, only one, Downs' analysis due to its widespread use, will be briefly described.

Downs (1948) suggested the angle formed by the intersection of the Facial plane (N-Pg) and Frankfurt horizontal plane (Figs 7.3, 4, 5) would provide a measure of the relationship of the chin position relative to the facial profile. He also chose two points, A and B, to represent the most concave points on the anterior outline of the maxilla and mandible respectively and measured the angle made between the line AB and the Facial plane. Riedel (1952) related points A and B to the Sella-Nasion plane. The angle SNA relates the maxilla and angle SNB the mandible to the Sella-Nasion plane. The size of angle ANB indicates the anteroposterior discrepancy or skeletal malrelationship between points A and B (Fig. 7.6). Although derived from small numbers, the original mean values for angles SNA, SNB and ANB have been shown to be reliable by subsequent population studies. Unfortunately, A and B points are not true indicators of skeletal bone. A point particularly may change its position during treatment. The size of angles SNA, SNB may be affected by abnormal positions of points N or S.

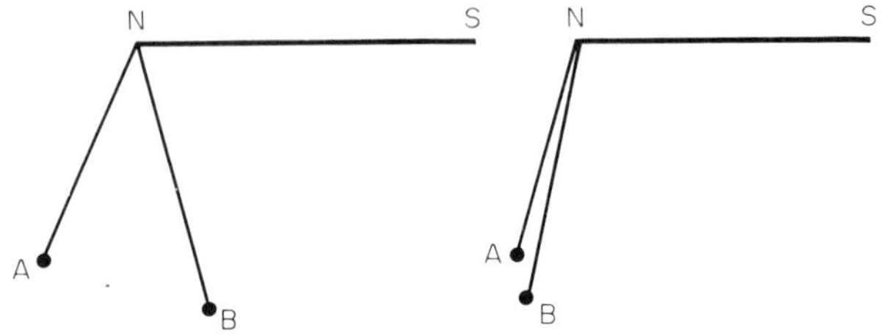


Fig. 7.6. Down's analysis. The larger the angle ANB, the more posteriorly placed is B point to A point (Class II dental base relationship). When B point is anterior to A point, a Class III dental base relationship is present. A Class I relationship is present when angle ANB is in the range + 2° to 4°.

### Cephalometric Serial Studies During Orthodontic Treatment

Cephalograms may be superimposed during treatment or at the completion of treatment to assess progress or to determine whether treatment objectives have been completed. The manner of superimposition varies, but three superimpositions are generally suggested (Fig. 7.7).

(A) An overall composite is usually suggested using the plane SN centred on S or on N or DeCoster's line.

(B) The maxillae are superimposed along the maxillary plane (ANS to PNS), getting best fit of the maxillary outlines favouring the inferior surface of the posterior curvature of the hard palate.

(C) The mandibles are superimposed after the manner described later by Björk (1969).

Overall growth changes can thus be visualized while the maxillary and mandibular superimpositions give a clearer indication of the tooth movements achieved and of remodelling and growth of maxillary and mandibular outlines.

## CEPHALOMETRIC STUDY OF FACIAL GROWTH

The early data for cephalometric growth studies were largely derived from cross-sectional or mixed cross-sectional and longitudinal material, and the constancy of facial growth suggested by this work has proved to be

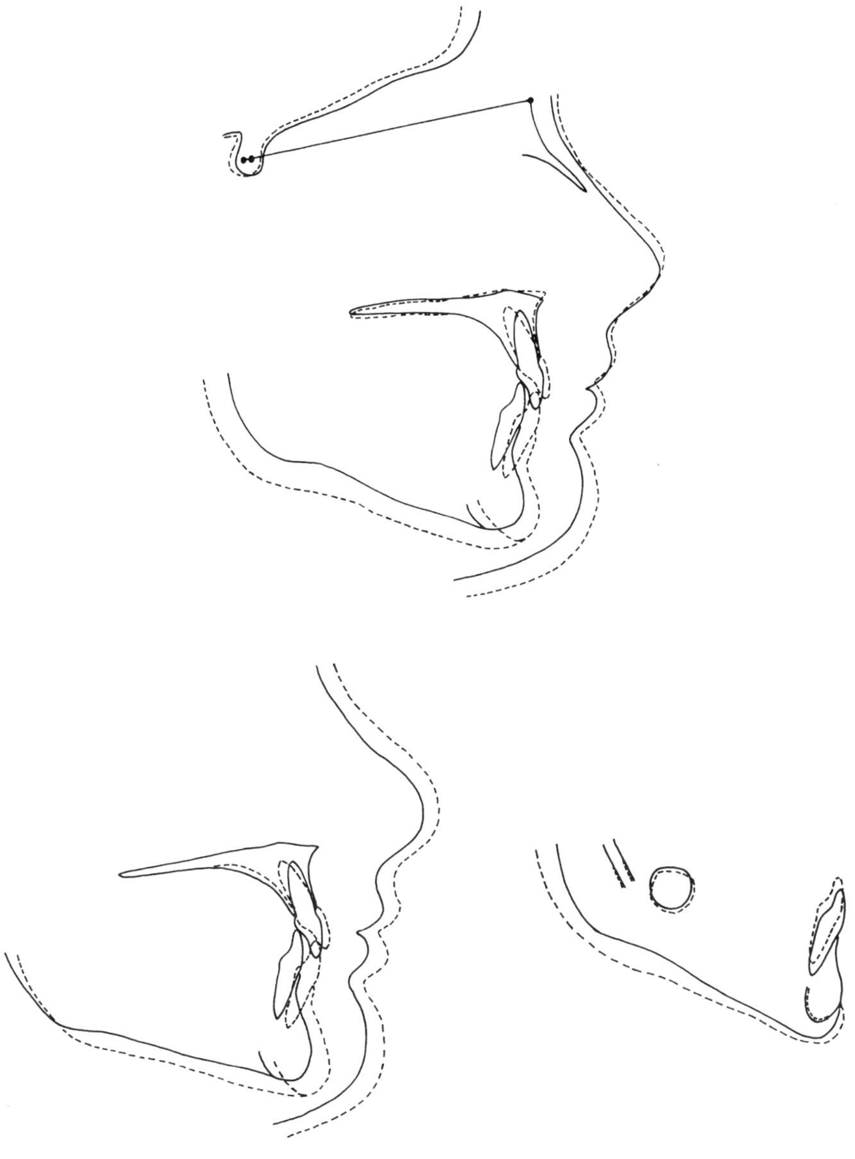

Fig. 7.7. Superimposition of the lateral cephalograms of a patient before (solid line) and after (broken line) orthodontic treatment. A, Superimposed on plane SN, centred on N. Note the downward and forward growth of the lower face and increasing mandibular prognathism. B, Superimposed on maxillary outlines. Note the change in angulation of the upper incisor produced by the treatment and the manner in which mandibular growth has carried forward the lower incisors. C, Mandibles superimposed in the manner of Björk (1969). Note growth of the mandible especially in the chin region.

misleading. For example, Broadbent (1937) and Brodie (1941), superimposing on the plane Nasion to Sella Turcica, found that the cranial base angle BSN varied only slightly during growth. The chin point appeared to move downwards and forwards along a constant axis, the palatal plane appeared to descend in a parallel manner. Björk and Palling (1955), examining cross-sectional data, showed that the average increase in mandibular length in boys from age 12 to 20 years was 17.2 mm. However, when the 12-year-old boys were examined later, at the age of 20 years, that is in a longitudinal study, a large amount of individual variability became apparent. However, they comment that much of the variability is masked because dentoalveolar compensation enables the occlusion to adapt to changes in facial proportions.

To examine individual variability, a number of longitudinal or serial growth studies were started so that a more accurate picture of individual growth could be obtained.

### Cephalometric Growth Studies

Major growth studies have derived their data in different ways. The Bolton standards (Broadbent *et al.* 1975) were obtained from healthy children with excellent occlusions and aesthetically pleasing facial proportions. None had undergone orthodontic treatment. Lateral annual standards from 1 year to 18 years have been produced. Frontal annual studies begin at 3 years and finish at 18 years. Though male and female data have been presented combined, sexual dichotomy in size, in growth timing and in the development of secondary sexual characteristics have been noted (Fig. 7.8). Many other studies have concentrated upon children with ideal occlusion, with the idea of creating mean or standard values for the ideal facioskeletal supporting structures.

However, the Burlington Growth Centre serial study attempted to capture an entire child community in Burlington, Canada. The racial origins of the Burlington population is Caucasian, and the major ethnic background is Anglo-Saxon. Thompson and Popovich (1977), who in constructing templates from the serial records of 120 boys and 90 girls between the age of 4 and 20 years reported that this represented approximately 85 per cent of all the children in the Burlington community at the start of the growth study. The data has been used to prepare standards of facial growth by age and sex and to produce distance and velocity charts of mandibular growth.

One of the most comprehensive growth studies is reported by Riolo *et al.* (1974, 1979), who listed cephalometric standards from the University School Growth Study, University of Michigan. The sample group was comprised of 47 males and 36 females, with continual attendance between the ages of 6 and 16 years, none of whom received orthodontic treatment before or during the study. Growth templates have been produced from this data.

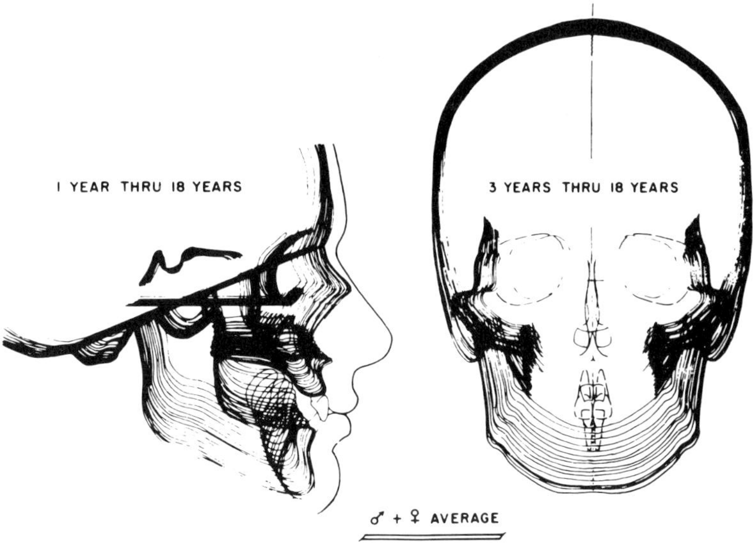


Fig. 7.8. Annual Bolton standards, sexes combined. Both lateral and frontal views superimposed in Bolton relation. (By kind permission of Drs B. H. Broadbent and W. H. Golden (1975) *Bolton Standards of Dentofacial Developmental Growth* and the C. V. Mosby Company.)

In Great Britain, longitudinal cephalometric growth studies were initiated in London (Leighton 1958) and Belfast (Adams 1960). Cephalometric reports on these studies have been made by Bhatia (1970) and Kerr (1979), and reference to their findings will be made later.

Apart from adding to the general knowledge of craniofacial growth, such studies provide statistical data which will allow comparison with other longitudinal growth data. Clinically, craniofacial norms and treatment goals may be established. Annual increments of growth change can be calculated with the possibility of predicting growth change over a period of time. Group data may be used as control groups to permit statistical analysis against treated groups.

However, before using the data from these studies, to make comparisons with the individual patient one must be aware of the manner in which the data has been compiled. For example, Broadbent (1973) commented that a more Class II mandibular relationship (see Chapter 9) was found in the computer derived norms of a random cross-sectional population sample than found in the Bolton standards. This is hardly surprising when the small number of ideal occlusions compared with Class II cases in a random population is considered.

Having established the nature of the data and therefore of the cephalometric norms reported, the clinician must ascertain that the individual patient that he wishes to compare comes from a similar population. At the very least, data should be drawn from children of the same age, sex and racial group.

The nature of the biologic and cephalometric norm has been dealt with at great length by Horowitz and Hixon (1966) and it is worth spending a moment considering their observations. They suggest that a norm is more than an average figure or mean, for a mean figure is derived from a range which includes the smallest and the largest. The variability around the mean is expressed as the standard deviation (see Statistical Appendix). Using this we can compare the relative position of the individual patient to the sample mean. The larger the sample the more reliable will be the mean and the standard deviation in describing the population. However, most cephalometric growth variables will show large standard deviations and thus populations with different mean values may overlap. Small mean growth changes with large individual variability often makes it impossible to differentiate statistically between population groups or to differentiate between growth change over a short period of time or in comparison with larger treatment changes.

### Cephalometric Approaches to Facial Growth Analysis

The vast majority of analyses have been carried out using the conventional superimposition techniques on the anterior cranial base area as described earlier. Ricketts (1972), however, favoured the Frankfurt plane and Pterygoid vertical to create the zero point of a coordinate system. The basicranial axis (BaN) is used as a base line for growth analysis (Figs. 7.3, 7.4, 7.5). Throughout the progress of research one sees continually different attempts to overcome the problem of analysing a growing face in the absence of stable non-growing reference planes. Björk (1955) used metallic implants inserted into the jaw bones. Superimposition on these implants demonstrated true change in bone growth or tooth eruption, without reference to craniofacial planes. In view of the function of the semicircular canals in assessment of spatial position, Delatire and Fenart (1958) propose that they might be used for the superimposition of cephalometric radiographs. Johnson (1960, 1978) has developed a method of orientating cephalograms upon centres of gravity used as mathematical fixed points. Walker (1972) used the computer to draw skulls averaged by age and sex with approximately 100 individuals in each group. An atlas of craniofacial development was thus produced and the growth changes examined both statistically and visually.

Moorrees and Yem (1955), doubting the reliance of intracranial reference planes, analysed skull growth changes using a mesh diagram analysis, based on the coordinate analysis method described by D'Arcy Thompson (1917). Grids are constructed based on core rectangles. These core rectangles are superimposed (that is a later cephalogram upon an earlier one), and the resultant distortion of the mesh lines shows the difference in the position of the various landmarks within the rectangles of the mesh diagram. A visual change in pattern, or computer analysis, illustrates the changes in growth which are occurring.

Moyers and Bookstein (1979), in a comprehensive explanation of the inappropriateness of conventional cephalometrics, propounded a method of biorthogonal grids or change coordinates. Instead of measuring change by subtracting measurement A from measurement B, the change in shape or distortion of the pattern or grid is analysed by computer programs.

### Cephalometric Appraisals of Facial Growth

It was suggested earlier that the important pioneering work of Broadbent (1937), which demonstrated a regular downward and forward growth direction of the facial complex, had been misleading. The mean pattern of facial growth was derived from cross-sectional data. This masked not only individual growth variability but tended to give an impression of an even growth rate. However, in serial work on growth of the calvaria, Brodie (1943) demonstrated an initial rapid period of growth to 4 years of age, after which only a small amount of sagittal cranial growth occurred. Woodside (1969) has shown that the mandible displays rest and spurt growth periods. The clinician must thus know not only the direction and quantity of facial growth, but also the velocity at which it is occurring at any particular time.

Our understanding of facial growth owes much to the cephalometric and implant studies of Björk (1961) (1963) and Björk and Skieller (1972, 1977). Metallic implants were inserted into the growing jawbones of children to provide more accurate reference landmarks for superimposition of serial cephalometric-radiographs. This work is complemented and supported by reports of other longitudinal growth studies.

*Cranial base.* Despite histological studies, which indicate extensive remodelling of the cranial base (Melsen 1974, Thilander and Ingervall 1973), the cranial base angle between anterior and posterior segments appears to remain constant between 12 and 20 years. However, individual variability is large with changes as measured by angle SN-Ba ranging from $+5°$ to $-5°$ in the 243 boys studied by Björk (1955). Kerr (1978) confirmed these findings, again reporting a large range of change from $-9.1°$ to $+10.2°$ in boys. However, there is growing evidence that changes in head posture caused, for example, by obstruction of the nasopharyngeal airway are capable of influencing cranial base flexure.

*Maxillary complex.* This is attached to the anterior cranial base. Björk (1947) has shown a statistical relationship between cranial base flexure and the position of the maxilla, a smaller than average cranial base angle being associated with increased maxillary prognathism, a larger than average angle resulting in reduced maxillary prognathism.

On average, the maxillary complex is displaced downwards and forwards at about 50° to the Sella-Nasion planes (Björk 1966). However, there is considerable individual variability. The implant studies also made apparent changes in the velocity of maxillary bone growth related to the pubertal growth spurt at age 14 years and 12½ years in boys and girls respectively. Kerr (1979) showed that the mean value of angle SNA did not change significantly between 5 years and 15 years, though variability was large, with a range of -7.9° to + 8.2°. On average, therefore, maxillary prognathism relative to nasion did not increase, but clearly in some individuals it did increase and in others it decreased. Kerr (1979) and Bhatia (1970) demonstrate broad agreement that there is, on average, a mean increase in the anterior cranial base/maxillary plane angle. Thus the maxillary plane does not descend in a parallel manner as described by Broadbent (1937). On occasions, environmental causes may be responsible, for the maxillary plane has been shown to dip occlusally at PNS in mouth breathers resulting from impairment of the nasal airway (Linder-Aronson 1979).

*Mandible.* During growth the mandible is spatially relocated away from the cranial base, its shape and size being modified by the eruption of the dentoalveolar structures and extensive resorption and deposition of bone. Woodside has shown from Burlington Growth Study data that the direction of growth may be horizontal, horizontal/vertical, or vertical, but rarely is the growth entirely horizontal or entirely vertical. The implant studies of Björk (1961, 1969) showed that mandibular displacement by condylar growth results in a rotation of the mandible. Investigation of 45 males demonstrated that the mandible rotates during growth in either a predominantly downward and backward or downward and forward manner.

A forward mandibular growth rotation occurs when condylar growth is upwards and forwards, the posterior part of the mandible being lowered more than the anterior part (Fig. 7.9). Type I is the most commonly occurring form of growth rotation. However, it may result in a deep overbite if the incisor teeth fail to make contact, whilst in type III the anterior section of the mandible rotates upwards around a point in the premolar region, increasing overbite.

A backward growth rotation will occur when the condyle grows in an upwards and backwards direction, displacing the mandible downwards and forwards (Fig. 7.10). Rotation may occur at the condyle or because the lowering of the posterior part of the mandible can be less than that of the anterior part, so that the mandible will rotate downwards and backwards around a point in the premolar region. If the incisor teeth fail to compensate by increased eruption, an incomplete or an anterior open bite will result.

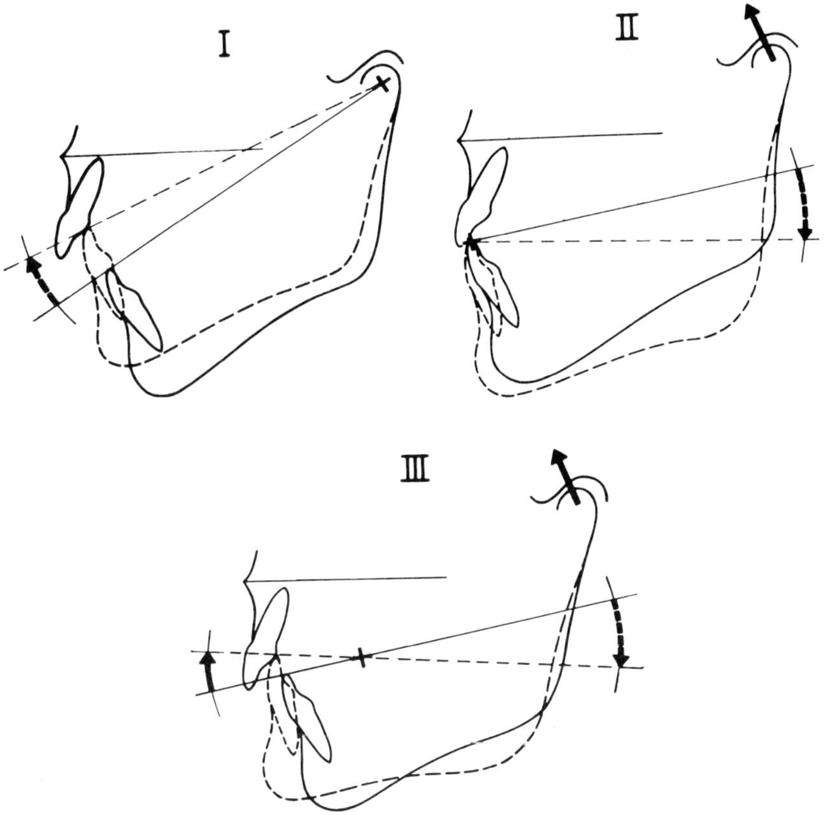


Fig. 7.9. Forward rotation of the mandible with the centre at the joints (I), with the centre at the incisal edges of the lower incisors (II), and with the centre at the premolars (III). (By kind permission of Professor A. Björk, Royal Dental College, Copenhagen, and *American Journal of Orthodontics*.)

Following the forward mandibular rotation there is marked resorption of the mandibular lower border in front of the gonial angle and apposition below the symphysis. This displays itself as a decrease in the gonial angle. Björk (1963) found a mean decrease of 6° in boys between 5 years and 22 years. Similar changes in 44 boys with a mean decrease of 6.7° was found by Kerr (1979). In the subjects with a backward mandibular rotation, the remodelling changes of the lower border do not occur and indeed apposition below the gonial angle may result in the development of an antigonial notch.

Kerr (1979) and Bhatia (1970) showed that the mean anterior cranial base-mandibular plane angle, decreased in their longitudinal studies, confirming Björk's (1963) view that in the majority of cases there is a forward mandibular rotation, concealed to some extent, as we have seen, by extensive remodelling of the mandibular lower border.

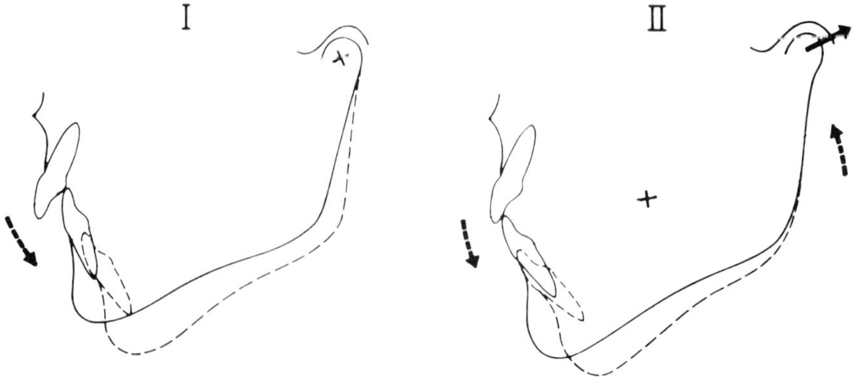


Fig. 7.10. Backward rotation of the mandible with the centre at the joints (I) and with the centre at the last occluding molars (II). (By kind permission of Professor A. Björk, Royal Dental College, Copenhagen and *American Journal of Orthodontics.*)

Based on his implant studies, Björk (1969) suggested four mandibular landmarks as fiducial markers or points of superimposition, when implants are not used. The suggested points are the inferior dental nerve canal, the inner cortical surface of the symphysis, the lower margin of the third molar tooth germ, prior to the commencement of root formation, and the tip of the chin.

Considerable interest has been expressed in the position of the inferior dental neurovascular bundle during growth. Koski (1973) found by superimposing lateral cephalograms scaled to correct differences in scale and size, that the position of the inferior dental nerve was very constant during growth. Moss and Selentijn (1970) and Moss *et al.* (1974), using metal implants to aid superimposition, proposed a curving path of mandibular growth, based on a logarithmic spiral. Three neurovascular foramina, the foramen ovale, mandibular and mental foramina, were found to lie on a logarithmic spiral. This is basically in agreement with Ricketts' (1972) theory that the mandible grows along an arc.

Woodside (1969) has prepared mandibular distance and velocity population standards from the Burlington data. The annual data obtained were computer smoothed to obtain mandibular length at every tenth of a year. The results were plotted against chronological age, according to sex (Fig. 7.11). Velocity curves (Fig. 7.12), however, indicate more clearly periods of growth, rest and spurt. The graphs indicate periods of rapid growth associated with circumpubertal growth between 10½ years and 13 years in girls and 13 years and 16 years in boys. However, important accessory periods of growth can be seen, particularly in males. Additionally, the slower but more prolonged mean velocity curve of male growth compared with the shorter and more clearly defined juvenile and pubertal growth acceleration of the female sample are apparent.

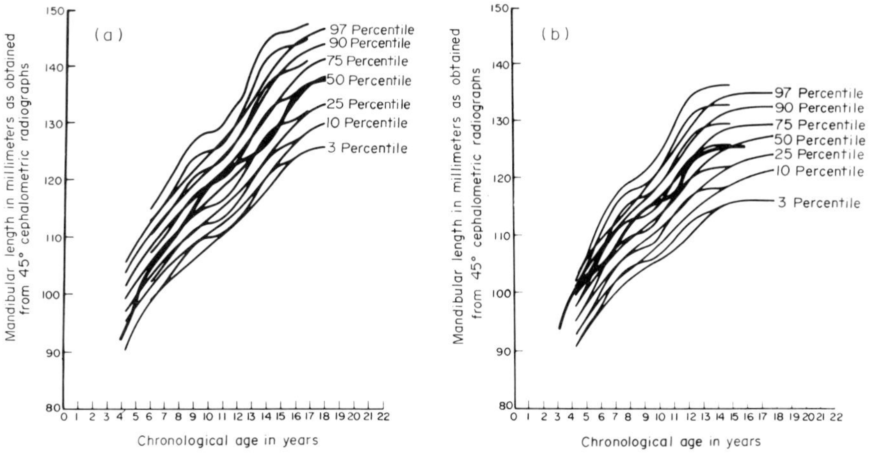


Fig. 7.11. The individual computer-smoothed mandibular distance curve superimposed on the population standards for A, Case No. 130 (male) and B, Case No. 416 (female). Periods of accelerated mandibular growth in both A and B are shown in areas of increased steepness on the individual distance curves. (By kind permission of D. G. Woodside, R. T. Reed, J. D. Doncet and G. W. Thompson, and *Transactions of the Third International Orthodontic Congress,* ed. J. T. Cook, Crosby Lockwood Staples, London.)

*Facial profile.* Comment was made earlier of Björk's (1947) cross-sectional study of males at age 12 years and 21 years, which indicated that both maxillary and mandibular prognathism appears to increase with age. In the longitudinal follow-up of the 12-year-old sample, Björk and Palling (1955) showed great individual variability. However, most of the boys displayed improved sagittal jaw relationships, though some were unchanged or even worsened. Lande (1972), in a longitudinal study from 7 to 18 years, also showed that the chin point became more prognathic relative to the cranial base, though the maxilla's relationship was little changed. Kerr (1979) confirmed these findings, but was able to demonstrate that relative mandibular prognathism appeared greater in the 5-10-year period than the 10-15-year period, rather earlier than shown by Björk (1947).

Serial cephalometric studies of growth changes of the soft tissues of the face have been carried out by a number of workers including Subtelny (1959), Posen (1967) and Wisth (1972). Subtelny used the Broadbent study data to examine the relationship of the soft tissue profile of the face to the underlying bony structures. He showed that from birth to 18 years the forward displacement of the soft tissues was minimal at nasion and maximal at the tip of the nose. Considerable forward soft tissue growth occurred at the levels of point A and pogonion. Clearly nasal growth increases midfacial prominence and is a facial feature which continues to grow after the completion of most orthodontic treatments.

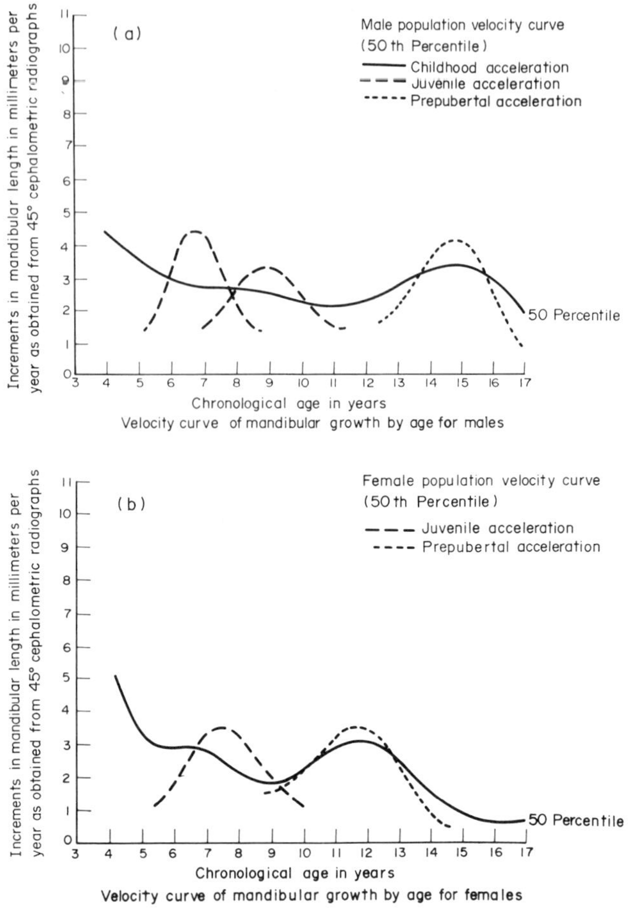


Fig. 7.12. The population standards for mandibular velocity for A, males, and B, females, obtained by mathematical derivation from the computer-smoothed distance curves. (By kind permission of D. G. Woodside, R. T. Reed, J. D. Doncet, and J. W. Thompson and *Transactions of the Third International Orthodontic Congress,* ed. J. T. Cook, Crosby Lockwood Staples, London.)

There are a number of studies of soft tissue changes in facial profile during treatment, including those of Burstone (1958), Wisth (1974), Huggins and McBride (1975) and Roos (1977). However, all the above work represents examination of a two-dimensional analysis of the mid-sagittal projection of the soft tissue. The use of short-base stereophotogrammetry (Burke 1980) or stereophotography (Robertson 1976) to produce contour maps of the soft tissues of the face, measuring changes by the application of aerial mapping techniques, enables a three-dimensional picture to be analysed.

This work confirms the clinical impression that Class II profiles improve with growth whilst Class III (see Chapter 9) profiles worsen, particularly when it is realized that mandibular growth generally continues after mid and particularly upper face growth has been completed. This has had important implications upon orthodontic treatment technique. Surgical correction of malocclusion was, and still is, generally postponed until the completion of mandibular growth. However, maxillary procedures particularly, and some mandibular surgical procedures, have been carried out with success before the cessation of growth. Orthodontists now may attempt to correct Class II skeletal cases by using orthopaedic forces, delivered either by headgears or functional appliances, in an attempt to restrain or redirect maxillary growth to enable mandibular growth to improve the sagittal jaw and tooth relationships. Alternatively, functional appliances may be employed to enable mandibular growth to express its full potential.

The orthodontist would thus like to know the amount and direction of remaining mandibular growth. Clearly, to make most rapid change, treatment procedures should be employed when growth is occurring most rapidly. Hence considerable effort has been made to predict mandibular growth direction and quantity, and to pinpoint the onset of the pubertal growth spurt.

### The Assessment of the Maximal Growth Period

It is not possible to forecast accurately from chronological age the timing of the adolescent growth spurt. The standard deviation from the mean is about 1 year, which means that about 30 per cent of children start their growth spurt 1 year before or after the mean for their sex (Houston *et al.* 1979).

However, the difference between boys and girls with respect to peak growth velocity in body height is well documented and has been discussed in Chapter 1.

An increase in the rate of growth of the jaws accompanies the rapid increase in body height at the time of puberty. Research findings are variable, but in general the correlation of a facial growth spurt and growth in body height is accepted (Bergersen 1972), though there is some evidence that the peak of facial growth occurs at a slightly later time from that of body height.

In an attempt to pinpoint more accurately the onset of the facial pubertal growth spurt, facial dimensions have been compared with the state of skeletal maturation as determined from wrist and hand radiographs. Björk and Helm (1967) demonstrated a correlation between the beginning of the maximum pubertal growth period and the onset of ossification of the sesamoid bone. They suggested that ossification of the adductor sesamoid preceded the peak of pubertal growth by approximately 1 year or coincided with it. In fact, in a later paper, Helm *et al.* (1971), did acknowledge far greater individual variability, and a number of papers have reported that the sesamoid can occur after the time of peak growth velocity. Houston *et al.* (1979) examined subjects drawn from the Harpenden Growth Study. The longitudinal records of 64 boys and 49 girls were examined, rather greater numbers than in previous studies. The relationship of the ossification events to peak velocity in height was examined. They found that the regression coefficients for ossification events, which on average occur more than 2 years in advance of peak height velocity, are low. The largest coefficients are those for events that take place at, or after, peak height velocity, which clearly are of no value for predicting peak height velocity. Taking a number of ossification events into account simultaneously did not significantly improve the correlations or prediction. They felt thus that ossification events are only of limited value in the prediction of the growth spurt.

In the present state of our knowledge, therefore, hand/wrist radiographs should not be used in isolation, but may be helpful in supporting evidence derived from serial lateral cephalometric radiographs, body height measurements and relating the individual's general bodily development to that of the average of the population and mid-parental height.

**Prediction of Facial Growth**

Comment has been made that the recognition of variations in facial growth, particularly of mandibular growth direction and rotation, together with changing treatment approaches, has caused the orthodontist to seek methods of growth prediction.

Tanner (1962) and Tanner *et al.* (1966, 1975) have been able to predict body height within quoted probability levels. Average values according to age and sex were derived from a longitudinal growth study of children. Despite individual variations, the level of prediction is good. Body height is, however, a single measurement taken from a well-defined reference plane, whereas facial profile and facial form is dependent upon many bones with widely different spatial relationships and without, as we have seen earlier, a satisfactory non-growing base line from which to make measurement. While, therefore, many attempts to predict facial form have been attempted, the results generally are disappointing (Balbach 1969, Houston 1979). A number of prediction templates showing average facial patterns at different ages have been derived, for example, by Broadbent *et al.* (1975) Johnstone (1975) and Popovitch and Thompson (1977). Growth changes between appropriate ages can be obtained by superimposing templates. However, criticisms of the method may be made on grounds of small sample size, the choice of the landmarks chosen for analysis, and that the templates are not always age or sex specific.

Ricketts (1972) has used the computer (Rocky Mountain data system) to store information of facial dimensions derived from population means according to ethnic grouping, age and sex. The individual patient may be compared with this data. However, Schulof *et al.* (1977) correctly described the method as "pattern extension", for starting with the patient's existing facial dimensions, average incremental values for age, sex and ethnic grouping are added in the same way as using a template. The data is applied to the patient's lateral skull radiograph tracing and an estimation made of the expected growth during an appropriate time period. The prediction is visually displayed on a computer-drawn plot of the skull. The effects of proposed orthodontic treatment may be shown in the same way. Print-outs are then available to the orthodontist, showing the predicted growth without treatment and with the proposed treatment effects.

Schulof *et al.* (1977) attempted to individualize the prediction of Class III malocclusions by using data derived from a Class III subgroup. The average increments for this group were added to the existing facial pattern; the level of prediction was increased in this way and it may be that by creating subgroups of other extreme malocclusion types that the accuracy of prediction will be increased.

Mitchell *et al.* (1975) studied eight cases in which actual growth assessed with the aid of implants was compared with the growth predicted by the Rocky Mountain Data System. Acceptable accuracy was achieved in six out of eight cases. Schulof and Bagha (1975) felt that the Rocky Mountain Data System was accurate in the 70-80 per cent range and that the method therefore constituted a useful clinical aid to treatment planning. However, Greenberg and Johnstone (1975) found that the programme was not more accurate than simply adding average growth increments and indeed was often less accurate than assuming that no change would occur.

Houston (1979) argues forcefully that at the present time accurate individualized growth prediction is not possible. He comments that the use of average values masks individual variability and feels that an accuracy of 70-80 per cent is not clinically useful.

Correlation studies to attempt to individualize prediction by relating the present size of skeletal structures to future increase in size have been reviewed by Hixon (1972). The relationships were all low and not considered to be of predictive value. A change in size over a period of time compared with a change in size over a subsequent period of time by Harvold (1963) investigating mandibular length in boys resulted in low correlations which were not statistically significant. Similarly multiple correlation studies relating the relationships of a large number of variables have proved equally unhelpful.

## BIBLIOGRAPHY

ADAMS, C. P. (1960) Belfast Growth Study, initiated 1960. Queen's University Belfast, Northern Ireland.

BALBACH, D. R. (1969) The cephalometric relationship between the morphology of the mandible and its future occlusal position. *Angl. Ortho.* **39,** 29.

BERGESEN, E. O. (1972) The male adolescent facial growth spurt, *Angl. Ortho.* **42,** 319.

BHATIA, S. N. (1970) A longitudinal study of the SN-mandibular, Frankfurt-mandibular and maxillary-mandibular plane angles, *Trans. Brit. Soc. Orthodont.* **169.**

BJÖRK, A. (1947) The face profile. An anthropological X-ray investigation on Swedish children and conscripts, *Sven. Tandlak-Tidskr.* **40,** Suppl.

BJÖRK, A. and M. PALLING (1955) Adolescent age changes in sagittal jaw relation, alveolar prognathy, and incisal inclination, *Acta Odont. Scand.* **12,** 201.

BJÖRK, A. (1955) Cranial base development. A follow-up X-ray study of the individual variation in growth occurring between the ages 12 and 20 years and its relation to brain case and face development, *Am. J. Ortho.* **41,** 198.

BJÖRK, A. (1961) The relationship of the jaws to the cranium, in *Introduction to Orthodontics,* ed. A. Lundstrom, McGraw-Hill, London.

BJÖRK, A. (1963) Variations in the growth pattern of the human mandible: longitudinal radiographic study by the implant method, *J. dent. Res.* **42,** 400.

BJÖRK, A. (1966) Sutural growth of the upper face, studied by the implant method, *Acta Odont. Scand.* **24,** 109.

BJÖRK, A., and S. HELM (1967) Prediction of the age of maximum pubertal growth in body height, *Angl. Ortho.* **37,** 134.

BJÖRK, A. (1969) Prediction of mandibular growth rotation, *Am. J. Ortho.* **55,** 585.

BJÖRK, A., and V. SKIELLER (1972) Facial development and tooth eruption, *Am. J. Ortho.* **62,** 339.

BJÖRK, A. and V. SKIELLER (1977) Growth of the maxilla in three dimensions as revealed radiographically by the implant method, *Brit. J. Ortho.* **4,** 53.

BROADBENT, B. H. (1931) A new X-ray technique and its application to orthodontics, *Angl. Ortho.* **1,** 45.

BROADBENT, B. H. (1937) The face of the normal child, *Angl. Ortho.* **7,** 183.

BROADBENT, B. H. Jr. (1973) Bolton Standards. Chronologic norms in clinical application, in *Transactions of the Third International Orthodontic Congress,* ed. J. T. Cook, Crosby Lockwood Staples, London.

BROADBENT, B. H., BROADBENT, B. H. Jr. and GOLDEN, W. H. (1975) *Bolton Standards of Dentofacial Development Growth,* C. V. Mosby, St. Louis.

BRODIE, A. G. (1941) On the growth pattern of the human head from the third month to the eighth year of life, *Am. J. Anat.* **68,** 209.

BRODIE, A. G. (1953) Late growth changes in the human face, *Angl. Ortho.* **23,** 146.

BURKE, P. H. (1980) Serial growth changes in the lips, *Brit. J. Ortho.* **7,** 17.

BURSTONE, C. J. (1958) The integumental profile, *Am. J. Ortho.* **56,** 403.

CHACONAS, S. J. (1969) A statistical evaluation of nasal growth, *Am. J. Ortho.* **56,** 403.

D'ARCY THOMPSON, W. (1917) *On Growth and Form,* Cambridge University Press, Cambridge.

DELATIRE, A. and F. FENART (1958) La méthode vestibulaire appliqué a l'étude du crâne. Son champ d'application, *Z. Morphol. Anat.* **1,** 90

DOWNS, W. B. (1948) Variations in facial relationships, their significance in treatment and prognosis, *Am. J. Ortho.* **34,** 812.

GREENBERG, L. Z. and L. E. JOHNSTONE (1975) Computerised prediction: the accuracy of a contemporary long-range forecast, *Am. J. Ortho.* **67,** 243.

HARVOLD, E. (1963) Some biologic aspects of orthodontic treatment in the transitional dentition, *Am. J. Ortho.* **49,** 1.

HELM, S., S. SKIERSBAEK-NIELSEN, V. SKIELLER and S. BJÖRK (1971) Skeletal maturation of the hand in relation to maximum pubertal growth in body height, *Tandlaegebladet,* **75,** 1223.

HIXON, E. H. (1972) Cephalometrics: a perspective, *Angl. Ortho.* **42,** 200.
HOFRATH, H. (1931) Bedeutung der roentgenfernuud abstandonfnahne fur die diagnostik der kieferanomolien, *Fortschr. der Orthod.* **1,** 232, after Brodie, A. G. (1931) Growth of the human head from 3 months to 8 years, *Am. J. Anat.* **68,** 209.
HOROWITZ, S. L. and E. H. HIXON (1966) Fundamental considerations in cephalometrics and Norms, classification and treatment goals, in *The Nature of Orthodontic Treatment,* C. V. Mosby, St. Louis.
HOUSTON, W. J. B., J. C. MILLER and J. M. TANNER (1979) Prediction of the timing of the adolescent growth spurt from ossification events in handwrist films, *Brit. J. Ortho.* **6,** 145.
HUGGINS, D. and L. McBRIDE (1975) Influences of the maxillary incisors on soft tissue profile, *Brit. J. Ortho.* **3,** 141.
JOHNSON, J. S. (1960) The uses of centres of gavity in cephalometric analysis, *Dent. Practit.* **10,** 107.
JOHNSON, J. S. (1978) A new approach to cephalometric analysis of the dental base relationship, *Angl. Ortho.* **48,** 23.
JOHNSTONE, L. E. (1975) A simplified approach to prediction, *Am. J. Ortho.* **67,** 253.
KERR, W. J. S. (1978) A method of superimposing lateral cephalometric films for the purpose of comparison: a preliminary report, *Brit. J. Ortho.* **5,** 51.
KERR, W. J. S. (1979) A longitudinal cephalometric study of dento-facial growth from 5 to 15 years, *Brit. J. Ortho.* **6,** 115.
KOSKI, K. (1973) Variability of the facial skeleton: an exercise in roentgencephalometry, *Am. J. Ortho.* **64,** 188.
LANDE, M. J. (1952) Growth behaviour of the human bony facial profile as revealed by serial cephalometric roentgenology, *Angl. Ortho.* **22,** 78.
LEIGHTON, B. C. (1958) Growth study initiated in 1958, King's College Hospital Medical School, University of London.
LINDER-ARONSON, S. (1979) Respiratory function in relation to facial morphology and the dentition, *Brit. J. Ortho.* **6,** 59,
MELSEN, B. (1974) The cranial base, *Acta Odont. Scand.* **32,** Suppl. 62.
MITCHELL, D. L., J. F. JORDAN and R. M. RICKETTS (1975) Arcial growth with metallic implants in mandibular growth prediction, *Am. J. Ortho.* **68,** 655.
MOORREES, C. F. A. and P. K.-J. YEM (1955) An analysis of changes in the dento-facial skeleton following orthodontic treatment, *Am. J. Ortho.* **41,** 526.
MOSS, M. L. and L. SALENTIJN (1970) The logarithmic growth of the human mandible, *Acta Anat.* **77,** 341.
MOSS, M. L. and L. SALENTIJN and H. P. OSTREICHER (1974) The logarithmic properties of active and passive mandibular growth, *Am. J. Ortho.* **66,** 645.
MOYERS, R. E., F. L. BOOKSTEIN and K. E. GUIRE (1979) The concept of pattern in cranio-facial growth, *Am. J. Ortho.* **76,** 136.
POPOVICH, F. and G. W. THOMPSON (1977) Cranio-facial templates for orthodontic case analysis, *Am. J. Ortho.* **71,** 406.
POSEN, J. M. (1967) Longitudinal studies of the nose, *Am. J. Ortho.* **53,** 746.
RICKETTS, R. M., R. W. BENCH, J. J. HILGERS and R. SCHULHOF (1972) An overview of computerised cephalometrics, *Am. J. Ortho.* **61,** 1.
RIEDEL, R. A. (1952) The relation of maxillary structures to cranium in malocclusion and in normal occlusion, *Angl. Ortho.* **22,** 142.
RIOLO, M. L., R. E. MOYERS, J. A. McNAMARA Jr., and W. S. HUNTER (1974) *An Atlas of Craniofacial Growth,* Center for Human Growth and Development, University of Michigan, Ann Arbor.
ROBERTSON, N. R. E. (1976) Contour photography, *Brit. J. Ortho.* **3,** 105.
ROOS, N. (1977) Soft tissue profile changes in Class II treatment, *Am. J. Ortho.* **72,** 165.
SCHULHOF, R. J. and L. BAGHA (1975) A statistical evaluation of the Ricketts and Johnstone growth forcasting methods, *Am. J. Ortho.* **67,** 258.
SCHULHOF, R. J., S. NAKAMURA and W. V. WILLIAMSON (1977) Prediction of abnormal growth in Class III malocclusions, *Am. J. Ortho.* **71,** 421.
SHAW, W. C. (1977) Problems of accuracy and reliability in cephalometric studies with implants in infants with cleft lip and palate, *Brit. J. Ortho.* **4,** 93.

SOLOW, B. (1980) The dento-alveolar compensatory mechanism; background and clinical implications, *Brit. J. Ortho.* **7,** 145.

SUBTELNY, D. (1959) A longitudinal study of soft tissue facial structures, *Am. J. Ortho.* **45,** 481.

TANNER, J. M. (1962) *Growth at Adolescence,* 2nd ed., Oxford, Blackwell.

TANNER, J. M., R. H. WHITEHOUSE and M. TAKAISHI (1966) Standards from birth to maturity for height, weight, height velocity and weight velocity; British children, 1965, *Archives of Disease in Childhood,* **41,** 454.

TANNER, J. M., R. H. WHITEHOUSE, W. A. MARSHALL, M. J. R. HEALY and H. GOLDSTEIN (1975) in *Assessment of Skeletal Maturity and Prediction of Adult Height (TW2 method),* Academic Press, London.

THILANDER, B. and B. INGERVALL (1973) The human spheno-occipital synchondrosis II. A histological and micro-radiographic study of its growth, *Acta Odont. Scand.* **31,** 323.

THOMPSON, G. W. and F. POPOVICH (1977) A longitudinal evaluation of the Burlington Growth Centre Data, *J. dent. Res. Special Issue C,* **56,** C71.

WALKER, G. F. (1972) A new approach to the analysis of craniofacial morphology, *Am. J. Ortho.* **61,** 221.

WISTH, P. (1972) Changes in soft tissue profile during growth, *Trans Eur. Ortho. Soc.* 123.

WISTH, P. (1974) Soft tissue response to incisor retraction, *Brit. J. Ortho.* **1,** 199.

WOODSIDE, D. G. Distance, velocity and relative growth rate standards for mandibular growth for Canadian males and females age three to twenty years. Unpublished manuscript 1969. Reported by D.G. Woodside, R. T. Reed, J. D. Doucet and G. W. Thompson. Some effects of activator treatment on the growth rate of the mandible and position of the midface, in *Transactions of the Third International Orthodontic Congress,* ed. J. T. Cook, Crosby Lockwood Staples, London.

CHAPTER 8

# *The Development and Structure of the Teeth and Their Supporting Tissues*

The development and structure of the teeth and their supporting structures clearly form an integral and important part of dentofacial development and growth. The teeth develop and erupt over a considerable period of time and in humans there are two generations, the deciduous and permanent dentition. The tooth germs are enclosed by the tissues of the developing jaws and in achieving a functional position they undergo a complex and coordinated series of physiological movement both before, during and after eruption. The deciduous teeth are smaller and fewer than the permanent, and as the deciduous teeth are shed they are gradually replaced by the permanent teeth. In order to accommodate the larger permanent teeth, considerable remodelling of the supporting bone takes place, accompanied by expansion of the tooth-bearing areas of the jaws; that is, the maxilla and mandible. A diagram of a tooth and its supporting and surrounding structures is shown in Fig. 8.1.

Anatomically a tooth consists of the crown, the roots and the pulp. The anatomical crown is that part of the tooth covered with a layer of enamel that ends at the cervical line or neck. The clinical crown is that part of the tooth which is exposed into the oral cavity and ends at the gingival line. The root is that portion of the tooth which is covered in cementum and located in the alveolus adjacent to the soft tissues. The roots begin at the cervical line and are covered in a layer of cementum. The pulp is the central portion of a tooth enclosed by dentine.

Enamel is a nonvital highly calcified acellular tissue and once lost cannot be replaced. Cementum is an avascular but cellular tissue similar in structure to bone. The bulk of the tooth consists of dentine, a vital tissue, which encloses the dental pulp except at the apical foramen, where nerves and blood vessels enter. Lining the surface of the pulp are the dentine-forming cells, the odontoblasts, which extend processes through the dentine and possibly to the amelodentinal junction. The dental pulp is a cellular fibrous tissue supporting the blood vessels and nerves which traverse it. The dentine and pulp, which have the same embryological origins, may be considered as a single functional unit, the dentine pulp complex.

When a tooth is fully developed it is suspended by a fibrous vascular structure, the periodontal ligament, in a bony socket formed by the alveolar

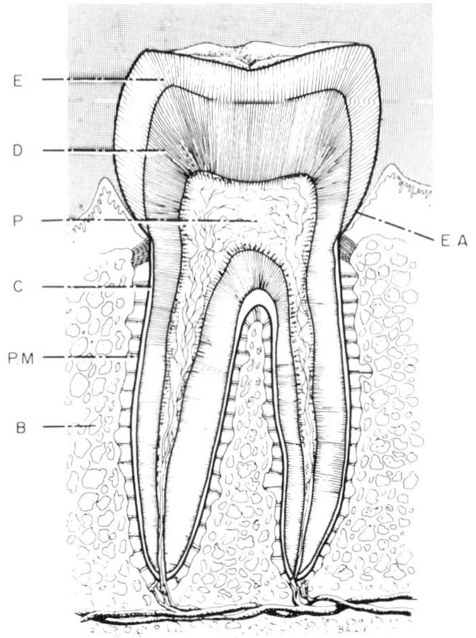


Fig. 8.1. Diagram of a longitudinal section through a molar tooth and its supporting structures showing (E) enamel, (D) dentine, (EA) epithelial attachment, (PM) periodontal ligament, (B) bone.

processes of the mandible or maxilla. The fibres are attached to the bone on one side and the cementum covering the root on the other. Such an arrangement is known as a gomphosis and is unique to mammals.

When the tooth erupts it perforates the lining of the oral cavity, the oral mucosa, so that a specialized junction is established between the oral epithelium and the tooth. The term periodontium is the collective term used to describe the junctional epithelium, the supporting alveolar bone, cementum and the periodontal ligament.

Advance in knowledge has been so extensive that numerous separate treatises exist on the individual dental tissues mentioned above. The objective of this chapter, therefore, is to provide a brief account of the development and structure of the dental tissues relevant to the other chapters in this text and to stimulate the reader to seek additional information through the use of the bibliography.

## TOOTH DEVELOPMENT

The morphological changes occurring throughout the complex process of human odontogenesis have been studied extensively. These morphological changes are, however, the result of more fundamental and complex biological processes which include embryonic induction, cell differentiation, histogenesis, extracellular matrix formation, matrix calcification and tooth eruption. Much of the experimental work on odontogenesis, however, has been carried out on amphibian eggs and embryos. Such work has suggested an important role for cells of neural crest origin, ectomesenchyme, in tooth development. Comparable experiments on mammalian embryogenesis have so far not been possible, however. What information is available would suggest that it is possible to cautiously extrapolate on the basis that mammalian teeth are homologous with non-mammalian forms.

**The Role of Ectomesenchyme in Tooth Development**

Ectomesenchyme arises when the margins of the neural plate elevate and eventually fuse in the midline to form the neural tube. Ectodermal cells derived from the edges of the neural plate which do not become part of the neural tube and are surrounded by mesenchyme remain on the dorsolateral surface to form ridges known as neural crests (Fig. 8.2). These cells rapidly divide

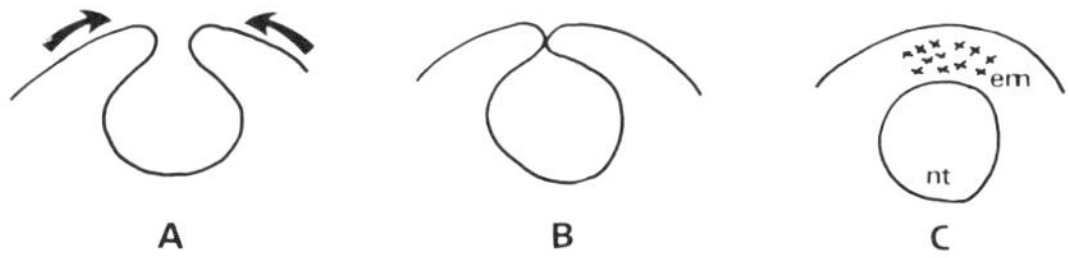


Fig. 8.2. Diagram showing stages in the formation of the neural tube (nt) and ectomesenchyme (em) following the fusion of ectodermally covered process.

and during and following cell division the ectomesenchyme of the neural crest migrates through the cephalic region of the embryo. The mechanism of this highly developed migratory capacity is unknown, but it can be closely followed in lower vertebrates, such as amphibians, since the ectomesenchymal cells contain yolk granules. Cells of neural crest origin can also be labelled with tritiated thymidine and their migrations followed by autoradiography, but only for a limited period, since successive divisions dilute the radiactive label. Interaction between ectomesenchyme cells and the epithelium of the primitive stomatodeum results in the induction of local epithelial thickenings known as the odontogenic epithelium or primary epithelial band. The earliest stages of tooth development take place internally and cannot be seen on external examination of the embryo. Therefore, a technique has been used in which the formation of the odontogenic epithelium and the resultant epithelial dental lamina were carefully investigated by the construction of three-dimensional models from serial sections of human embryos. At 28 days odontogenic epithelium develops on the inferior margins of the maxillary processes and the superior margins of the mandibular arch (Fig. 8.3). The proliferating odontogenic epithelium is about four cells in thickness and is carried along by the ventromedial growth of the maxillary process. Similarly,

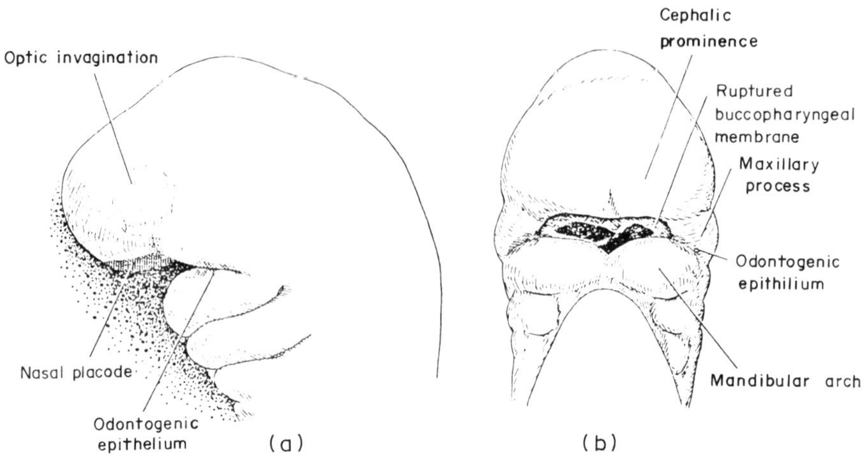


Fig. 8.3. A 28-day human embryo. Lateral (A) and frontal (B) views of the cephalic portion (by kind permission of Dr E. B. Nery *et al.* and *Archives of Oral Biology).*

the odontogenic epithelium over the mandibular arch develops and extends medially.

At 33 days the odontogenic epithelium associated with the maxillary processes extends as far as the nasal fin. When the two epithelial layers of the nasal fin break down at 35 days the convergence of the nasal and maxillary processes is advanced. The odontogenic epithelium of the upper jaw can now be recognized in four separate zones. Two zones are situated on the maxillary process and two on the lateral borders of the frontonasal process adjoining the former site of the nasal fin. In the mandible there are only two areas of odontogenic epithelium, left and right, extending to the midline which may also have fused by 35 days (Fig. 8.4).

At 37 days the odontogenic lamina may be observed as a single plate of epithelium in both the upper and lower jaws. Therefore, the odontogenic epithelium arises from six separate zones, the medial portion of the maxillary dental lamina taking its origin from the frontonasal rather than the maxillary process (Fig. 8.5).

## The Formation of the Tooth Germ

Odontogenesis is a continuous process, but for the purposes of description the morphological changes are usually divided into a series of well-defined stages. The major stages in human odontogenesis will therefore be described as a foundation for discussing the more fundamental aspects of tooth development.

There is proliferation of the odontogenic epithelium resulting in its invagination into the underlying ectomesenchyme. The odontogenic

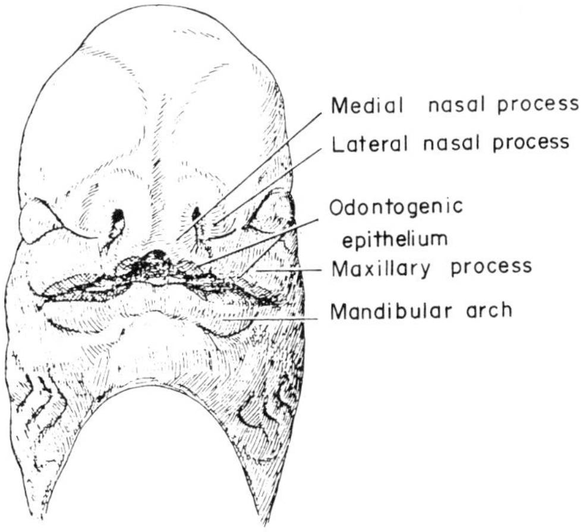


Fig. 8.4. A 35-day human embryo, frontal view, showing the six zones of odontogenic epithelium (by kind permission of Dr. E. B. Nery *et al.* and *Archives of Oral Biology*).

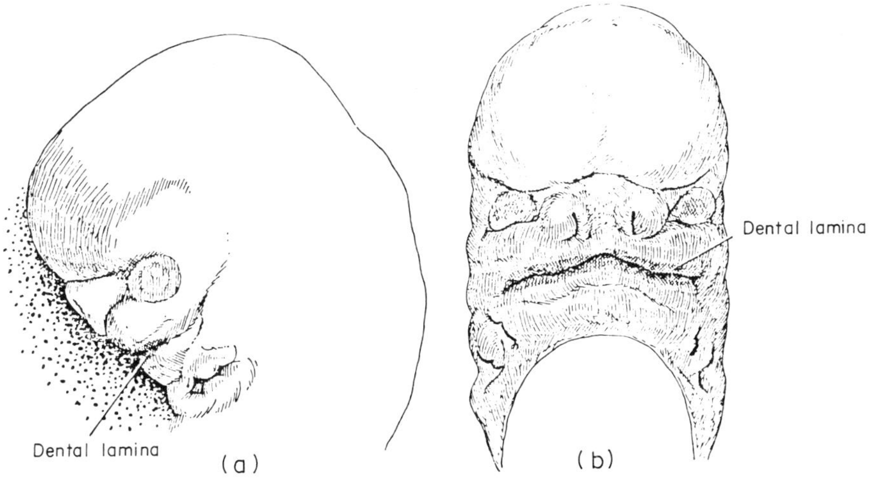


Fig. 8.5. A 37-day human embryo. Lateral (A) and frontal (B) views of the head showing the location of the dental lamina (by kind permission of Dr E. B. Nery *et al.* and *Archives of Oral Biology).*

epithelium divides into two branches, the dental lamina and labial part the vestibular lamina, which will separate the lip from the oral cavity. The vestibular lamina follows a curve parallel to the dental lamina.

Increased mitotic activity at specific locations along the dental lamina, initially in the anterior portion of the maxillary and mandibular arches, results in knob-like structures appearing on the labial surface of the dental lamina. These structures are associated with distinct condensations of ectomesenchymal cells and together are known as tooth germs (Fig. 8.6). There is a bilateral symmetry and a definite anterior posterior gradient in the development of the tooth germs.

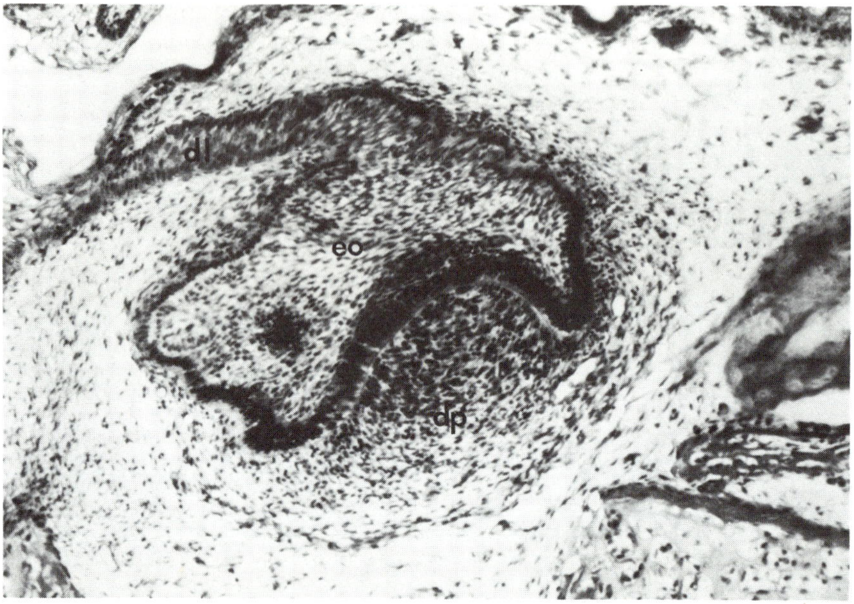


Fig. 8.6. Photomicrograph showing the early "cap stage" of tooth development. dl, dental lamina; eo, enamel organ; dp, dental papilla.

**The "Cap" and "Bell" Stages of Tooth Development**

*"Cap" stage.* The knob-like invaginations of the oral epithelium continue to grow principally by cell division at their periphery and invade underlying ectomesenchyme. As a result the inferior surfaces of the epithelial downgrowth becomes concave and partially enclose the condensation of ectomesenchymal cells now termed the dental papilla (Fig. 8.6). The tall cells of the concave surface are in a single layer and form the internal dental epithelium. This layer is continuous with the cuboidal cells of the convex dental epithelium in an area known as the cervical loop. These epithelial layers enclose the cells of the stellate reticulum, so called because they are star-shaped and widely separated with long processes connected by desmosomes. The cells become separated by the intercellular accumulation of acidic mucopolysaccharides which are very hydrophilic, hence the whole enamel organ becomes turgid. This turgidity probably protects the crown during development, and since the stellate reticulum disappears during tooth development it may have a nutritive role.

Enclosed by the cells of the enamel organ, the ectomesenchymal cells of the dental papilla, or primitive dental pulp, continue to divide and condense. There is an ingrowth into the dental papilla of capillaries. Nerve fibres form a plexus around the base of the dental papilla but do not enter yet. It is not until dentinogenesis commences that pioneer nerve fibres enter the dental papilla. These pioneer nerves are adrenergic; cholinergic nerves do not appear until later. There is also a marginal condensation which is probably ectomesenchymal extending from the papilla to partially envelop the enamel organ. This is the layer of ectomesenchyme, from which the periodontal ligament, cementum and alveolar bone will develop. Enclosing the whole tooth germ is the fibrous mesodermal dental follicle or sac.

*"Bell" stage.* With further growth at the cervical loop the enamel organ assumes a bell shape and almost completely encloses the dental papilla (Fig. 8.7). The cells of the internal dental epithelium have increased in size and are now up to 40 μm in length and 4 μm in width. Overlying the internal dental epithelium, several layers of flattened cells appear to form the stratum intermedium. The stellate reticulum continues to enlarge by an increase in intercellular material. In all the developing teeth, except the permanent molars, the dental lamina proliferates and extends lingually to produce the lamina for the permanent teeth. The internal dental epithelium is separated from the adjacent cells of the dental papilla by a basement membrane—the membrane preformativa. Differential growth of the internal dental epithelium in a genetically predetermined manner maps out the shape of the future enamel-dentine junction and hence the shape of the crown of the tooth. The flattened cuboidal cells of the external enamel epithelium become folded. Between the folds are cores of mesenchyme tissue which contain capillary loops from the dental follicle.

The tooth germ at the bell stage, therefore, consists of the following cell layers: outer dental epithelium, stellate reticulum, stratum intermedium, internal dental epithelium and dental papilla (Fig. 8.8). The dental lamina breaks down the connection with the oral epithelium at the end of the bell stage of tooth development. Sometimes the epithelium remnants proliferate and form structures known as the Glands of Serres. They usually all degenerate, but occasionally give rise to cysts.

At the end of the second month of intrauterine life all the deciduous dentition has started to develop. The teeth of the permanent dentition are produced by proliferation at the free end of the dental lamina lingual to the deciduous tooth germ. The tooth germs for the permanent incisors are complete after 7 months of intrauterine life and after 8 months for the second permanent premolar. Extension of the dental lamina distally produces the development of the permanent molars. The development of the first permanent molar tooth germ is complete at 6 weeks, the second permanent molar

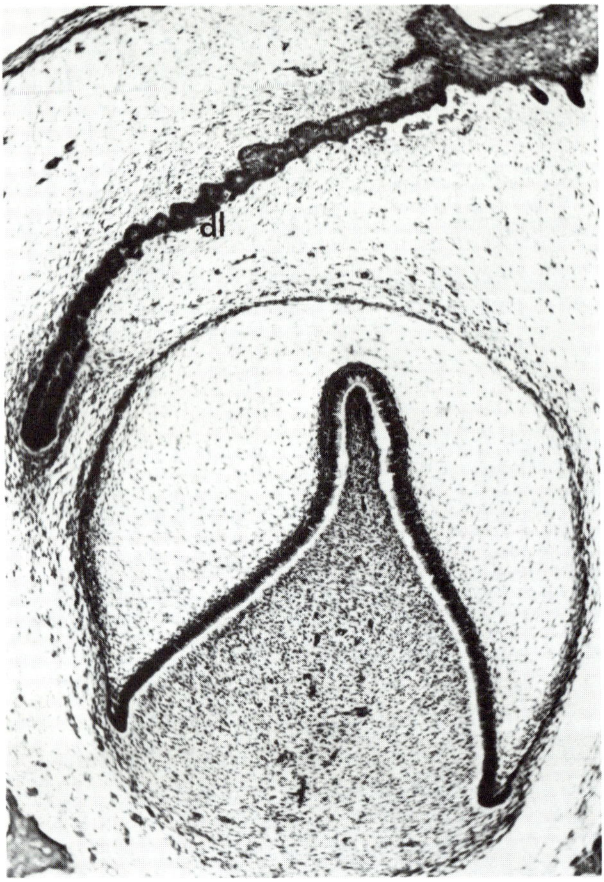


Fig. 8.7. Photomicrograph showing the "bell stage" of tooth development. The dental lamina (dl) is about to disintegrate.

tooth germ at 6 months after birth and the third permanent molar tooth germ at the 5th or 6th year after birth.

### The Control of Tooth Development

The factors involved in determining tooth shape, number, class and the timing of initiation are complex. Two different control mechanisms have been suggested, the so-called "field model" and the "clone model" (Fig. 8.9 a and b). The role of biological fields or gradients in odontogenesis was first proposed by Huxley and deBeer (1934) and later used by Butler (1939) to account for gradients in tooth shape. In the field model the development of the dentition is controlled by an external source, but in the clone model the pattern is self-generated.

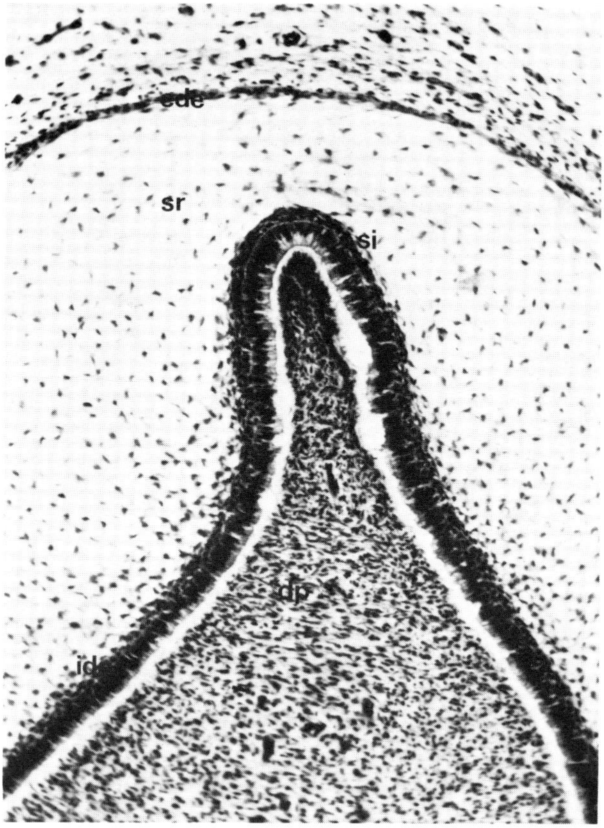


Fig. 8.8. Photomicrograph showing in detail the cell layers of the tooth germ at the "bell stage" of tooth development. ede, external dental epithelium; sr, stellate reticulum; si, stratum intermedium; ide, internal dental epithelium; dp, dental papilla.

In the field model consider several different structures the shape of which constitutes a gradient. Early in development an area is differentiated, the field generator, which secretes a substance, the field substance. This substance then diffuses through the growing region. As the field substance diffuses through the tissues it is destroyed, so that further away from the field generator the lower the concentration of field substance. Identical primordia differentiate from the growing tissues and become surrounded by field substance. Therefore, any gradient in structure is the result of the reaction of primordia to different concentrations of field substance.

In the clone model all the structures develop from a single clone of cells. The clone grows posteriorly and after cell division becomes competent to initiate a primordium. As new primordia appear, a surrounding area develops in which the initiation of new primordia is inhibited. With successive

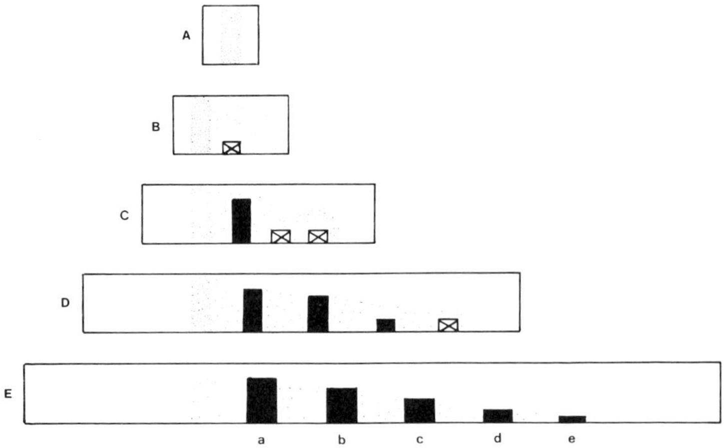


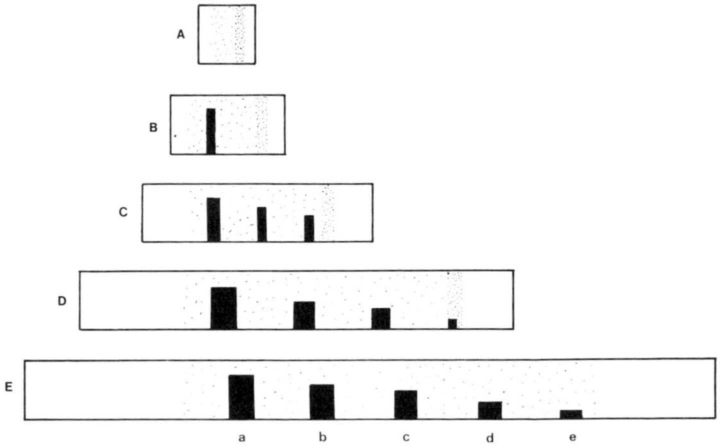


Fig. 8.9 (a). An explanation in terms of fields for the development of five structures whose shapes are graded a to e in E. A field generator (heavy stipple) is differentiated in A and produces a gradient of field substance (light stipple). All primordia (e.g. a in B, b and c in C and d in D) are identical. Each primordium develops into a shape determined by the concentration of field substance. This correspondence is indicated by matching the height of each structure (black rectangles) to the level of the field substance. (By kind permission of Professor J. W. Osborn, University of Alberta, Canada from *Development, Function and Evolution of Teeth,* ed. P. M. Butler and K. A. Joysey, 1978, Academic Press, London.)

Fig. 8.9 (b). An explanation in terms of a clone model for the development of the gradient of structures. All the structures develop from a clone of cells (stippled in A). The clone grows to the right (its growing edge is heavily stippled). New primorida are initiated when space becomes available inside the clone (light stipple). When a primordium differentiates out of the clone (a in B, b and c in C, d in D) its shape (represented by the height of the rectangle) is already determined. (By kind permission of Professor J. W. Osborn, University of Alberta, Canada from *Development, Function and Evolution of Teeth,* ed. P. M. Butler and K. A. Joysey, 1978, Academic Press, London.)

primordia the cells will have divided more times and there will be a gradient of cell ancestry. Therefore, until growth starts, the gradient does not exist and when growth stops is complete.

If all tooth primordia are equivalent, as proposed by the field model, then each must contain a full complement of incisor, canine and molar targets to respond to the field gradient. Osborne (1978), however, has developed a model for tooth shape which does not depend on targets. The model requires that the internal enamel epithelium grows over the dental papilla at a constant rate in all directions, with viscous drag restraining the internal enamel epithelium from sliding over the dental papilla. Detailed analysis has shown that the shape into which the internal enamel epithelium folds depends on the initial growth rate. Therefore, to account for a gradient in tooth shape, or size, etc., a mechanism is required for providing a gradient in the growth rates of successive primordia. Support for the clone model is provided by the fact that when tooth germs are cultured *in vitro* away from any possible field substance they develop normally. Also Glasstone (1952) has shown that if a tooth germ is halved at the cap stage each half produces a full complement of cusps. This result is fully consistent with the clone model, which proposes the rates of cell division within the primordia determine tooth shape, and this is not altered by halving the tooth germ.

Therefore, the evidence suggests that the development of a tooth depends on internal factors determined when the tooth primordium differentiates. Experimental evidence shows that there is reciprocal interaction between the epithelially derived enamel organ and the ectomesenchymal dental papilla.

## Epithelial Ectomesenchymal Interactions

It can be shown experimentally using rodent embryonic teeth that odontogenesis is the result of reciprocal interaction between the oral epithelium and the papillary ectomesenchyme. Dissociation of these components *in vitro* prevents cell differentiation and the development of the dental tissues. Recombination will allow tooth development to proceed, suggesting that "developmental information" is passed between the cell layers. Furthermore, these experiments show that the papillary ectomesenchyme is responsible for determining the form of the tooth. For example, incisor papillary ectomesenchyme when combined with epithelium from the molar region will induce the development of an incisor. The papillary ectomesenchyme will also induce tooth development in non-tooth oral epithelium and in non-oral epithelium. Cultured dental papilla cells also retain their morphogenetic capabilities. Therefore, the ectomesenchyme carries the genetic information for producing a tooth as well as for whether the tooth is to be a molar or an incisor.

Contact between the cell layers is not necessary for development. Tooth rudiments have been dissociated *in vitro* and with tissues separated by a filter development proceeds. Electron microscope investigations suggest, but do not confirm, that there is no cell contact with the cell processes that pass into the filter. However, the inductive influence can be retarded by increasing the thickness of the filter and decreasing the pore size, indicating that a diffusable agent of some kind is involved. It has been shown experimentally, for example, that reducing the pore size of a 25-μm thick Millipore filter from 0.5 to 0.1 μm significantly retards the inductive influence. Thus if a diffusable agent is involved, it requires a pore diameter of 0.1 μm or more which is massive when compared with most macromolecules or viruses but smaller than the cell processes.

It has been suggested that the collagen of the dental papilla or other specific macromolecules play an important role in controlling the developmental process. For example, if lathyritic agents are administered to developing tooth germs, then morphogenesis is disrupted. However, this effect is reversible and when returned to the control media normal development proceeds.

Another possible explanation is that the information is packaged in membrane-bound vesicles transported through the extracellular matrix situated between the epithelium and mesenchyme. This matrix can be isolated and stripped of adherent cells. If either epithelium or mesenchyme are cultured in association with the matrix as a xenograft on the chick chorioallantoic membrane for up to 10 days they become like ameloblasts or odontoblasts. Culture experiments using radioactive precursors for RNA indicate that RNAs are synthesized *de novo* within each cell type and transferred to the extracellular matrix. The RNAs within the matrix are of low molecular weight.

Ultrastructural examination of the extracellular matrix shows that vesicles are present and are between 0.5 and 0.1 μm in diameter with a characteristic trilaminar membrane. These vesicles may be biochemically separated from the matrix and some have been shown to contain RNA by direct chemical analysis. Ultrastructural evidence suggests that the matrix vesicles are produced and secreted into the organic matrix by ectomesenchymal cells by a process of budding. The vesicles are then incorporated into the internal enamel epithelium by pinocytosis or ingestion. It is possible, therefore, that the dental papilla is synthesizing and packaging "instructional macromolecules" which are secreted into the extracellular matrix and transferred to a competent epithelium.

## The Development of the Roots

The end of the bell stage of tooth development is marked by the beginning of hard tissue formation in the crown. The roots begin to develop after the shape of the crown has been mapped out but before the hard tissues are fully developed.

At the cervical margins of the developing crown the external and internal dental epithelia come together, with the exclusion of the stratum intermedium and stellate reticulum. This double layer is referred to as the epithelial rooth sheath of Hertwig and it grows downward to mark the beginning of root formation. As it grows the root sheath turns horizontally to form the epithelial diaphragm. The epithelial diaphragm by its further growth determines the number of roots (Fig. 8.10).

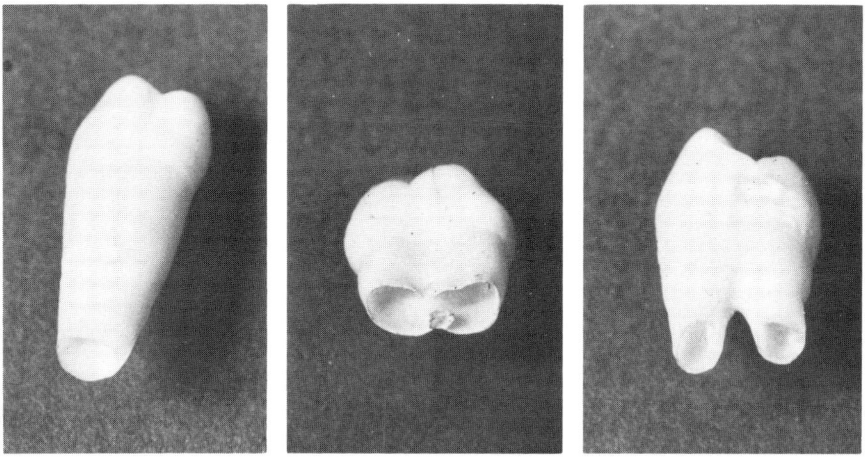

Fig. 8.10. The developing roots of three teeth indicated by the wide apex. In life the root surface is covered by Hertwig's epithelial root sheath which in a multirooted tooth grows inwards to map out the shape of the root.

There are said to be two phases in root development, the eruptive phase and the penetrative phase. The eruptive phase begins with root development and ends when the tooth is in occlusion with about two-thirds of the root developed. During this eruptive phase the level of the epithelial diaphragm remains fairly constant. When the tooth is in occlusion the penetrative phase begins and the level of the diaphragm is displaced towards the alveolar base. These phases are reflected in the external appearance; the apical third of the penetrative is rough compared to the smooth surface of the eruptive phase.

During development the tooth becomes enclosed in a bony crypt formed by extensions of the mandible or maxilla. Until the onset of root formation the tooth germ and its follicle expand in all directions and is accompanied by a uniform resorption of bone lining the crypt. With the onset of root formation the tooth migrates in an occlusal direction to its functional position within the oral cavity, that is the tooth erupts.

## DENTINE

Dentine is more logically considered together with the dental pulp, since these tissues form a single functional unit. They both develop from the ectomesenchyme of the primitive dental papilla and the odontoblasts which cover the pulpal surface are responsible for dentinogenesis. In addition, the pulp by virtue of its blood and nerve supply is both nutritive and sensory to the dentine. By its ability to react to stimuli the pulp is also protective and reparative.

### Dentinogenesis

Dentine is the first hard tissue to form in the developing tooth and its appearance marks the end of the bell stage of tooth development. Dentine formation commences in relation to the future incisal edges or cusps. The odontoblasts which produce dentine differentiate from the ectomesenchyme cells of the primitive dental pulp which lie adjacent to the basement membrane or membrana preformativa of the internal dental epithelium. The differentiation of the odontoblasts in coronal dentine is preceded by specific histological changes in the cells of the internal dental epithelium. These cells cease to divide and elongate and the nucleus moves from a central position to the future non-secretory end of the cell. The newly differentiating odontoblasts are widely separated, but later come together to be attached by junctional complexes (Fig. 8.11).

Initially the odontoblast has numerous blunt projections at the secretory end, but as dentine formation begins one of the projections becomes dominant and will form the odontoblast process. Associated with the odontoblasts is a subodontoblastic layer and a capillary plexus. These subodontoblastic cells are positive for the enzyme alkaline phosphatase. Later the odontoblast cell surface becomes positive for this enzyme which may be associated in these instances with membrane transport.

The odontoblast has the typical ultrastructural characteristics of a matrix synthesizing and secreting cell. There is a large amount of endoplasmic reticulum, numerous mitochondria, a complex juxtanuclear Golgi region and large numbers of secretory granules. Throughout the cytoplasm is a complex system of microtubules. In the odontoblast process secretory granules are located principally beneath the plasma membrane, but the other cell organelles do not usually extend beyond the level of the junctional complexes (Fig. 8.12).

Collagen is the principle organic matrix component of dentine. In the matrix of the first formed dentine Von Korff (1905) described agyrophilic fibres which extended from the primitive pulp between the odontoblasts and fanned out against the basement membrane (membrana preformativa) of the internal dental epithelium. Since these fibres had a corkscrew appearance, they were termed the corkscrew fibres of Von Korff (Fig. 8.13). In 1925

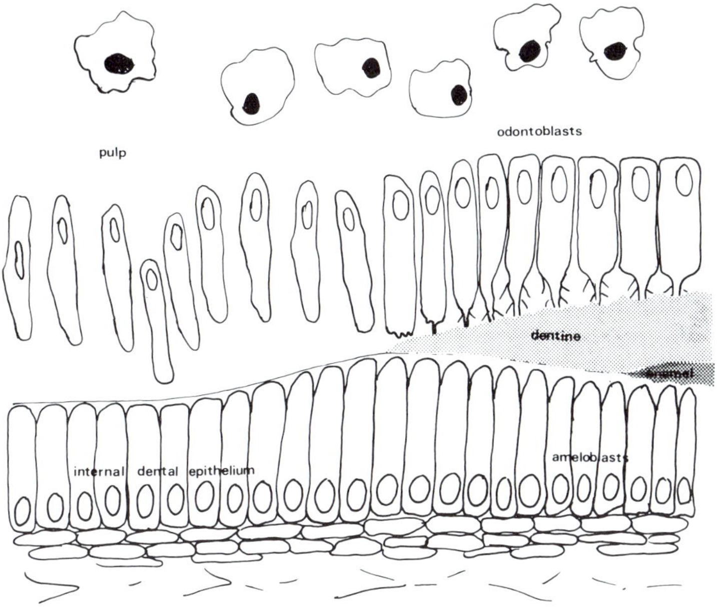


Fig. 8.11. Diagram illustrating the stages in differentiation of odontoblasts and ameloblasts from the cells of the primitive dental pulp and internal dental epithelium respectively.

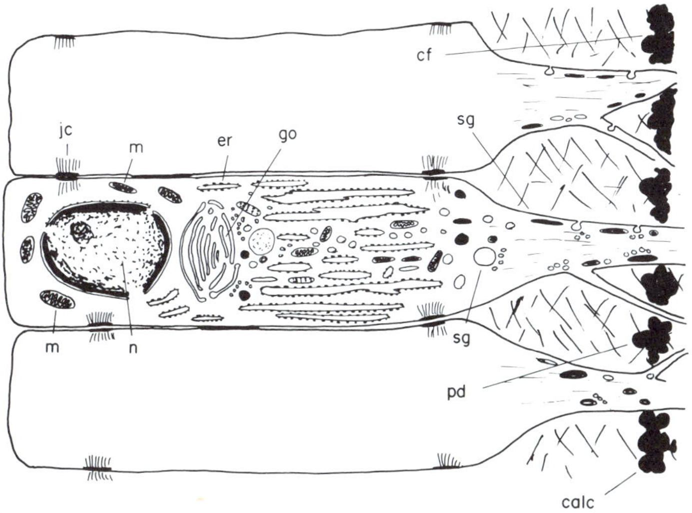


Fig. 8.12. The ultrastructural organization of the odontoblast and odontoblast process shown diagramatically. calc, calcospherites; cf, calcifying front; er, endoplasmic reticulum; go, Golgi region; jc, junctional complex; m, mitochondria; n, nucleus; pd, predentine; sg, secretory granule.

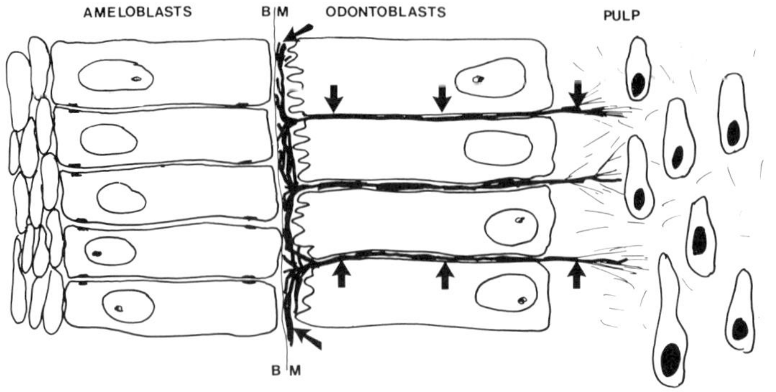


Fig. 8.13. Von Korff fibres are shown in this diagram extending from the pulp, passing between the newly differentiated odontoblasts and fanning out against the basement membrane, or membrane preformativa (BM).

Weidenreich termed this first formed layer of dentine, containing the so-called corkscrew fibres, mantle dentine, and the remainder circumpulpal dentine.

The presence of matrix fibres, as described by Von Korff, has been disputed. It was initially suggested that the silver stain was not staining fibres but pooling in the spaces between the differentiating odontoblasts. Later in dentine formation when the odontoblasts came together silver was excluded. Indeed with silver staining, the Von Korff fibre contribution is less as dentine formation proceeds. However, electron microscopic observations have supported the view that collagen fibres were present between the newly differentiated odontoblast as described by Von Korff.

Recently it has been shown that the silver staining is probably an artifact due to neutral carbohydrates in the interfibrillar matrix and that collagen fibres are indeed present but not as specifically defined by Von Korff. Fibres do not extend completely from the primitive pulp between the odontoblasts and almost all the electron micrographs are probably a misrepresentation of the plane of section. There are, however, fibres present in the first formed dentine which are at right angles to the membrana preformativa. Therefore, two types of dentine may be distinguished, but not on the basis as formerly defined.

If collagen fibres, as defined by Von Korff, did exist, this would suggest some role for the subodontoblastic cells of the primitive dental pulp. However, autoradiographic studies indicate that the odontoblast alone has the role of collagen production. These studies show that precursor material synthesized in the endoplasmic reticulum of the odontoblast cell body is transported to the odontoblast process where it is liberated into the organic matrix.

The collagen fibres of the mantle dentine are coarse and in bundles and at right angles to the basement membrane. This appearance may be related to the spatially restricted environment in which they develop. By contrast, the remainder of the dentine which forms the bulk of the tooth, the circumpulpal dentine, has a matrix of fine fibrils orientated at right angles to the odontoblast process (Fig. 8.14). The odontoblast process, therefore, becomes enclosed in a tubule, the dentinal tubule. The other matrix components are also synthesized by the odontoblast and have been identified biochemically and histochemically. They are chiefly proteoglycans with some glycoproteins and constitute the matrix ground substance.

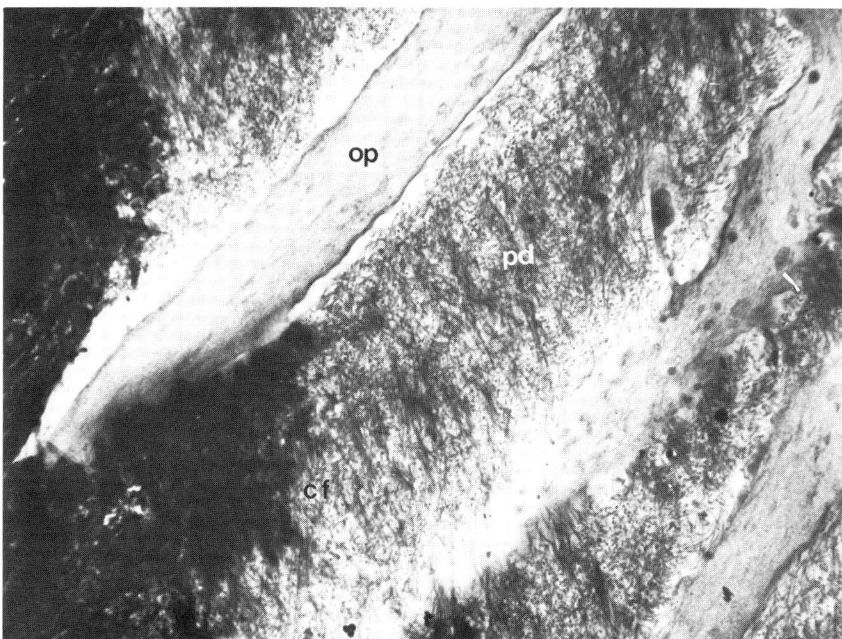


Fig. 8.14. Electron micrograph of the odontoblast process (op) extending through the collagen fibres of the predentine (pd) and into the calcified dentine. The calcifying front (cf) is represented by calcospherites at the light microscope level.

As the odontoblasts retreat towards the future dental pulp they leave behind the odontoblast process with its terminal branches in mantle dentine. It produces fine lateral branches and traces out an S-shaped curvature, the first convexity of which is directed towards the apex of the tooth (Fig. 8.19). It has been shown, using experimental models, that this curvature is probably a function of the odontoblasts becoming more crowded and jostling for position as they approach the future pulpal surface. The so-called secondary curvatures, which consists of small undulations with greater frequency, may be produced by the buckling of the process in situations where the growth in its length is greater than the distance moved by the odontoblast.

### Calcification of Dentine

Dentine formation is always associated with a distinct layer of uncalcified matrix, the predentine (Figs. 8.12 and 8.14). It has been suggested that calcification may be iniated in relation to the matrix collagen fibres, or some other macromolecule. Alternatively, the odontoblasts may produce the so-called matrix vesicles by a process of budding. At the histological level, calcification proceeds by the formation of mineral globules or calcospherites which fuse at the calcifying front giving it a somewhat irregular appearance (Fig. 8.12). Sometimes the fusion of calcospherities is incomplete so that uncalcified areas remain as the calcification front advances. Such areas are known as interglobular dentine (Fig. 8.15).

During dentine formation it is the matrix fibrils surrounding the odontoblast process which become calcified to form intertubular dentine. Near the predentine junction a hypercalcified layer develops on the inner wall of the tubule to form peritubular dentine (Fig. 8.16). The matrix of the peritubular dentine has few, if any, collagen fibres. As dentine formation proceeds, the layer of peritubular dentine becomes thicker. The source of this additional mineral is uncertain, it may arrive via the odontoblast process or by the redistribution of mineral already present in the intertubular matrix. Peritubular dentine, however, is absent in interglobular areas where intertubular dentine is also uncalcified.

### Structure of Dentine

The dentinal tubule traverses the dentine occupied by the odontoblast process and tissue fluid. The tubule branches terminally in the mantle dentine and there are also lateral branches at regular intervals of 1-2 $\mu$m along its length; these branches may extend into the adjacent tubule (Fig. 8.17). Near the pulp the dentinal tubules are wider than at the amelodentinal junction. There are about twice as many per unit area because the tubules become more crowded into a smaller surface area at the pulpal surface. The lumen of the tubule also becomes reduced by the formation of a layer of peritubular dentine which is thicker near the amelodentinal junction. As a result of pathological change, or age, the peritubular layer may become so thick as to completely occlude the tubules and form translucent or sclerotic dentine. As an age change this process is seen particularly in relation to the apices of the anterior teeth.

The odontoblast process is thicker where it leaves the odontoblast at the pulpal surface than at the amelodentinal junction. Near the odontoblast the process is characterized by microfibrils, large numbers of vesicles which may be fused with the plasma membrane, and possibly a few mitochondria. More remote from the odontoblast cell body, these organelles become less evident. Indeed the odontoblast process may be completely translucent or hyalinized. Sometimes the process may be vacuolated so that cytoplasm only occupies the

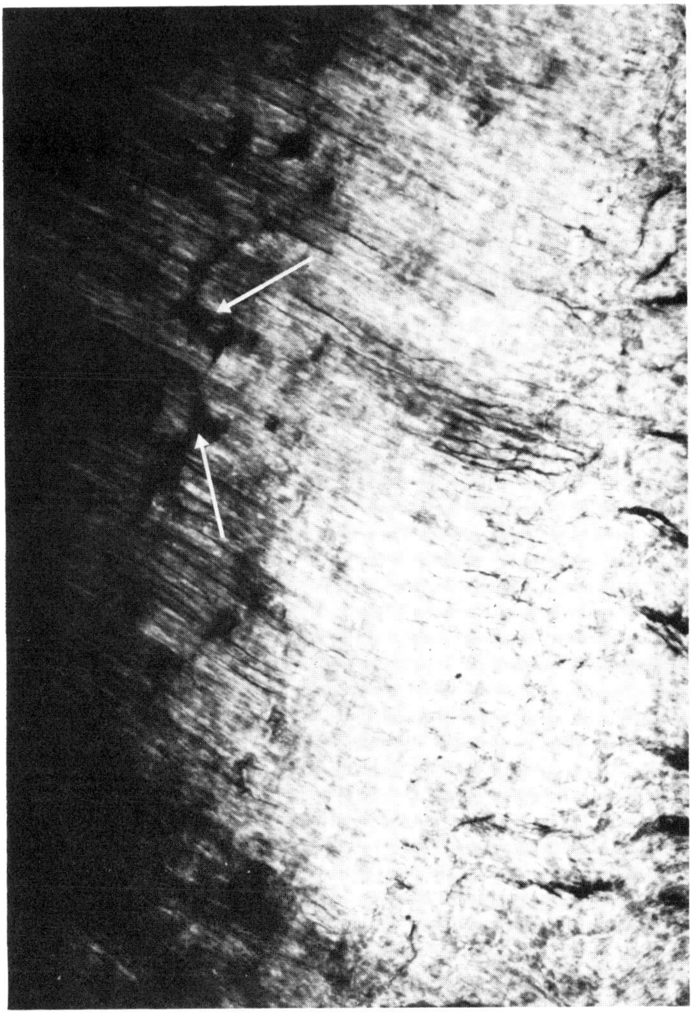

Fig. 8.15. Photomicrograph of a ground section through coronal dentine beneath the amelodentinal junction. The interglobular areas are arrowed.

periphery (Fig. 8.12 and 8.16). However, doubt has recently been cast on the idea that the odontoblast process normally extends across the whole width of the dentine, at least in some animal species.

The formation of hypocalcified interglobular dentine has already been described. Such areas are found chiefly in the coronal dentine near the amelodentinal junction (Fig. 8.15). Another area which was thought to be hypocalcified is the so-called granular layer of Tomes. As the term implies, this layer has a distinct granular appearance and extends beneath the cement dentine junction in the apical two-thirds of the roots (Fig. 8.18). It can be

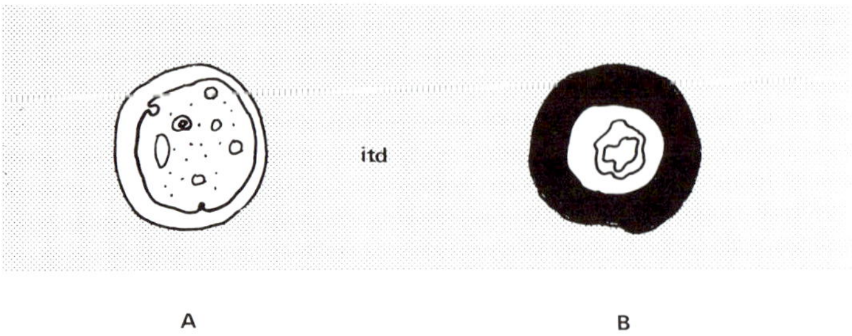


Fig. 8.16. Diagramatic section through the odontoblast process and tubule in (A) the predentine, (B) coronal dentine. In predentine the odontoblast process contain some organelles and the wall of the tubule is formed by intertubular dentine (itd). More remote from the odontoblast in coronal dentine the cell process is vacuolated and the tubule is lined by hypercalcified peritubular dentine.

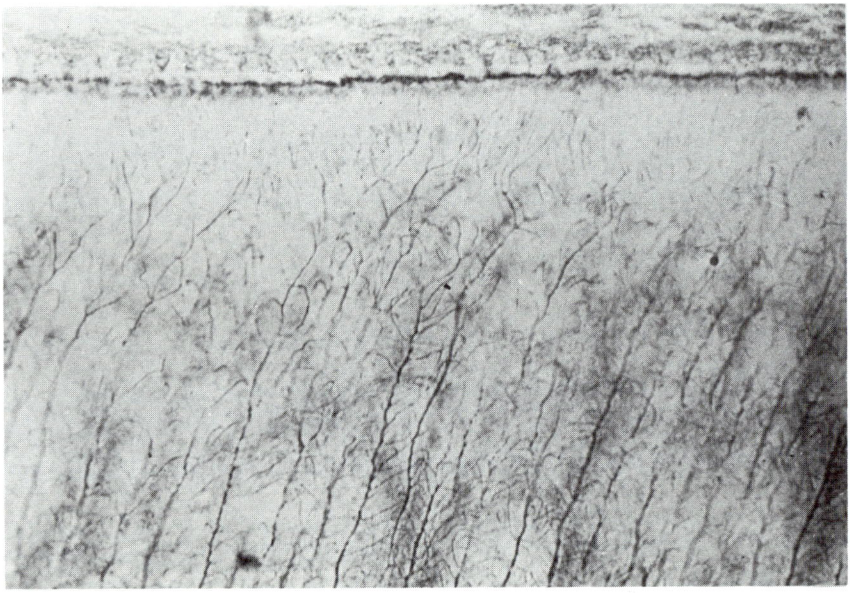

Fig. 8.17. Photomicrograph of a transverse section through root dentine showing the branching of the dentinal tubules and their secondary curvature.

clearly seen only in ground sections and not in decalcified sections or the electron microscope. Current ideas suggest, therefore, that this appearance represents the looping of the terminal odontoblast process and not true hypocalcification of the dentine matrix.

Between the dentine surface and cementum is a thin, but distinct, hyaline layer which may function to attach the cementum and dentine. It is probably produced by the cells of the epithelial root sheath.

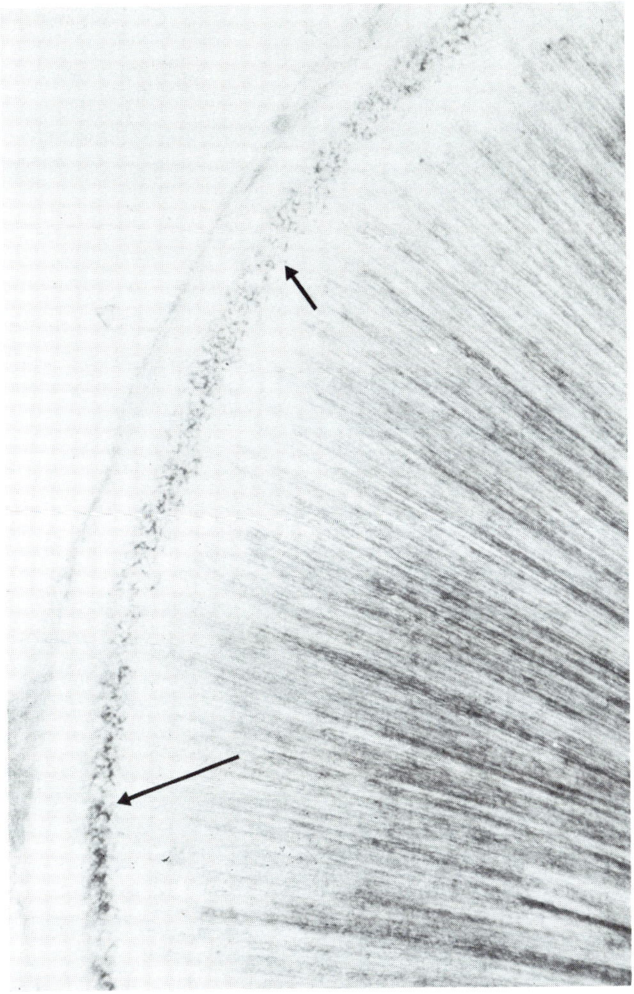

Fig. 8.18. Photomicrograph of a transverse ground section through the root showing Tomes granular layer (arrowed) and the dentinal tubules.

Like all hard tissue, dentine is deposited in increments, that is there are phases of active dentine formation followed by rest. This is reflected by the presence of incremental lines which may be clearly seen in ground sections orientated at right angles to the dentinal tubules (Fig. 8.19). Generally two types of incremental lines are described, the incremental lines of Von Ebner and the incremental lines of Owen. Using tetracycline as a label, it has been shown that the lines of Von Ebner represent the daily incremental growth of the dentine. The lines of Owen, however, may not be true incremental lines, but merely represent the congruence of the secondary curvature of the

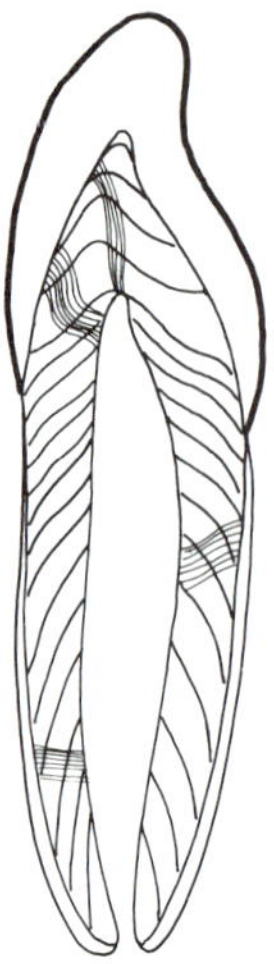

Fig. 8.19. Diagrammatic longitudinal section of an anterior tooth showing the orientation of the incremental lines in dentine and indicating the primary curvature of the dentinal tubules in various parts of the dentine.

dentinal tubules. In teeth that are calcifying at birth, there will be an exaggerated incremental line, the neonatal line, resulting from the physiological disturbance which occurs at this time. Other exaggerated incremental lines may represent disturbances in dentine formation as a result of illness.

Recent work has suggested that the incremental pattern in dentine is more complex than previously imagined. There are probably finer increments of growth than those represented by the Von Ebner lines.

*Secondary dentine.* The formation of dentine does not cease when the root of the tooth is fully formed, but continues throughout life. Therefore, dentine formed subsequently to the completion of the tooth is known as secondary dentine. Its formation is not necessarily related to functional stress, since it may be deposited in unerupted teeth. Secondary dentine may be deposited over the whole dentinal surface so that the pulp chamber becomes progressively reduced. In molars particularly, however, secondary dentine is deposited on the roof and floor of the pulp chamber.

Histologically, this type of secondary dentine is very similar to the first formed or primary dentine. There may be fewer and less regular tubules since the surface area the odontoblasts occupy is becoming progressively reduced as additional dentine is formed.

Irregular secondary dentine is formed as the result of a direct stimulus, such as dental caries, and involves therefore only relatively few odontoblasts. The number of dentinal tubules may be considerably reduced and irregular.

Since it can be deposited in response to a strong stimulus, and form very rapidly, cells may become included.

### Dental Pulp

Dental pulp is derived from the ectomesenchyme of the dental papilla to become primitive connective tissue. This consists of cells, matrix, blood vessels and nerves normally enclosed within the pulp cavity of the tooth except at the apical foramen where nerves and blood vessels enter. However, dental pulp differs from other connective tissues in that its surface is formed by the odontoblasts which are specialized for the production of dentine and the pulp is completely enclosed by the incompressible dentine walls of the pulp chamber.

The dental pulp is both sensory and nutritive to the dentine by virtue of the enclosed nerves and blood vessels. In reaction to stimuli reaching the pulp, as a result of damage to the substance of the tooth, the pulp may produce secondary dentine or an inflammatory response may result within the confines of the pulp chamber; the resultant increase in the amount of tissue fluid, associated with inflammation, produces pain.

The pulp cavity consists of a pulp chamber lying within the crown of the tooth completely enclosed by dentine and root canals which leave from the floor of the pulp chamber. The pulp chamber is box-shaped, with the walls parallel to the amelodentinal junction (Fig. 8.1). In deciduous teeth the pulp chamber is relatively larger than in permanent teeth. Extending occlusally or incisally from the pulp chamber pulpal horns or cornua which are sharp and long in young teeth, but become obliterated as the pulp chamber decreases in size with age and the formation of secondary dentine. There may be lateral branches from the root canals and these can be numerous around the apex to form an apical delta.

*Structure of dental pulp.* The highly specialized dentine-forming cell, the odontoblast, has to be considered as part of the dental pulp. The variation in the position of the nucleus gives these cells a stratified appearance. In a mature tooth, the odontoblasts are normally more elongated in the pulp chamber, becoming cuboid or eventually flattened towards the root apex. Beneath the odontoblasts is the so-called "cell-free zone of Weil". Electron microscopical examination of this area shows it can be more properly termed a cell-sparse zone.

If a healthy tooth is fractured in a vice, the pulp may be removed intact without damage. The pulp is pinkish-white in appearance and resilient on handling. This probably is due to the presence of gelatinous ground substance bound together by a network of fine reticulin and collagen fibres. Also giving the pulp mechanical strength are the fibres which support blood vessels and nerve fibres. The principle cell of the normal pulp is the fibroblast, which is responsible for producing the fibrous components. There are also pluripotential mesenchyme cells, macrophages and lymphocytes present. With increasing age the number of fibres increases but the number of cells decreases.

*Innervation.* The detailed distribution of nerve fibres has been studied by electron microscopy and with the light microscope by the use of silver stains. Nerve fibres enter the tooth through the apical foramen and are closely associated with blood vessels. Within the pulp chamber the nerve fibres branch, forming a plexus beneath the cell sparse zone, the so-called Plexus of Raschkow. As nerve fibres approach the odontoblast layer some lose their myelin sheaths and pass through the intercellular spaces while some are diverted back towards the pulp. Most of these fibres will be diverted by the predentine and only a very few will enter the dentine via the space between the odontoblast process and the wall of the tubule. In fact, only about 1 in 10,000 tubules are so innervated, but fibres do not extend through the full width of the dentine. However, using electron microscopy terminal nerve fibres have been demonstrated near the surface of the odontoblast process within the dentinal tubule. Nerve endings have also been described in the subodontoblastic plexus both at the light and electron microscope level.

*Blood supply.* Dental pulp is highly vascularized by a system of afferent and and efferent blood vessels with a network of capillaries interposed. Blood vessels enter and leave through the apical foramen and traverse the long axis of the root canal. There is little branching in the root canal, but within the pulp chamber branching occurs to form a distinct subodontoblastic plexus.

Arteriovenous anastomoses, which are direct connections between arteries and veins, have been observed, almost exclusively, in the coronal pulp. The veins are distinguished from the other vessels by their thin walls and large lumina. The tunica intima consists solely of a layer of endothelium and the tunica media is made up of a very thin layer of muscle. An adventitia is lacking in these veins. The presence of an arteriovenous anastomosis means that blood may be taken directly from the afferent to the efferent channel, thereby avoiding the capillary circulation. During the functioning of tissue supplied by the capillary bed the arteriovenous anastomoses shut down, precapillary sphincters relax and blood is transported to the tissue via the capillaries.

*Calcifications in pulp.* These are common, but their incidence increases with age, caries and other pathological changes affecting the pulp. However, it is known that teeth, not obviously affected by any histological change, for example, unerupted teeth and teeth extracted for orthodontic reasons, often show pulpal calcification.

The histologically detectable calcifications are of three types; denticles with laminations, without laminations and diffuse calcification. The laminated types are round or ovoid with a smooth surface. There is a distinct centre of origin around which the concentric layers of organic matrix and mineral are deposited, indicating incremental growth. The denticles without laminations are irregular in shape and are usually associated with smaller surrounding denticles.

The denticles are usually free within the pulp chamber, but they may eventually fuse with the dentine of the pulp cavity as they enlarge and as secondary dentine is formed. Therefore, the denticles often become surrounded by odontoblast-like cells from the pulp and are often permeated by some of the odontoblast processes of the dentine. Blood vessels and nerves are diverted rather than enclosed by the denticles, but in some instances a blood vessel or nerve may become surrounded by a denticle.

Diffuse calcification consists of numerous foci scattered throughout the fibrous matrix of the pulp. This type of calcification is predominant in the pulp canals.

The increased resolution of the electron microscope shows that most pulps have some calcifications. Small foci of calcification are seen in relation to the collagen fibres, interfibrillar matrix and connective tissue cells of the pulp. The fully formed denticles consist of hydroxyapatite crystallites and collagenous organic matrix. The laminated denticles appear to grow by addition of layers of collagen to the surface, leaving an uncalcified border zone which gradually calcifies. The matrix of non-laminated denticles is formed by collagen fibres orientated in the long axis of the pulp and no border zone is present. These denticles grow by the addition of mineral to the adjacent matrix fibres. The smaller denticles do not have a collagen fibre matrix.

The non-laminated denticles also contain areas devoid of fibres in which crystallites are larger but give a diffraction pattern indictive of hydroxyapatite. Irregular crystal size, shape and distribution is typical of pathological calcification in which there is no specialized preformed organic matrix.

## ENAMEL

Like all the other hard tissues, enamel forms by the incorporation of mineral salts into a preformed organic matrix (Chapter 2). However, unlike other hard tissues the ameloblasts which form enamel are not mesodermal but ectodermal in origin, and this is reflected in the unique composition of the organic matrix. Also there is a relatively high proportion of inorganic material in enamel. This consists of untypically large hydroxyapatite crystallites which are specifically ordered to form the enamel rods or prisms. Furthermore, the rapid increase in the proportion of inorganic material during enamel development and maturation is not due simply to an influx of mineral but involves the withdrawal of specific amino acids.

## Amelogenesis

The ameloblasts differentiate from the internal dental epithelium of the enamel organ (Fig. 8.11). These epithelial cells are cuboidal with a central nucleus and they rest on a basement membrane (membrana preformativa) which separates them from the primitive dental pulp. Like all epithelial cells they are joined by desmosomes both at their future secretory end and non-secretory ends. As odontoblasts differentiate from the dental papilla, the epithelial cells lengthen and the nucleus moves to the non-secretory end of the cell. This is followed by a shortening of the cells which are now adjacent to the first formed mantle dentine since the membrana preformativa has disappeared. These epithelial cells may now be termed ameloblasts and are ready to begin enamel formation.

Ameloblasts are invariably associated with a covering of several layers of flattened cells, the stratum intermedium (Fig. 8.8). The extent of the internal dental epithelium and its accompanying stratum intermedium determines the cervical line of the tooth where enamel formation ends. It is evident, therefore, that the stratum intermedium is necessary for enamel formation. Since the newly differentiated ameloblast is separated from the blood vessels of the dental papilla by a layer of dentine, and from the capillaries surrounding the external dental epithelium by the stellate reticulum, it needs to be energetically independent. This is reflected by the intracellular stores of glycogen which will be utilized until the blood supply above the external dental epithelium becomes available with the subsequent reduction of the stellate reticulum. Histochemically the ameloblasts demonstrate RNA and oxidative enzymes and the stratum intermedium is positive for the enzyme alkaline phosphatase. Alkaline phosphatase has been involved with membrane transport and in this capacity it may be associated with the transfer of material into the ameloblast layer during enamel formation. Ultrastructurally the ameloblast is packed with rough endoplasmic reticulum. There is a large central Golgi complex and numerous mitochondria are situated around the nucleus (Fig. 8.20). All of these characteristics clearly indicate a cell capable of synthesizing and secreting organic macromolecules for export. In the newly differentiated ameloblast there is a ruffled cell border adjacent to the mantle dentine. Beneath this border vesicles accumulate containing stippled material. This indicates the onset of matrix synthesis and subsequently it is suggested that the vesicles fuse with the cell membrane to release their contents into the extracellular space. As soon as enamel matrix production commences, the secretory end of the ameloblast produces a triangular-shaped process, the so-called Tomes process, in place of the ruffled border. This gives the developing front of the enamel a saw-toothed appearance.

Using labelled matrix precursors such as $H^3$ tyrosine, $H^3$ proline, $H^3$ methionine, $H^3$ galactase and $S^{35}$ sulphate, the pathway of intracellular syn-

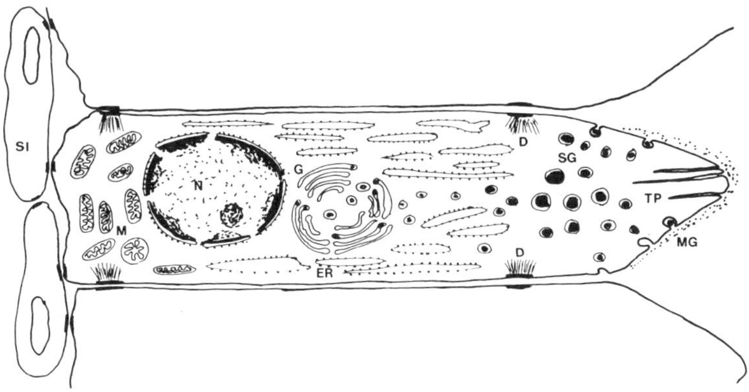


Fig. 8.20. The ultrastructural organisation of the ameloblast shown diagramatically. D, desmosome; ER, endoplasmic reticulum; G, Golgi region; M, mitochondria; MG, matrix granules; N, nucleus; SG, secretory granule; SI, stratum intermedium; TP, Tomes process.

thesis and secretion of proteins, glycoproteins and proteoglycans has been well established. Enamel protein is rapidly synthesized from the available amino acids in the rough endoplasmic reticulum. The short polypeptide chains are then transferred to the cisternae of the immature face of the Golgi apparatus. The protein passes through the several stacks of cisternae being concentrated and packaged into mature secretory granules to leave the Golgi apparatus on the mature face. Molecules such as the terminal sugar galactose, sulphate and phosphate are added to the enamel protein as it passes through the Golgi apparatus. The secretory granules migrate towards the secretory end of the cell, probably under the guidance of cytoplasmic microtubules. Large numbers of granules collect in Tomes process, but the exact method by which these granules are released is uncertain, since classical excytosis has not been well demonstrated.

In the electron microscope the uncalcified organic matrix which accumulates around the Tomes process has a stippled appearance similar to that in vesicles. Apatite crystallites appear within the matrix only a short distance from the membrane of the Tomes process (Fig. 8.21). The true physical nature of this organic material is unknown and its appearance in the electron microscope can be altered according to the methods of tissue preparation that are used. In some instances it may appear fibrous, but X-ray diffraction analyses of untreated matrix do not indicate an organized fibrous structure. The general view is that the physical state of the organic matrix is a gel with the ability to flow under pressure, that is it is thixotropic.

Proteins make up about 20 per cent by weight of the organic phase in enamel. This is unusually high in proline, about 25 per cent glutamic acid, leucine and histidine. The complete absence of hydroxyproline, low glycine

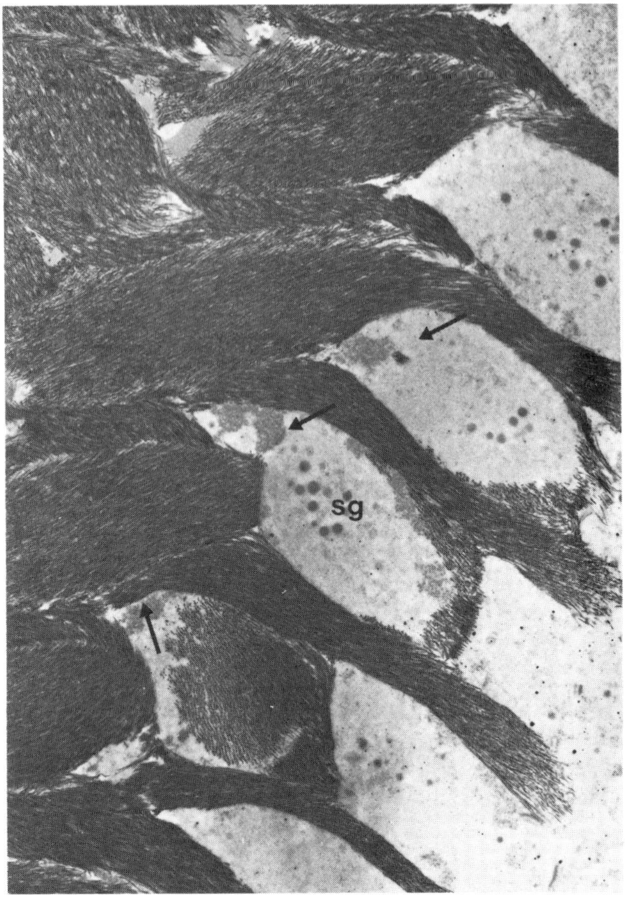


Fig. 8.21. Electron micrograh of rat enamel showing enamel prisms and triangular-shaped Tomes processes containing secretory granules (sg). A fine granular organic matrix is present between the membrane of Tomes process and the calcifying front (arrowed).

and the high ratio of aspartic-to-glutamic acid distinguish it from collagen. The overall composition, especially the low cystine unusually high methionine and high ratio of histidine to other basic amino acids, clearly exclude the protein from the keratin family. Some 40 per cent of the organic matrix is lipid and the remainder protein carbohydrate complexes.

### Calcification of Enamel

The first crystallites appear in the organic matrix after a layer about 50 nM in thickness has been deposited by the ameloblasts (Fig. 8.21). The ribbon-like crystallites grow rapidly in thickness as the ameloblasts retreat, therefore rapidly occupying more space in the enamel matrix which has a physical nature enabling it to be displaced by the crystallites. The first formed enamel contains about 27 per cent by volume inorganic material, but at 0.5 mm from the ameloblasts it contains 88 per cent (Fig. 8.22). This rapid increase is not achieved simply by an influx of inorganic material, but also by removal of specific amino acids from the organic matrix. Both the secretion of enamel matrix and the withdrawal of specific parts of it are presumably under the control of the ameloblast layer.

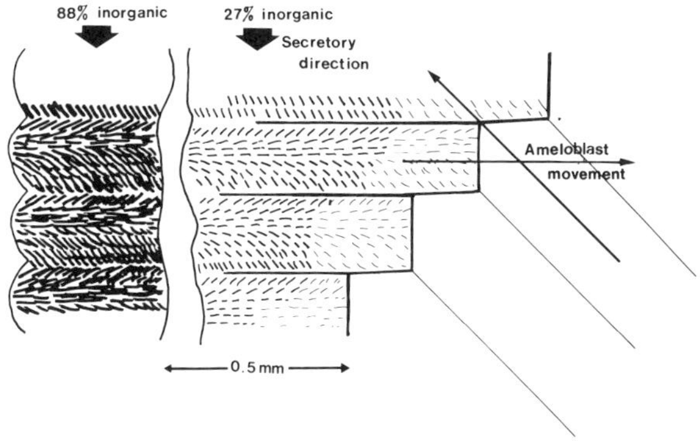


Fig. 8.22. Diagram illustrating the rapid accummulation of mineral in the forming enamel. (By kind permission of Professor J. W. Osborn, University of Alberta, Canada, and *Calcified Tissue Research,* 1970, Vol. 5, Springer Verlag, Heidelberg.)

There is some contention concerning the initiation of calcification in the enamel matrix. It has been suggested that since there is no collagen in enamel the crystallites first appear in relation to collagen fibres or the matrix vesicles of the mantle dentine. If, however, nucleation is related to some organic macromolecule in enamel matrix only a few nucleation sites will be required since the individual enamel crystallites become so large.

The rapid growth of crystallites requires an influx of the necessary elements. There is considerable evidence to indicate, however, that the ameloblast does not concentrate calcium. It has been suggested, therefore, that the enamel organ is responsible for critically regulating the passage of calcium into the developing enamel.

In the initial stages of enamel formation the ameloblast has no Tomes process and the enamel is aprismatic, but as the pyramidal process develops the enamel becomes prismatic. The enamel crystallites are clearly orientated at right angles to the membrane of the Tomes process and the resultant changes in the orientation of the crystallites produces boundaries and the subsequent organization of enamel into rods or prisms. It has been suggested that the material leaving the tip or sides of the Tomes process becomes enamel rod, while that leaving the surface between adjacent cells becomes interrod material. Accordingly it can be argued that no one prism is related to a single ameloblast and may be formed by several.

The question arises, however, as to how this specific crystallite orientation during prism formation is achieved. It has been suggested that crystallites are orientated along a concentration gradient and that their orientation is further influenced by the streaming of organic macromolecules. Boyde (1965) considers an additional stroking factor may occur in regions where there is relative sliding movements between the Tomes process membrane and the mineralizing front, so that the crystallites are orientated slightly in this direction (Fig. 8.23).

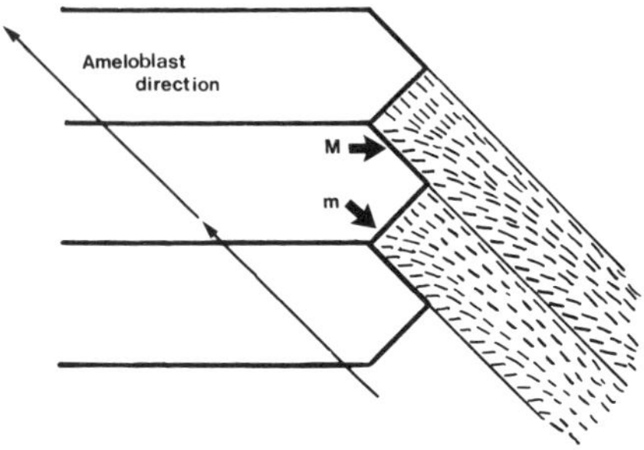


Fig. 8.23. Diagram indicating that crystallite orientation is influenced by shear which is at a maximum at (M) and a minimum at (m).

Alternatively it has been proposed by Osborne (1970) that the crystallites are orientated along flow lines. Since the stellate reticulum of the enamel organ is turgid, there will be a pressure build-up between Tomes process and the mineralizing front as the ameloblasts retreat. This, it is suggested, will produce flow in the organic matrix around the pyramidal-shaped Tomes process. The crystallites become orientated along these flow lines and shearing effects may be produced by the angulation of the ameloblasts to the forming enamel. In reptiles where there is no stellate reticulum, the enamel is aprismatic. According to the above hypothesis, the formation of a prism is accomplished by a single ameloblast and not by several as suggested earlier.

Also, since material flows back towards the ameloblast, it is possible that one surface may be absorptive and one secretive. Indeed autoradiographic studies confirm an influx of amino acids back into the ameloblasts during the maturation of the enamel. This could indicate that the stippled vesicles which accumulate in the Tomes process result from the absorption of the organic matrix and not secretion.

Towards the end of enamel formation the ameloblasts shorten, decrease in volume and lose many of their intracellular organelles. The ameloblasts gradually lose their Tomes processes and as the enamel undergoes maturation the ameloblasts acquires a ruffled border beneath which are numerous vesicles containing material of variable electron density. There is some evidence that organic material is still being removed from the organic matrix as well as mineral being added. At the final phase of its life cycle the ameloblast loses its ruffled border and produces a structure similar in appearance to a basement membrane. The ameloblasts become attached to this layer by hemidesmosomes.

### Enamel Structure

Enamel is formed of rods or prisms in which the large enamel crystallites have a specific orientation. As has been seen, the boundaries between prisms are formed where crystallites change their orientation to form the prism sheath. There are millions of enamel prisms in the enamel of each tooth and they extend from the amelodentinal junction out towards the surface of the enamel.

The structure of enamel is difficult to investigate using microscopic techniques. Decalcification totally removes the enamel and undecalcified or ground sections are thick when compared with conventional histological sections. This leads to internal reflection and loss of resolution. Also, since the enamel prisms are essentially cylinders, the plane of section in which they are cut influences the apparent shape of the prism. With transmission and scanning electron microscopy the sample is relatively small and there may be loss or translocation of the inorganic phase during sample preparation. All of these factors make the interpretation of images more difficult.

However, three types of prism, as outlined by the prism sheath, have been described in sections of mammalian enamel. These are briefly: (1) Circular prisms, separated by interprismatic enamel, (2) Parallel rows of prisms alternating with interprismatic enamel in which the prisms are continuous with interprismatic enamel at the cervical aspect, (3) The so-called keyhole-shaped prisms with a head directed towards the crown or incisal edge and tail towards the cervix (Fig. 8.24). This latter configuration has been disputed, but it is clear that the description of the prism shape and the extent of interprismatic enamel depends entirely on the construction of arbitrary boundaries.

These various prism shapes may be seen at specific phases of enamel formation. The first-formed prisms have a circular profile, but as enamel formation proceeds the prisms with an arcade or keyhole form predominate. Towards the end of enamel formation the circular profiles are evident again and as the enamel matures and the ameloblasts lose their Tomes processes the enamel becomes aprismatic.

Within the prism head or body the bulk of crystallites are orientated with their long or $C$-axis parallel to the long axis of the prism. It is at the open cervical aspect and beneath the prism boundary that the crystallites deviate from this orientation. Where there is an abrupt change in crystallite orientation, the prism sheath is formed and it can be argued that this is what the prism

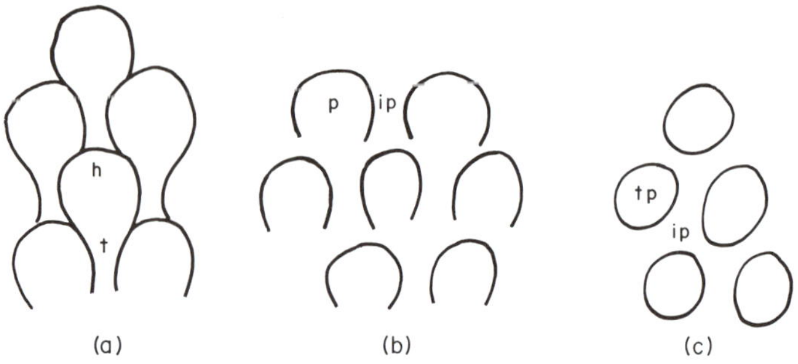


Fig. 8.24. Diagrammatic cross-section of various types outlined by the prism sheath. A, keyhole prisms; h, head; t, tail. B, parallel rows of prisms (p) alternating with interprismatic substance (ip). C, circular prisms of forming enamel (tp, Tomes process).

sheath represents (Figs. 8.21, 8.23 and 8.24). However, it has been suggested that most of the organic material of the enamel is contained within the prism sheath region.

The prisms extend from the amelodentinal junction to the surface of the enamel and are arranged in rows circumferentially and approximately perpendicular to the surface of the enamel. In the transverse plane the prisms bend to the right and then the left, while in the vertical plane they undulate. A change of angulation of about 2° occurs between successive rows.

*Incremental lines.* The cross-striations which are seen in ground sections of enamel prisms at intervals of approximately 4 μm may represent incremental lines at the prism level (Fig. 8.25). In the scanning electron microscope some enamel prisms show regular constrictions which may represent the banding at the light microscope level. However, it has been suggested that these lines may often represent bundles of prisms which have been cut obliquely.

The incremental lines in enamel are the brown striae of Retzius which are so named because they appear as a series of brown lines of different widths and intensities (Fig. 8.26). These may be seen both in transverse and longitudinal ground sections of most teeth running approximately at right angles to the enamel prisms. The precise physical nature of these lines is uncertain, they may be bands of hypomineralization or they may represent a regular bending of the prisms. A neonatal line will be present in those teeth which are calcifying at birth.

*Hunter-Schreger bands.* These are an optical phenomena observed when reflected light is used to examine a longitudinal ground section. They are a series of alternating light and dark bands found in the inner three-quarters of the enamel. The bands result from changes in orientation of the prisms so that light may be reflected or transmitted.

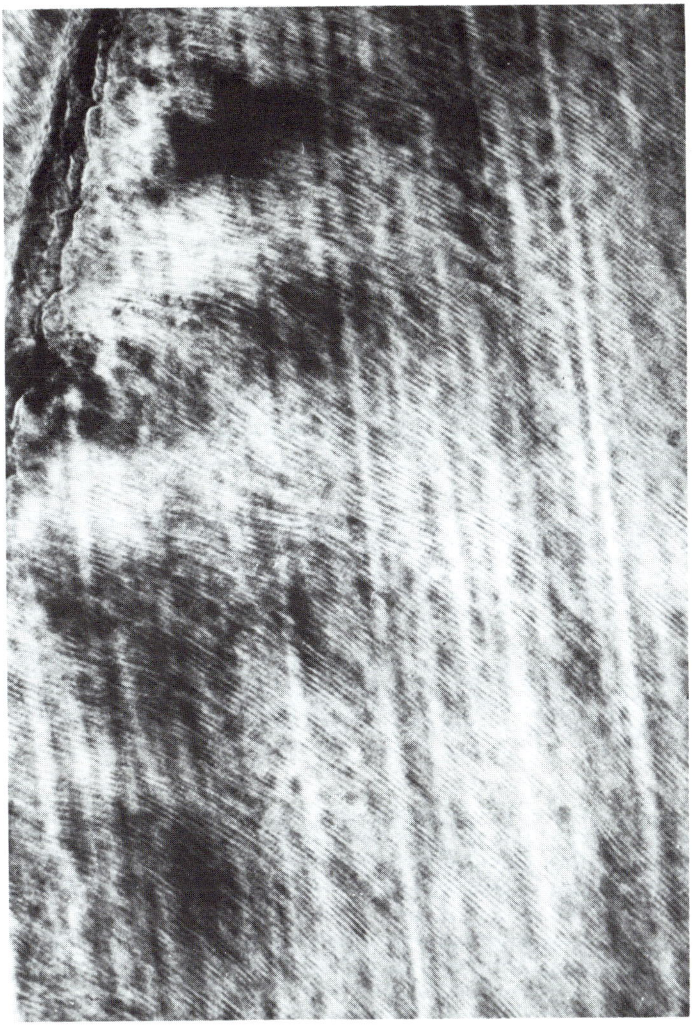

Fig. 8.25. A photomicrograph of a longitudinal ground section of enamel near the amelodentinal junction. Enamel prisms are clearly visible and in some cross-striations may be seen. Incremental lines are present orientated at right angles to the prisms.

*Surface enamel.* This is the final part of the enamel to be laid down during tooth formation. It is an aprismatic layer and is more highly calcified than the enamel beneath. The tightly packed crystallites are at right angles to the enamel surface. Reaction with elements such as fluoride take place principally in the surface layer. An organic pellicle is also rapidly acquired by the enamel surface on exposure to the oral environment.

Parallel ridges and grooves are seen particularly in the cervical third of the

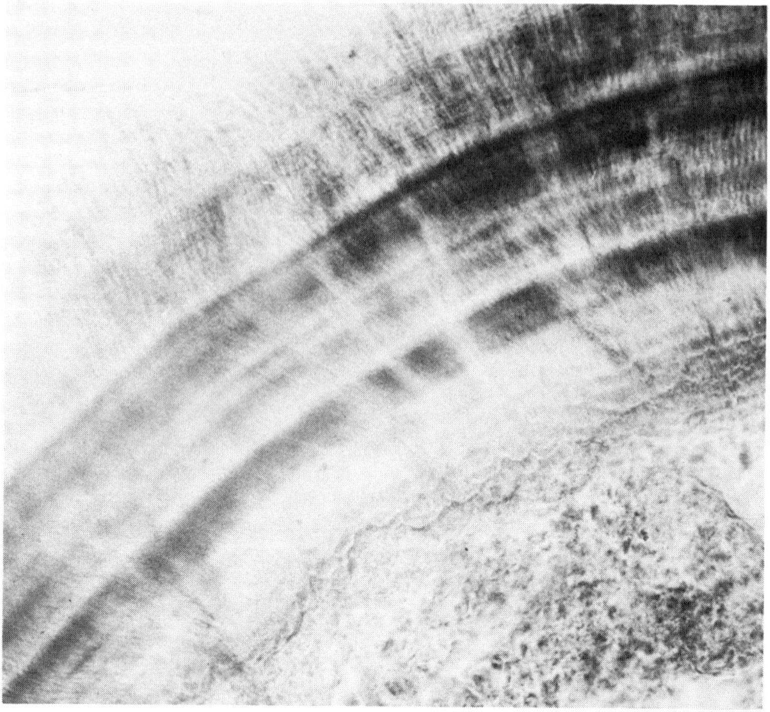

Fig. 8.26. A photomicrograph of a transverse section of enamel showing brown striae of Retzius of various widths and intensities.

enamel. They are known as the imbrication lines of Pickerill or perikymata, and are the external manifestation of the incremental lines. The ridges represent areas where the aprismatic surface layer is intact, but in the grooves it is absent. In some places the surface enamel may be missing over the top of a projection above the general level of the surface. Such features have been termed brochs and are confined to the cervical margin. The distribution of these features appears to be genetically determined. In some broch-like structures the surface enamel is present but overlaps the surface layers at the periphery. The appearance of these structures is a developmental defect in calcification which is filled in by adjacent cells. Many of these surface projections break off to leave deep pits, the possible clinical significance of which is the retention of cariogenic organisms. These defects are often found along the ridges of the perikymata.

Several structures are routinely seen in ground sections of enamel, the enamel lamellae, tufts and spindles.

*Enamel lamellae.* These represent organic material or hypocalcified enamel. They are best seen in tranverse section since they are longitudinally and radially orientated, so forming vertical sheets extending from the enamel surface to the amelodentinal junction and beyond. Lamellae develops as splits in the enamel which may result from the release of tension built up during amelogenesis. Since the splits extend across prisms it is suggested that they prevent calcification and some also become filled with cells from the enamel organ. Another type of lamella develops as a result of stress in erupted teeth and becomes filled with organic material from the saliva (Fig. 8.27).

*Enamel tufts.* These structures have the appearance of a tuft of grass and are also best seen in transverse sections. They represent hypomineralized areas extending from the amelodentinal junction into the enamel. It has been suggested that they represent a widening of the prism sheaths in this area (Fig. 8.27).

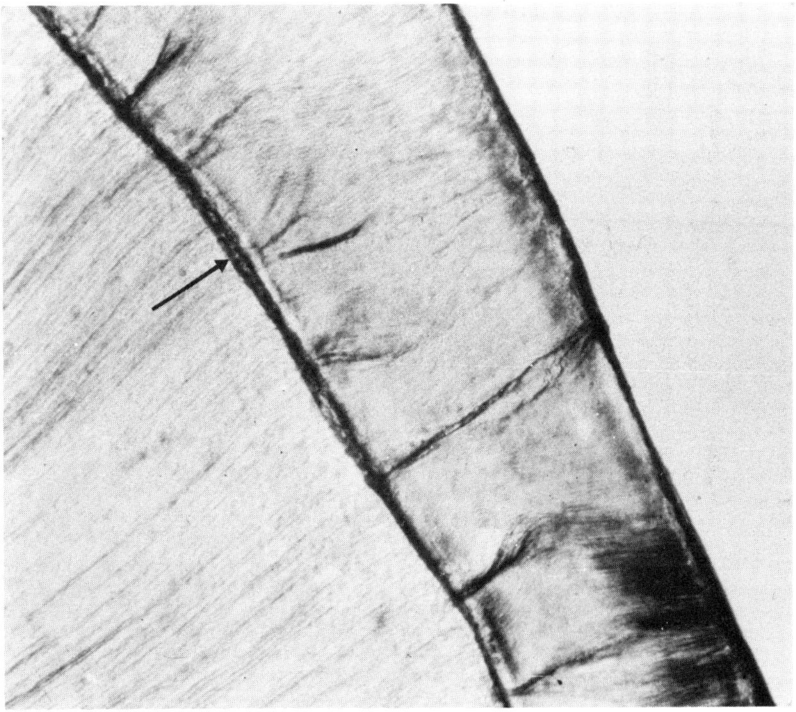

Fig. 8.27. A photomicrograph of a transverse section of enamel with enamel tufts extending a short distance from the amelodentinal junction (arrowed). An enamel lamella extends through the whole width of the enamel.

*Enamel spindles.* During the early stages of dentine formation some odontoblast processes penetrate the layer of newly differentiated ameloblasts. These processes become enclosed in the forming enamel to produce hypocalcified areas known as enamel spindles. They can be seen most frequently beneath the tips of cusps (Fig. 8.28).

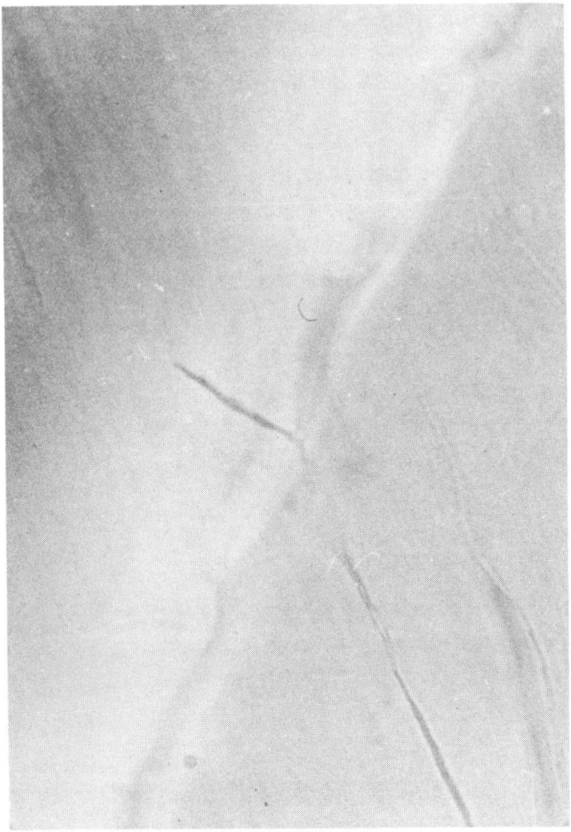

Fig. 8.28. A photomicrograph of an enamel spindle extending into the enamel from the amelodentinal junction.

## THE PERIODONTIUM

The term periodontium is used to describe the tissues which support and surround the tooth, that is alveolar bone, cementum, periodontal ligament, junctional and sulcular epithelium. Experimental work suggests that the bone, cementum and periodontal ligament all develop from the layer of ectomesenchyme which invests the tooth germ and not from the fibrous dental follicle.

### Alveolar Bone

The tooth germs develop in a trough of bone which also encloses the blood vessels and nerve fibres which will supply the teeth. Bony septa develop between adjacent tooth germs so that each becomes enclosed in a separate crypt (alveolus). With the eruption of the dentition the alveolar bone develops to form the sockets. This bone is continuous with the bone of the mandible or maxilla so that no definable junction exists. If the tooth germs fail to develop or the teeth do not erupt, the alveolar bone likewise does not develop. In other words the existence of alveolar bone is dependent upon the presence of teeth. There is considerable variation in the anatomy of the alveolar process which is dependent on the site and the functional demands placed on the teeth. For example, the alveolar bone of the molar teeth is more robust than that of the incisors. However, a generalized alveolar process consists of an inner layer of bone adjacent to the periodontal membrane and an outer layer continuous with the cervical plate of the mandible or maxilla. Between these layers are bony trabeculae the extent and precise arrangement of which depends upon the site (Fig. 8.29).

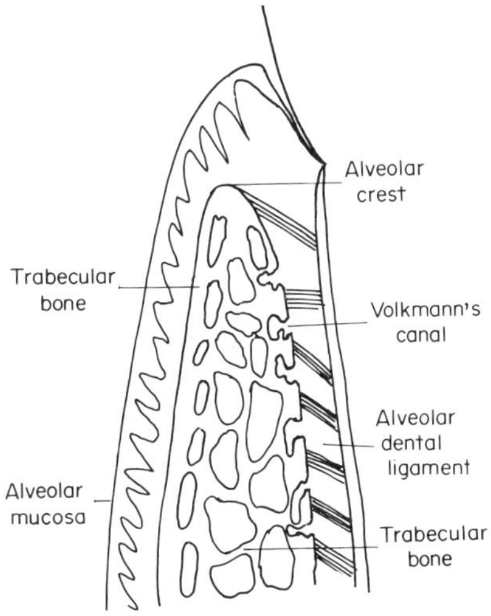


Fig. 8.29. A diagrammatic section of a generalized alveolar process.

The collagen fibre bundles of the periodontal ligament are inserted into the adjacent bone as Sharpeys fibres and, therefore, this layer of bone has been termed bundle bone. Its intrinsic fibres are at right angles to the Sharpeys fibres and are widely separated by ground substance. Furthermore, this bone is heavily calcified and from its appearance in radiographs has been termed the lamina dura.

Blood vessels and nerve fibres enter the periodontal ligament via openings or canals (Volkmann's canal) in the bone and hence another descriptive term, the cribriform plate, is used to describe the bone which lines the alveolus

(Fig. 8.29). In some areas bundle bone alone is present, but in others it rests on lamellar bone arranged circumferentially or into Haversian systems.

Alveolar bonc is constantly remodelled during tooth eruption and growth of the jaws. In doing so it responds to functional stress so that where tensional forces are transmitted new bone is deposited and where there are no such forces bone is resorbed (see Chapter 2). Such bone deposition and resorption is also responsible for the normal physiological mesial drift of the dentition. As wear occurs interproximally, contact is maintained by the mesial movement of the dentition. This is accomplished by the deposition of bone on the distal aspect of the socket and resorption on the mesial aspect.

### Periodontal Ligament (Alveolar Dental Ligament)

The periodontal ligament is the ligament, normally between 0.1 mm and 0.2 mm in thickness, which serves to suspend the tooth in the socket or alveolus (Fig. 8.1). Its principal fibres are collagenous and are attached to the cementum of the root and the bone forming the alveolus. These fibres are often described and grouped according to their orientation.

Collagen fibre bundles are orientated both horizontally and obliquely and the oblique fibres have their attachment to the cementum apical to the bone. There are groups of fibres orientated irregularly around the apex and interradicular fibres extending from the tip of the radicular process onto the cementum at the bifurcation of the roots. Fibres also extend from the tip of the alveolar process onto the cementum, and there are also groups of specifically orientated fibres in the lamina propria of the gingiva (Fig. 8.30).

Elastic fibres are confined to the walls of blood vessels where they help to maintain patency. However, another type of fibre, the oxytalan fibre, is found in the periodontal ligament. These fibres stain with silver after oxidation with periodic acid and in the electron microscope they appear similar to elastric fibres. Oxytalan fibres are found chiefly around the apical region of the tooth, running at right angles to the collagen fibres. Since they are closely associated with blood vessels and are also attached to the cementum of the tooth, they may be involved in both maintaining vascular patency and the physical position of the blood vessels. All the fibrous and cellular elements of the ligament are embedded in a ground substance which consist chiefly of proteoglycans and glycoproteins.

The orientation of the collagen fibre bundles may be clearly seen in haematoxylin and eosin-stained sections because of the closely associated fibroblasts (Fig. 8.31). The fibroblast is the most frequent cell present and has been clearly identified with the synthesis of collagen, elastic fibres and oxytalan fibres. It has also been shown to be capable of fibre breakdown as well as synthesis, and numerous electron micrographs have been published illustrating this capacity. This dual capability provides an explanation for the

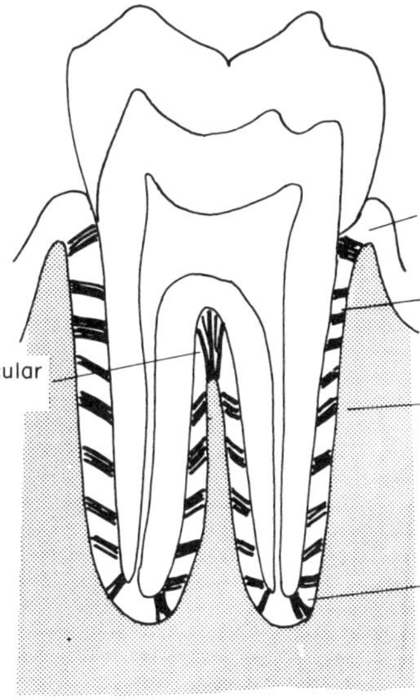


Fig. 8.30. A diagrammatic longitudinal section through a molar tooth indicating the various group of fibres in the alveolar dental ligament.

rapid turnover of collagen which can occur during tooth eruption and in functional stress.

Other cellular components of the periodontal membrane include osteoblasts, osteoclasts, cementoblasts, cementoclasts, mast cells, macrophages and undifferentiated mesenchyme cells. There may also be the epithelial remnants of Hertwig's root sheath which form clumps of cells known as the epithelial cell rests of Malassez.

The role of the principal collagen fibres in supporting the teeth during masticatory stress is uncertain. It is most likely that the fluid components of the periodontal ligament act as a damper when a force is applied to a tooth and are then displaced according to the space available in other parts of the ligament. Such a displacement would cause dilation of the socket margin, which would appear to accord with the observed facts. The role of the fibres in such circumstances could be to limit excessive dilation.

The periodontal ligament also has an important sensory and nutritive function.

## Cementum

Cementogenesis commences with the breakdown of Hertwig's epithelial root sheath. This allows the ectomesenchymal cells of the fibrous dental follicle to migrate through the spaces so that they come to lie on the surface of the dentine of the newly formed root. Direct contact with the dentine is not

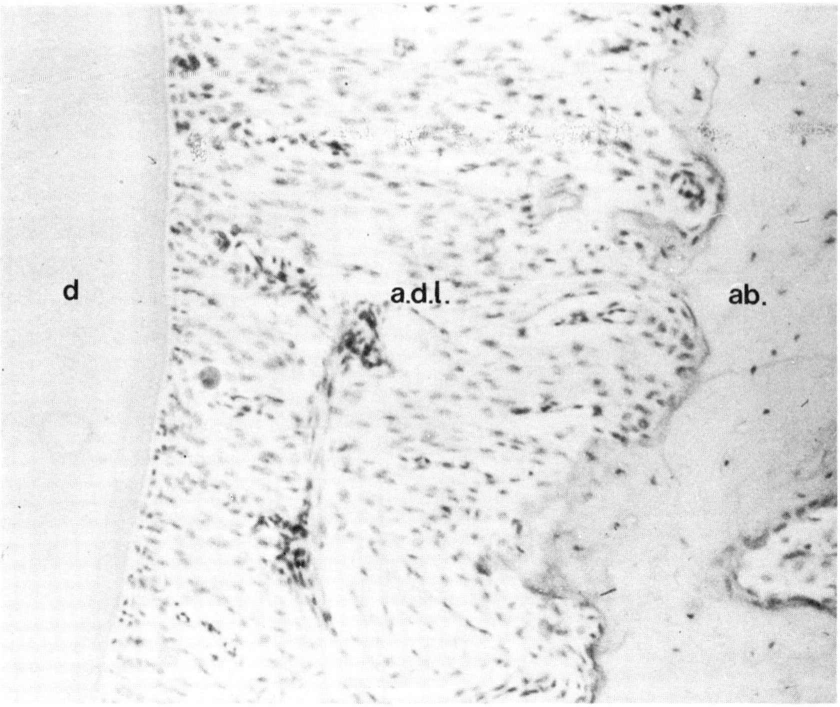


Fig. 8.31. Photomicrograph of a transverse section through the alveolar dental ligament (adl). Fibroblasts can be seen closely associated with the principal collagenous fibres. ab, alveolar bone; d, dentine.

made, since there is an intervening layer of so-called hyaline material probably deposited by the epithelial cells before they fragment. This layer may attach the newly forming cement onto the surface of the root.

The ectomesenchyme cells differentiate to become cementoblasts which are secretory cells similar histologically and ultrastructurally to osteoblasts. The cementoblasts secrete an organic matrix or cementoid consisting of collagen fibres and ground substance onto the surface of the root and around the existing fibres of the periodontal ligament. The cementoid calcifies by an extension of the calcification already present in the dentine. The cementoblast may remain on the surface of the forming cementum which is acellular. Alternatively the cementoblasts may become enclosed to form cementocytes and cellular cementum.

*Structure of cementum.* Cementum normally covers the whole root of the tooth except in about 10 per cent of cases where there is a gap at the cement-enamel junction, thereby exposing the underlying dentine. In 60 per cent of teeth the cementum extends onto the surface of the enamel and in the remaining 30 per cent abutts precisely with the enamel.

Two types of cementum are described, acellular and cellular. Acellular cementum covers the whole root where it may be up to 60 μm in thickness. Towards the apical third of the root, however, the cementum is up to 260 μm in thickness because of the deposition of cellular cementum. This layer may extend into the apical foramen of the tooth.

Where formation of cementum is taking place, actively secreting cementoblasts, as described above, may be seen. When they become incorporated into the cementum to form cementocytes they lie in lacunae, appear to have less cytoplasm, and develop fine processes enclosed within canaliculi. The processes invariably point towards the vascular periodontal ligament even where they emanate from the opposite side of the cementocyte (Fig. 8.32). It is suggested that the cementocytes obtain nutrition from the blood vessels of the ligament. Cementocytes most remote from the ligament die, however, leaving empty spaces which may eventually become filled with mineral.

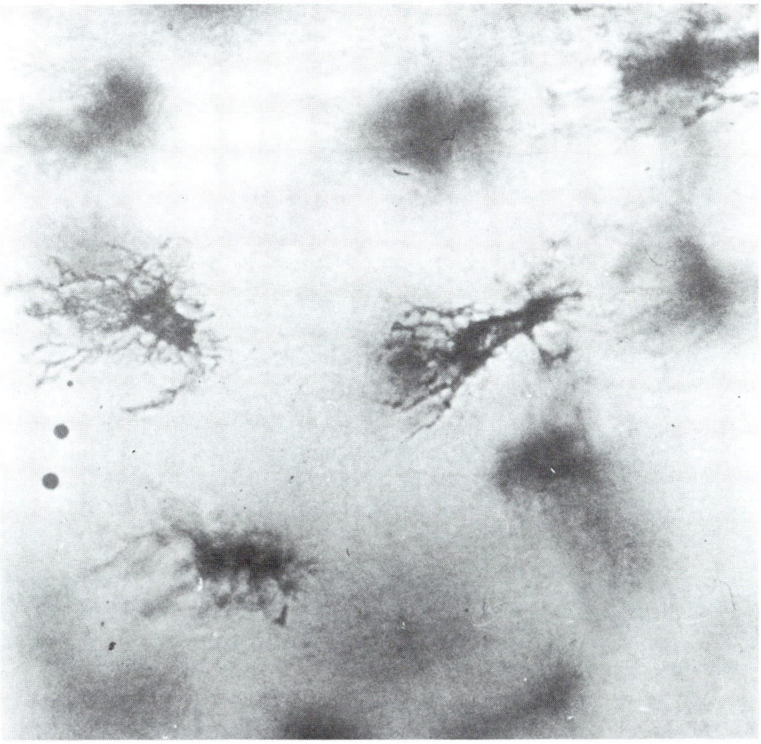

Fig. 8.32. Photomicrograph of a ground section of cementum showing cementocytes with their process pointing towards the alveolar dental ligament.

Cementum is clearly important in forming an attachment for the collagen fibres of the periodontal ligament. Unlike bone, it is avascular and, therefore, not resorbed under normal physiological conditions. It is continuously laid down throughout life to maintain attachment and also the occlusal height of the tooth. Should supporting bone be lost as a result of disease, additional cementum will be deposited to stabilize the tooth. Cementum will also attempt to repair damage such as fractures to the root surface.

### The Dentogingival Junction

When the crown of the tooth has been completed, the redundant enamel organ covers its surface. The innermost layer of the enamel organ is formed by the reduced enamel epithelium. These cells, like all epithelial cells, are joined by desmosomes and connected to the enamel surface by a basal lamina into which are attached hemidesmosomes.

As the tooth erupts through the overlying connective tissue the outer layer of the reduced enamel organ and the basal cells of the oral epithelium proliferate. This results in a mass of epithelial tissue forming between the crown of the tooth and the oral epithelial surface. It is through this mass of epithelial tissues that the tooth erupts. Consequently the connective tissues are never exposed to the oral environment.

The relationship of the surrounding soft tissues to the newly erupted tooth may be seen in Fig. 8.33. The epithelium in contact with the enamel of the crown is known as the junctional epithelium or epithelial attachment. Above is a space, the gingival sulcus or crevice, which is lined with sulcular or crevicular epithelium. This is continuous at the gingival crest with the gingival epithelium. Between the gingival and junctional epithelium are groups of collagen fibres which help to maintain the relationship between the soft tissues and the enamel surface in this area (Fig. 8.34).

The gingival sulcus is a narrow fluid-filled trough, the sides of which are formed by the tooth surface and the stratified squamous non-keratinized sulcular epithelium. It is up to 3 mm in depth and extends from the free gingival margin, where it is widest, apically to where its base is formed by the contact of junctional epithelium with the tooth surface. Its migrates apically with age, so that eventually the junctional epithelium may be in contact with the cementum. The crevicular fluid contains desquamated epithelial cells and neutrophils which have migrated through the junctional epithelium.

The junctional epithelium has a high rate of cell turnover and consists of a layer of flattened cells parallel to the tooth surface. The epithelium is attached to the tooth surface by hemidesmosomes which are inserted into a basement membrane-like structure. The cells are quite different from sulcular epithelium principally in having few intracellular organelles and desmosomal attachments so that wide intercellular spaces are present. It is through these

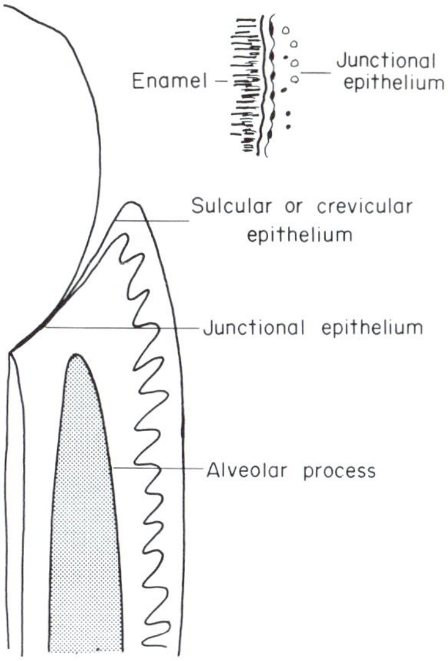


Fig. 8.33. Diagram of the dentogingival junction.

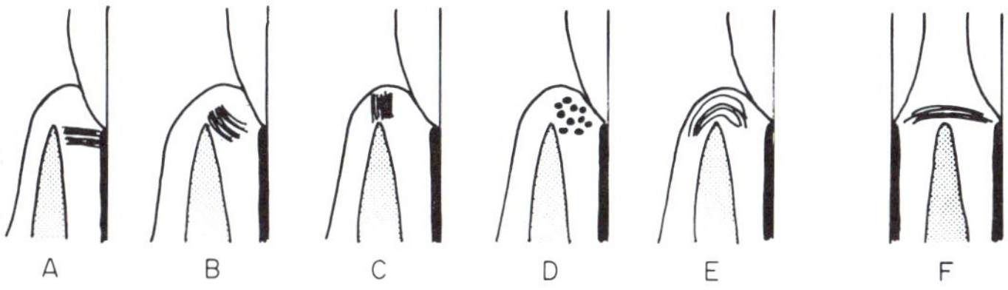


Fig. 8.34. Diagram indicating the orientation of the fibre groups in the gingival ligament.

spaces that inflammatory cells and antigens readily pass. These inflammatory cells are present in the underlying connective tissue even when the tissues appear clinically normal. However, the connective tissue is further distinguished by fewer collagen fibres and atypical fibroblasts.

The "col" is the appearance presented by the interdental tissues when seen in buccolingual section. It is not different in structure from the junctional epithelium, and the vulnerability of this area to periodontal disease is due to the accumulation of debris and plaque.

## BIBLIOGRAPHY

### Tooth Development

BEER, G. R. de (1947) The differentiation of neural crest cells into odontoblasts in Ablystoma *and re-examination of the germ layer theory, Proc. Roy. Soc.* **134B,** 377.

BUTLER, P. M. (1939) Studies of the mammalian dentition, *Proc. Zool. Soc. Lond.* **109,** 1.

BUTLER, P. M. (1956) The ontogeny of molar pattern, *Biol. Rev. Camb. Phil. Soc.* **31,** 30.

BUTLER, P. M. (1967) Dental merism and tooth development, *J. Dent. Res.* **46,** 845

FLEISCHMAJER, R. and R. E. BILLINGHAM (1968) *Epithelial Mesenchymal Interactions,* Williams & Williams, Baltimore.

GAUNT, W. A. (1959) The vascular supply to the dental lamina during early development, *Acta Anat.* **37,** 232.

GAUNT, W. A. and A. E. W. MILES (1967) Fundamental aspects of tooth morphogenesis, in *Structural and Chemical Organisation of Teeth,* Vol. 1, ed. A. E. W. Miles, Academic Press, New York.

GLASSTONE, S. (1952) The development of halved tooth germs. A study in experimental embryology, *J. Anat.* **86,** 12.

HUXLEY, J. S. and G. R. de BEER (1934) *The Elements of Experimental Embryology,* Camb. Univ. Press, Cambridge.

JOHNSTON, M. C. and R. M. PRATT (1975) The neural crest in normal matrix influences of gene expression, in *Extracellular Matrix Influences on Gene Expression,* ed. H. C. Slavkin and R. Greulich, Academic Press, New York.

KOLLAR, E. J. (1969) The influence of the dental papilla on the development of tooth shape in embryonic tooth germs, *J. Emb. exp. Morph.* **21,** 131.

KOLLAR, E. J. and G. R. BAIRD (1970) Tissue interactions in embryonic mouse tooth germs, *J. Emb. exp. Morph.* **24,** 159.

KOLLAR, E. J. and G. R. BAIRD (1970) Tissue interactions in embryonic mouse tooth germs, *J. Emb. exp. Morph.* **24,** 173.

KOLLAR, E. J. (1978) The role of collagen during tooth morphogenesis: Some genetic implications, in *Development, Function and Evolution of Teeth,* ed. P. M. Butler and K. A. Joysey, Academic Press, London.

LUMSDEN, A. G. S. (1979) Pattern formation in the molar dentition of the mouse, *J. Biol. buccale* **7,** 77.

LUNT, R. C. and D. B. LAW (1974) A review of the chronology and calcification of deciduous teeth, *J. Am. dent. Ass.* **89,** 599.

NERY, E. B., B. S. KRAUS and M. CROUP (1970) Timing and topography of early human tooth development, *Arch. oral. Biol.* **15,** 1315.

OSBORN, J. W. (1973) The evolution of dentitions, *Am. Scient.* **61,** 548.

OSBORN, J. W. (1978) Morphogenetic gradients: Fields versus clones, in *Development, Function and Evolution of Teeth,* ed. P. M. Butler and K. A. Joysey, Academic Press, London.

SCHOUR, I. and M. MASSLER (1940) Studies on tooth development: the growth pattern of human teeth, *J. Am. dent. Ass.* **27,** 1785.

SCOTT, J. H. (1967) *Dento-facial Growth and Development,* Pergamon Press, Oxford.

SCOTT, J. H. and N. B. B. SYMONS (1977) *Introduction to Dental Anatomy,* 8th ed., Churchill Livingstone, London.

SICHER, H. (1980) *Orban's Oral Histology and Embryology,* C. V. Mosby, St. Louis.

SLAVKIN, H. C. and L. A. BAUETTA (1972) *Developmental Aspects of Oral Biology,* Academic Press, New York.

SLAVKIN, H. C. (1974) Embryonic tooth formation: a tool for developmental biology, *Oral Sci. Rev.* **4,** 7.

TONGE, C. H. (1953) The early development of teeth, *Proc. R. Soc. Med.* **46,** 313.

TONGE, C. H. (1971) The role of mesenchyme in tooth development, in *Dental Morphology and Evolution,* ed. A. A. Dahlberg, Univ. Chicago Press, Chicago.

TONGE, C. H. (1976) The time structure relationship of tooth development in human embryogenesis, *J. dent. Res.* **48,** 745.

WESTON, J. A. (1970) The migration and differentiation of neural crest calls, *Advances in Morphography,* **8,** 41.

## Dentinogenesis, Dentine and Dental Pulp

APPLETON, J. and M. J. R. WILLIAMS (1973) Ultrastructural observations on the calcification of human dental pulp, *Calc. Tiss. Res.* **11,** 222.

APPLETON, J. and D. C. MORRIS (1979) An ultrastructural investigation of the role of the odontoblast in matrix calcification using the potassium pyroantimonate osmium method for calcium localization, *Arch. oral Biol.* **24,** 467.

BERNICK, S. (1948) Innervation of the human tooth, *Anat. Rec.* **101,** 81.

BERNICK, S. (1967) Age changes in the blood supply to human teeth, *J. dent. Res.* **46,** 544.

BEVELANDER, G. (1941) The development and structure of the fiber system of dentine, *Anat. Rec.* **81,** 79.

BEVELANDER, G. and H. NAKAHARA (1966) The formation and mineralization of dentine, *Anat. Rec.* **156,** 303.

BOYDE, A. and K. S. LESTER (1966) An electron microscope study of fractured dentinal surfaces, *Calc. Tiss. Res.* **1,** 122.

BRADFORD, E. W. (1967) Microanatomy and histochemistry of dentine, in *Structural and Chemical Organisation of Teeth,* ed. A. E. W. Miles, Academic Press, New York.

BRÄNNSTRÖM, M. and R. GARBEROGLIO (1972) The dentinal tubules and odontoblast processes: a scanning electron microscope study, *Acta Odont. Scand.* **30,** 291.

DAHL, E. and I. A. MJÖR (1973) The fine structure of the vessels in human dental pulp, *Acta Odont. Scand.* **31,** 223.

DAHL, E. and I. A. MJÖR (1973) The structure and distribution of nerves in the pulp-dentin organ, *Acta Odont. Scand.* **31,** 349.

EISENMANN, D. R. and P. L. GLICK (1972) Ultrastructure of initial crystal formation in dentine, *J. Ultrastruct. Res.,* **41,** 18.

FEARNHEAD, R. W. (1957) Histological evidence for the innervation of human dentine, *J. Anat.* **91,** 267.

FEARNHEAD, R. W. (1963) The histological demonstration of nerve fibres in human dentine, in *Sensory Mechanisms in dentine,* ed. D. J. Anderson, Pergamon Press, Oxford.

FRANK, R. M. (1959) Electron microscopy of undecalcified sections of human adult dentine, *Arch. oral Biol.* **1,** 29.

FRANK, R. M. (1966) Étude au microscope électronique de l'odontoblaste et du canalicule dentaire humain, *Arch. oral Biol.* **11,** 179.

FRANK, R. M. Attachment sites between the odontoblast process and the intradentinal nerve fibre, *Arch. oral Biol.* **13,** 833.

FURSETH, R. (1971) The fine structure of the odontoblasts/predentin area in the root, *Scand. J. dent. Res.,* **79,** 141.

FURSETH, R. (1974) The structure of peripheral root dentin in young human premolars, *Scand. J. dent. Res.* **82,** 557.

GRIFFIN, C. J. and R. HARRIS (1966) Ultrastructure of collagen fibrils and fibroblasts of the developing human dental pulp, *Arch. oral. Biol.* **11,** 659.

HARRIS, R. and C. J. GRIFFIN (1968) Fine structure of nerve endings in the human dental pulp, *Arch. oral Biol.* **13,** 773.

HARRIS, R. and C. J. GRIFFIN (1971) The ultrastructure of small blood vessels of the normal human dental pulp, *Austral. dent. J.* **16,** 220.

HOLLAND, G. R. (1976) The extent of the odontoblast process in the cat, *J. Anat.* **121,** 133.

KATCHBURIAN, E. (1977) Initiation of mineral deposition in dentine, *Calc. Tiss. Res. (Supp.),* **22,** 179.

KAWASAKAI, K. (1975) On the configuration of incremental lines in human dentine as revealed by tetracycline labelling, *J. Anat.* **119,** 61.

KORFF, K. VON (1905) Die Entwicklong der Zahnbeim ond Knochengrondsubstanz der Sangetiere, *Archiv. für Mikroskipische Anatomie und Entwicklongsmechanik,* **67,** 1.

LESTER, K. and A. BOYDE (1968) The question of Von Korff fibres in mammalian dentine, *Calc. Tiss. Res.* **1,** 273.

MJÖR, I. A. (1972) Human coronal dentine: structure and reactions, *Oral Surg.* **33,** 810.

MOSS, M. L. (1974) Studies on dentin. I. Mantle dentin, *Acta Anat.* **87,** 481.

MUNHOZ, O. G. and C. P. LEBLOND (1974) Deposition of calcium phosphate into dentin and enamel as shown by radioautography of sections of incisor teeth following injection of $Ca^{45}$ into rats, *Calc. Tiss. Res.* **15,** 221.

NAGAI, N. and R. M. FRANK (1974) Electron microscope autoradiography of $Ca^{45}$ during dentinogenens, *Cell. Tiss. Res.* **155,** 513.

NALBANDIAN, J. (1968) The ultrastructure of odontoblasts and dentinogenesis, in *Biology of the Dental Pulp Organ,* ed. S. B. Finn, Univ. Alabama Press, Alabama.

NOBLE, H. W., A. F. CARMICHAEL and D. M. RANKINE (1962) Electron microscopy of human developing dentine, *Arch. oral. Biol.* **7,** 395.

OSBORN, J. W. (1967) A mechanistic view of dentinogenesis and its relation to the curvatures of the processes of the odontoblast, *Arch. oral. Biol.* **12,** 275.

OSBORN, J. W. and A. R. TEN CATE (1976) *Advanced Dental Histology, Dental Practitioner Handbook,* 3rd ed., J. Wright, Bristol.

REITH, E. J. (1968) Ultrastructural aspects of dentinogenesis, in *Dentine and Pulp, their Structure and Reactions,* ed. B. Symons, Livingstone, Edinburgh.

REITH, E. J. (1968) Collagen formation in developing molar teeth of rats, *J. Ultrastruct. Res.* **21,** 383.

REITH, E. J. (1976) The binding of calcium within the Golgi saccules of the rat odontoblast, *Ann. J. Anat.* **147,** 267.

ROSENBERG, G. D. and D. J. SIMMONS (1980) Rhythmic dentinogenesis in the rabbit incisor: Circadian ultradian and infradian periods, *Calc. Tiss. Res.* **32,** 29.

SELVIG, K. A. (1963) Electron microscopy of Hertwigs epithelial sheath and of early dentin and cementum formation in the mouse incisor, *Acta Odont. Scand.* **22,** 105.

SISCA, R. F. and D. V. PROVENZA (1971) Initial dentine formation in human deciduous teeth. An electron microscope study, *Calc. Tiss. Res.* **9,** 1.

SLAVKIN, H. C. (1975) The isolation and characterisation of calcifying and non calcifying matrix vesicles from dentine, *Coll. Int. CNRS* **230,** 161.

SYMONS, N. B. B. (1967) The microanatomy and histochemistry of dentinogenesis, in *Structure and Chemical Organisation of Teeth,* ed. A. E. W. Miles, Academic Press, New York.

TAKUMA, S, (1960) Electron microscopy of the structure around the dentural tubule, *J. dent. Res.* **39,** 973.

TAKUMA, S. and N. NAGAI (1971) Ultrastructure of rat odontoblasts in various stages of their development and maturation, *Arch. oral Biol.* **16,** 993.

TAKUMA, S., T. YANAGISAWA and W. L. LIN (1977) Ultrastructural and microanalytical aspects of developing osteodentine in rat incisors, *Calc. Tiss. Res.* **24,** 215.

TEN CATE, A. R. (1972) An analysis of Tomes' granular layer, *Anat. Rec.* **172,** 137.

TEN CATE, A. R. (1978) A fine structural study of coronal and root dentinogenesis in the mouse: observations on the so-called "von Korff fibres" and their contribution to mantle dentine, *J. Anat.* **125,** 183.

TSATSAS, B. G. and R. M. FRANK (1972) Ultrastructure of the dentinal tubular substance near the dentino-enamel junction, *Calc. Tiss. Res.* **9,** 238.

WEIDENREICH, F. (1925) Uber den Bau die Entwicklung des Zahnbeins in der Reihe der Wirbeltiere, *Ergebrisse der Anatomie und Euntwicklungsgeschuchte,* **76,** 218.

WHITTAKER, D. K. and D. ADAMS (1972) Electron microscopic studies on von Korff fibres in the human developing tooth, *Anat. Rec.* **174,** 175.

YILMAZ, S., H. N. NEWMAN and D. F. G. POOLE (1977) Diurnal periodicity of Van Ebner growth lines in pig dentine, *Arch. oral. Biol.* **22,** 511.

## Amelogenesis and Enamel

ARENDS, J. and W. L. JONGEBLOED (1978) Crystallite dimensions of enamel, *J. Biol. Buccale* **6,** 161.

BOYDE, A. (1964) The structure and development of mammalian enamel, Ph. D. thesis, Univ. London.

BOYDE, A. (1965) The structure of developing mammalian dental enamel, in *Tooth Enamel,* ed. M. V. Stack and R. W. Fearnhead, J. Wright, Bristol.

BOYDE, A. (1970) The contribution of the scanning microscope to dental histology*J. dent. Res.* **49,** 15.

BOYDE, A. and E. J. REITH (1976) Scanning electron microscopy of the lateral cell surfaces of rat incisor ameloblasts, *J. Anat.* **122,** 603.

BOYDE, A. and E. J. REITH (1977) Scanning electron microscopy of rat maturation ameloblasts, *Cell Tiss. Res.* **178,** 221.

DACULSI, G. and B. KEREBEL (1978) High resolution electron microscopy study of human enamel crystallites: size, shape and growth, *J. Ulrastruct. Res.* **65,** 163.

DEPORTER, D. A. and A. R. TEN CATE (1976) Fine structural localization of alkaline phosphatase in relation to enamel formation in the mouse, *Arch. oral Biol.* **21,** 7.

DEPORTER, D. A. (1977) The early mineralization of enamel, *Calc. Tiss. Res.* **24,** 271.

EASTOE, J. E. (1979) Enamel protein chemistry—past, present and future, *J. dent. Res.* **58,** 753, Special Issue B.

FEARNHEAD, R. W. (1979) Matrix mineral relationships in enamel tissue, *J. dent. Res.* **58,** Special Issue B.

FRANK, R. M. (1978) Les stries brunes de Retzius en microscopie électronque á balayage, *J. Biol. Buccale* **6,** 139.

FRANK, R. M. (1979) Tooth enamel: current state of the art, *J. dent. Res.* **58,** 684, Special Issue B.

JOSEPHSON, K. and O. FEJERKOV (1977) Ameloblast modulation in the maturation zone of the rat incisor enamel organ. A light and electron microscope study, *J. Anat.* **124,** 45.

MECKEL, A. H., W. S. GRIEBSTEIN and R. J. NEAL (1965) Structure of mature human dental enamel as observed by electron microscopy, *Arch. oral Biol.* **10,** 775.

NYLEN, M. U., E. D. EANES and K. A. OMNELL (1963) Crystal Growth in the rat, *J. Cell Biol.* **18,** 109.

NYLEN, M. U. (1979) Matrix-mineral relationships, a morphologist's viewpoint, *J. dent. Res.* **58,** 922, Special Issue B.

OSBORN, J. W. (1970) The mechanism of prism formation in teeth, *Calc. Tiss. Res.* **5,** 155.

OSBORN, J. W. (1971) A relationship between the striae of Retzius and prism directions in the transverse plane of the human tooth, *Arch. oral Biol.* **16,** 1061.

OSBORN, J. W. (1973) Variations in structure and development of enamel, *Oral Sci. Rev.* **3,** 3.

OSBORN, J. W. and J. HILLMAN (1979) Enamel structure in some Therapsids and Mezozoic mammals, *Calc. Tiss. Res.* **29,** 47.

PALMARA, J., P. P. PHAKEY, W. A. RACHINGER and H. J. ORAMS (1980) Electron microscopy of surface enamel of human unerupted and erupted teeth, *Arch. oral Biol.* **25,** 715.

REITH, E. J. (1970) The stages of amelogenesis as observed in the molar teeth of young rats, *J. Ultrastruct. Res.* **30,** 111.

SPEIRS, R. L. (1971) The nature of surface enamel in human teeth, *Calc. Tiss. Res.* **8,** 1.

TAKANO, Y. and M. A. CRENSHAW (1980) The penetration of intravascularly perfused lanthanum into the ameloblast layer of developing rat molar teeth, *Arch. oral Biol.* **25,** 505.

TRAVIS, D. F. and M. J. GLIMCHER (1964) The structure and organisation of the relationship between the organic matrix and the organic crystals of embryonic bovine enamel, *J. Cel Biol.* **23,** 447.

WEBER, D. F. and D. R. EISENMANN (1971) Microscopy of the neonatal line in developing human enamel, *Am. J. Anat.* **132,** 375.

WEBER, D. F., D. R. EISENMANN and P. L. GLICK (1974) Light and electron microscope studies of Retzius lines in human cervical enamel, *Am. J. Anat.* **141,** 91.

WEBER, D. F. and P. L. GLICK (1975) Correlative microscopy of enamel prism orientation, *Am. J. Anat.* **144,** 401.

ROBINSON, C., H. D. BRIGGS, P. J. ATKINSON and J. A. WEATHERALL (1979) Matrix and mineral changes in developing enamel, *J. dent. Res.* **58,** 871, Special Issue B.

RONNHOLM, E. (1962) An electron microscopic study of the amelogenesis in human teeth. I. The fine structure of ameloblasts, *J. Ultrastruct. Res.* **6,** 229.

RONNHOLM, E. (1962) The amelogenesis of human teeth as revealed by electron microscopy. II. The development of the enamel crystallites, *J. Ultrastruct. Res.* **6,** 249.

RONNHOLM, E. (1962) The amelogenesis of human teeth as revealed by electron microscopy. III. The structure of the organic stroma of human enamel during amelogenesis, *J. Ultrastruct. Res.* **6,** 368.

SKOBE, Z. (1980) Scanning electron microscopy of the mouse incisor enamel organ in transition between secretory and maturation stages of amelogenesis, *Arch. oral Biol.* **25,** 395.

WEINSTOCK, A. and R. C. GREULICH (1971) Elaboration of the matrix glycoprotein of enamel by the secretory ameloblasts of the rat incisor as revealed by radioautography after galactose—$H^3$ injection, *J. Cell Biol.* **51,** 26.

WHITTAKER, D. K. and D. RICHARDS (1978) Scanning electron microscopy of the neonatal line in human enamel, *Arch. oral Biol.* **23,** 45.

## The Periodontium

ATKINSON, M. E. (1972) The development of the mouse molar periodontium, *J. Periodont. Res.* **7,** 255.

BEERSTON, W. (1980) Junctions between fibroblasts in mouse periodontal ligament, *J. Periodont. Res.* **15,** 655.

BERNICK, S. (1957) Innervation of teeth and periodontium after enzymatic removal of collagenous elements, *Oral Med., Oral Surg., Oral Path.* **10,** 323.

BERNICK, S. (1972) The organisation of the periodontal membrane fibres of the developing molars of rats, *J. Periodont. Res.* **7,** 255.

BLACKWOOD, H. J. J. (1957) Intermediate cementum, *Brit. dent. J.* **102,** 345.

DARYBEGI, P., C. H. PAMEIJER, M. P. RUBEN and P. A. RICCHETTI Jr. (1980) Root surface—soft tissue interface, Part I: A review, *J. Periodont.* **51,** 77.

DEPORTER, D. A. and A. R. TEN CATE (1980) Collagen resorption by periodontal ligament fibroblasts at the hard tissue—ligament interfaces of the mouse periodontium *J. Periodont.* **51,** 429.

FREEMAN, E. and A. R. TEN CATE (1971) Development of the periodontium an electron microscope study, *J. Periodont.* **42,** 387.

FREEMAN, E., A. R. TEN CATE and J. DICKINSON (1975) Development of a gomphosis by tooth germ implants in the parietal bone of the mouse, *Arch. oral Biol.* **20,** 139.

FULLMER, H. M. and W. A. GIBSON (1966) Collagenolytic activity in the gingiva of man, *Nature,* **209,** 729.

FULLMER, H. M., J. H. SHEETZ and A. J. NARKATES (1974) Oxytalan connective tissue fibres: a review, *J. Oral Path.* **3,** 291.

FURSETH, R. (1969) The fine structure of the cellular cementum of young human teeth, *Arch. oral Biol.* **14,** 1147.

FURSTMAN, L. and S. BERNICK (1965) Early development of the periodontal membrane, *Am. J. Ortho.* **51,** 482.

GRANT, D. A. and S. BERNICK (1972) Formation of the periodontal ligament. *J. Periodont.* **43,** 17.

GRIFFIN, C. J. and R. HARRIS (1967) The fine structure of the developing human periodontium, *Arch. oral Biol.* **12,** 971.

GRIFFIN, C. J. and R. HARRIS (1968) Unmyelinated nerve endings in the periodontal membrane of human teeth, *Arch. oral Biol.* **13,** 1207.

KARRING, T. and H. LÖE (1970) The three dimensional concept of the epithelial connective tissue boundary of gingiva, *Acta Odont. Scand.* **28,** 917.

LISTGARTEN, M. A. (1966) Phase contrast and electron microscope study of the junction between reduced enamel epithelium and enamel in unerupted human teeth, *Arch. oral Biol.* **11,** 999.

LISTGARTEN, M. A. (1966) Electron microscope study of the dento-gingival junction of man, *Am. J. Anat.* **119,** 147.

LISTGARTEN, M. A. (1967) Electron microscopic features of the newly formed epithelial attachment after gingival surgery, *J. Periodont. Res.* **2,** 46.

LISTGARTEN, M. A. (1972) Ultrastructure of the dentogingival junction after gingivectomy *J. Periodont. Res.* **7,** 151.

LISTGARTEN, M. A. (1972) Normal development structure physiology and repair of gingival epithelium, *Oral Sci. Rev.* **1,** 3.

LÖE, H. (1967) The structure and physiology of the dento-gingival junction, in *Structure and Chemical Organization of the Teeth,* Vol. II, ed. A. E. W. Miles, Academic Press, New York.

MALASSEZ, M. L. (1884) Sur l'existence de masses epithéliales dans le ligament alvéodentaire, *Comptes Rendus des Seances de la Société de Biologie et des Ses Filiales,* **36,** 241.

MANSON, J. D. (1963) The lamina dura, *Oral Surg., Oral Med., Oral Path.* **16,** 432.

McHUGH, W. D. (1971) The interdental gingivae, *J. Periodont. Res.* **6,** 227.

PICTON, D. C. A. (1965) On the part played by the socket in tooth support, *Arch. oral Biol.* **10,** 945.

SABAG, N., R. SAGLIE and C. MERY (1981) Ultrastructure of the normal human epithelial attachment to the cementum root surface, *J. Periodont.* **52,** 94.

SAGLIE, R., N. SABAG and C. MERY (1979) Ultrastructure of the normal human epithelial attachment, *J. Periodont.* **50,** 544.

SCHROEDER, H. E. (1969) Ultrastructure of the junctional epithelium of the human gingiva, *Helv. Odont. Acta* **13,** 65.

SCHROEDER, H. E. and M. A. LISTGARTEN (1971) Fine structure of the developing epithelial attachment of human teeth, in *Monographs in Development Biology,* ed. A. Wolsky, S. Karger, Basel.

SELVIG, K. A. (1965) The fine structure of human cementum, *Acta Odont. Scand.* **23,** 423.

SIMS, M. R. (1973) Oxytalan fibre system of molars in the mouse mandible, *J. dent. Res.* **52,** 797.

SMITH, C. J. (1969) Gingival epithelium, in *Biology of the Periodontium,* ed. A. H. Melcher and W. H. Brown, Academic Press, New York.

SPOUGE, J. D. (1980) A new look at the Rests of Malassez, a review of their embryological origin, anatomy and possible role in periodontal health and disease, *J. Periodont.* **51,** 437.

TEN CATE, A. R. and D. A. DEPORTER (1974) The role of fibroblast in collagen turnover in the functioning periodontal ligament of the mouse, *Arch. oral Biol.* **19,** 339.

TEN CATE, A. R. (1975) The dento-gingival junction: an interpretation of the literature, *J. Periodont.* **46,** 475.

YAJIMA, T., G. G. ROSE and C. J. MAHAN (1980) Human gingival fibroblast cell lines *in vitro.* II. Electron microscopic studies in fibrogenesis, *J. Periodont. Res.* **15,** 267.

## CHAPTER 9

# *Establishment of the Dental Arch*

At birth there are normally no teeth present in the mouth, although occasionally so-called natal or neonatal teeth may appear. These can actually be present initially or erupt within a few weeks. Sometimes they are very loose and need to be extracted as there may be risk of inhalation; other times they are rather firm, but may cause trouble with breast feeding. They are usually lower incisors of the deciduous dentition, but may be extra ones or so-called supernumeraries (see later).

In the normal situation there are just upper and lower gum pads. The former exhibit certain obvious anatomical features, one of which being a gingival groove on the lingual side of what will become the tooth-bearing area and also lateral sulci which pass over this area laterally into the buccal sulcus (Fig. 9.1). This separates the area containing the canine anteriorly from the first molar, and the pads also show segmentation elsewhere corresponding to the future deciduous teeth. Less easy to see is the dental groove which corresponds to the site of the former dental lamina.

The upper gum pad is wider than the lower and protrudes anteriorly to it. The mean overlap or protrusion when the pads are in light contact is about 5 mm with a range of 1-10 mm. Similarly the vertical overlap, that is the amount the upper pad covers the lower, varies from -4 to +5 mm with a mean of less than 1 mm (negative overlap means a so-called open bite, that is a space between the upper and lower gum pads).

Thus it may be seen there is a wide variation in size and relationships of the gum pads at birth and it is generally agreed the future occlusion of the child cannot be predicted at this stage. This is perhaps not surprising as there is little permanent contact between the gum pads, and then only in the future molar area, at this stage and rather limited occlusal movements apart from those involved in sucking.

The maxilla and mandible at birth contain all the deciduous teeth awaiting eruption and also the tooth germs of the permanent incisors, canines and premolars as well as the partially calcified germ of the first permanent molars.

Thus there is considerable overcrowding of tooth material. This is, of course, partially relieved by the subsequent emergence of the deciduous teeth starting at about 6 months and continuing until about 2 years.

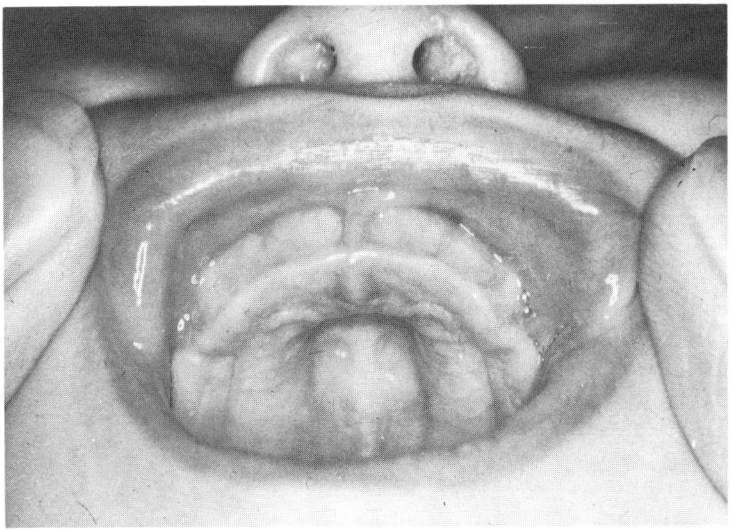

Fig. 9.1. Upper gum pad of a child of about 3 months. Note gingival groove and lateral sulcus.

## ERUPTION

Before dealing with these changes, however, something must be said about the mechanism of eruption. This term is sometimes used to mean the process of a tooth appearing through the gingiva into the mouth. However, this is better referred to as emergence, since eruption is a more or less continuous movement of the developing tooth from the depth of the alveolar bone, through the gingiva and into occlusion. That is to say, it is a continuing process from early on to its final position in the mouth and, of course, in the case of continuously growing teeth such as the incisors of rats the process goes on permanently as the tip of the tooth is worn away.

There have been many theories of the cause of eruption, such as the growth of the root or pulpal proliferation, local increased blood pressure, bone deposition below the tooth and the traction effect of the periodontal ligament. Unfortunately it is not an easy subject to investigate in man. It would be rather unethical to do any actual experiments during tooth eruption on children; the most that can be done is to follow the process radiographically and relate the position of the moving tooth to certain fixed points.

Study of abnormal cases such as in cleidocranial dysostosis or of teeth in ovarian teratomas may shed some light on the process, but are complicated by other factors.

Finally, animal experiments have been mainly carried out for convenience on continuously erupting teeth and therefore the results may not be totally applicable to man.

### Growth of the Root and Pulpal Soft Tissue

This has been shown to be unlikely as a mechanism, at least in continuously growing teeth, since when the forming end of a rat's or rabbit's incisor is resected, or the tooth is transected to separate its formative and incisal parts, the unimpeded* incisal portion erupts in a similar manner to an intact tooth after a period of time (Berkovitz 1976).

Clinically in man the length of the root is not enough to account for the amount of eruption in all teeth, for example the canines; teeth without roots may erupt, as has been seen in the case of neonatal teeth. Even teeth with fully formed roots can erupt. Thus it appears that root formation is not a vital factor in the process of eruption.

The effect of growing cells at the base of the pulp pushing against the so-called "cushioned hammock ligament" surrounding the end of the root has been suggested as a mechanism of eruption. This ligament, however, has not been generally identified, although some credence was given to this theory by the finding that substances stopping mitosis, for example demecolcine, did reduce eruption. However, this only proves that cells are involved in the eruptive process and they might, of course, be elsewhere such as in the periodontal ligament (see later).

All in all then, the role of the root and pulpal tissue may be no more than the filling up of the space left by the actively erupting tooth.

### Tissue Fluid Pressure

The apical region of an erupting tooth is very vascular and it has been proposed that tissue fluid pressure could build up here and cause eruption. Removal in animals of the appropriate sympathetic nerve supply, which results in vasodilation, is followed by an increased rate of eruption, but of course this is only indirect proof, as other factors may also be altered, such as tissue nutrition. Hypotensive drugs given to rats have provided contradictory results and cannot be said to support this theory.

More direct evidence has been shown in dogs by measuring tissue fluid pressures between resorbing deciduous teeth and the corresponding erupting permanent teeth and also within the pulp of the permanent teeth. There were found to be pressure differentials of about 13 mm Hg which could produce the force required in eruption (van Hassel and McMinn 1972).

### Bone Growth

It has been postulated that eruption could occur by means of selective deposition and resorption of bone in relation to the teeth. However studies

*The incisal tip is ground away to avoid the complication of occlusion.

with tetracyclines, which become incorporated in new bone and can be identified by their fluorescence, show that there is resorption of bone at the base of the socket at the beginning of eruption (Manson 1967). This is then followed by deposition and the amount of bone deposited plus the amount of root growth is the same as that of the movement of the tooth, indicating a filling in of space after the tooth has moved. Radiographic studies in children support this finding in that when root growth begins there is a downward movement first before eruption commences.

### Periodontal Ligament

The experiments mentioned earlier on root resection or transection indicate that eruption, anyway in the continuously growing incisor of the rat, is mediated by the periodontal ligament in some way since neither root proliferation nor cellular division from the pulp could be active. In addition, as there was no closed system it was unlikely that raised capillary pressure could be operative. This was even more unlikely in another type of experiment in which only the part of the odontogenic base producing enamel was removed. There are two possible origins of the source of movement within the periodontal ligament. The extracellular substance, or the cells themselves.

It is true that when collagen fibrils are formed and covalent cross-linkage bonds develop, a contraction occurs which may further be increased by shrinkage due to dehydration, and this could provide the eruptive force necessary. Experiments of giving animals substances which produce lathyrism, in which collagen synthesis is disturbed, showed retardation of eruption although root growth continued. This then seemed to prove that collagen was the important substance in the eruptive process. However, these early results have not been confirmed and it now seems less certain that this is the mechanism.

What about the cells within the periodontal ligament? The fact that demecolcine, which interferes with mitosis, slows down eruption points to proliferating cells as the possible force involved. Since those in the basal region of the tooth have been shown by the resection experiments to be inoperative in eruption, it may indicate that cells in the periodontal ligament are the active ones. It seems then possible that fibroblasts in the ligament may have contractile properties which could cause tooth eruption, but more work will need to be done to elucidate the exact mechanism.

Finally it must be admitted that it is unlikely that one causative agent only will be found in eruption, that is to say it is probably a multifactorial process.

### The Emergence of the Deciduous Dentition

Much of the earlier work on this was based on rather small samples and often non-representative material, so before dealing with details it will be as well to consider how, in fact, one can compare emergence between individuals or groups. For example, one may wish to see whether boys are behind girls in this respect or what effect serious neonatal disturbances might have. This presupposes two things, firstly that there are adequate standards against which to measure the findings of a particular group and secondly, that there is a reasonably simple method of statistical comparison. In fact neither of these conditions are altogether met. Particularly with regard to the deciduous dentition, there are not all that many studies which can be regarded as satisfactory for comparison. In addition, the statistical methods are neither simple nor entirely comparable in different investigations.

It could be said that all that is necessary is to count the number of teeth at particular ages and compare the mean number between groups (Fig. 9.2).

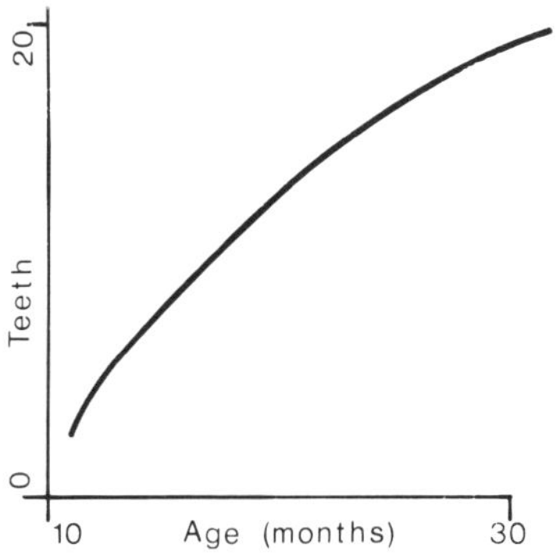


Fig. 9.2. Graph showing the number of erupted deciduous teeth at different ages up to 30 months.

However, although this is occasionally done for the deciduous dentition, partly to assess age in countries in which registration of births is not satisfactory, it is immediately apparent that alteration in the order of eruption will lead to the comparison between unlike events. For example, in one group canines may erupt earlier than the deciduous first molars but not in another. However, this is probably not a serious error in the deciduous dentition which is less variable in this respect than the permanent one.

Another problem is that one relatively rarely alights on an emerging tooth and therefore any particular child might have some teeth erupted, one or two emerging and others unerupted. This data does not, therefore, easily yield to simple methods of comparison. The order of eruption may be easy enough to describe, but the date of actual emergence of any particular tooth needs a different approach.

In the case of longitudinal studies, the date of tooth emergence is best calculated as the age of the child at the inspection when the tooth is present less half the time which has elapsed from the previous inspection when the tooth was unerupted. Quite often this correction has not been made, thus leading to figures which are too high.

In cross-sectional data things are more complicated and it may be best to look at the permanent dentition for an example since more work has been done here. Suppose one wishes to look at the maxillary second permanent molar in a sample of children of ages between 10 and 16 years, some of whom have the tooth and some who have not. First one calculates from this data the percentage of children at each age who have the tooth, then the cumulative percentage at each age (by adding in the previous children of the former ages, so one ends up with a final age where everyone has the tooth, that is 100 per cent). This can be shown graphically as a curve and the age where 50 per cent of the children have their second permanent molar can easily be read off (Fig. 9.3). A more sophisticated way of dealing with this problem is by means of the probit transformation whereby the curve is converted to a straight line. Means and standard deviations may then be calculated, allowing different populations to be compared statistically (Finney 1951).

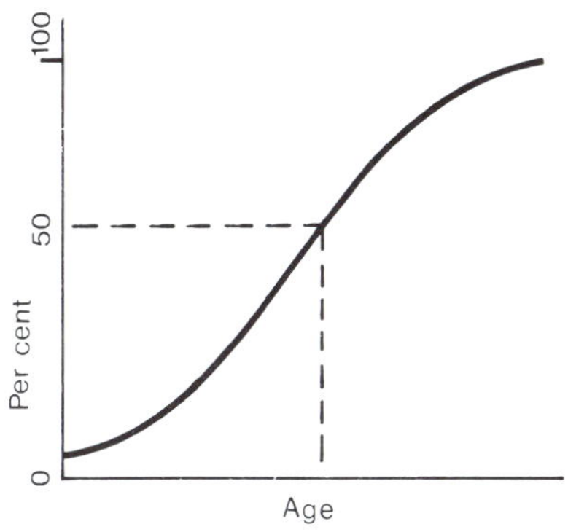


Fig. 9.3. Cumulative distribution of the number of children in which the second permanent molar has erupted at different ages. The broken lines indicate the age at which half the children have the tooth in their mouths.

Although conventionally one says that the deciduous teeth erupt between 6 months and 2 years, there is considerable variation; for example, some children not having their first tooth until up to 13 months or so. Similarly, only a minority actually have all their deciduous teeth by 2 years.

There appears to be no statistically acceptable evidence of a difference between sexes in dates of emergence for deciduous teeth, although some investigators have found boys first. There is no difference between left and right sides, but there is a tendency for the lower central incisors to appear before the upper.

The conventional order of eruption is $I_1$, $I_2$, $M_1$, C, $M_2$ in both jaws, although there may be variations around this. The incisors usually appear from 6 to 10 months, the first molars from 12 to 15 months, the canines about 18 months, followed by the second molars between 2 years and 30 months. Some racial differences have been found earlier in life, but in general any delay is caught up by 18 months to 2 years. Severe malnutrition may cause delayed eruption, but it affects other aspects of the child's growth much more. "Small for dates" babies seem to have delayed eruption, and this may be part of their general setback in early development.

### The Permanent Dentition

Only the permanent molars erupt without displacing deciduous predecessors, and normally the initial permanent tooth to appear is the first permanent molar. This often confuses parents who presume it is still one of the "milk set". The deciduous predecessors for incisors and canines are similar in form, but the molars are different in morphology from their successors which are two cusped premolars.

Shedding of deciduous teeth is due to the resorption of their roots associated with the eruption of their permanent successors (Fig. 9.4). This is caused by pressure from the erupting tooth on the overlying tissues which leads to resorption of the bony crypt. The resorption is mediated by osteoclasts and when the roots of the deciduous teeth are reached giant cells lying in concavities known as Howships lacumae continue the resorption (Fig. 9.5). Firstly it affects cementum and then dentine and proceeds intermittently so that a certain amount of repair occurs. Sometimes shedding is delayed resulting, for example, in a permanent incisor erupting into a bad position behind the deciduous one. In extreme cases fusion of the deciduous tooth may occur to the alveolar bone (ankylosis), preventing further eruption of the permanent successor. The normal position of permanent teeth in relation to their deciduous predecessors is well seen in Fig. 9.6 of a child of about 5 years of age.

Girls tend to shed their deciduous teeth earlier than boys, but the study of the timing of shedding is rather complicated by dental extractions. Although early exfoliation of deciduous teeth may advance the emergence of the permanent ones, premature extraction of deciduous teeth may actually delay eruption of permanent successors if these are at an early stage of development.

Usually the first incisor (in the case of the lowers it may appear before the first permanent molar) appears next in the mouth and Fig. 9.7 (Moorrees 1977) shows the ages of emergence of permanent teeth of a group of girls in the U.S.A. Boys are generally later by a few months and this is particularly marked for the canine. There are no differences between sides, but as can be seen from the figures the mandibular teeth are in advance by a few months over the maxillary ones.

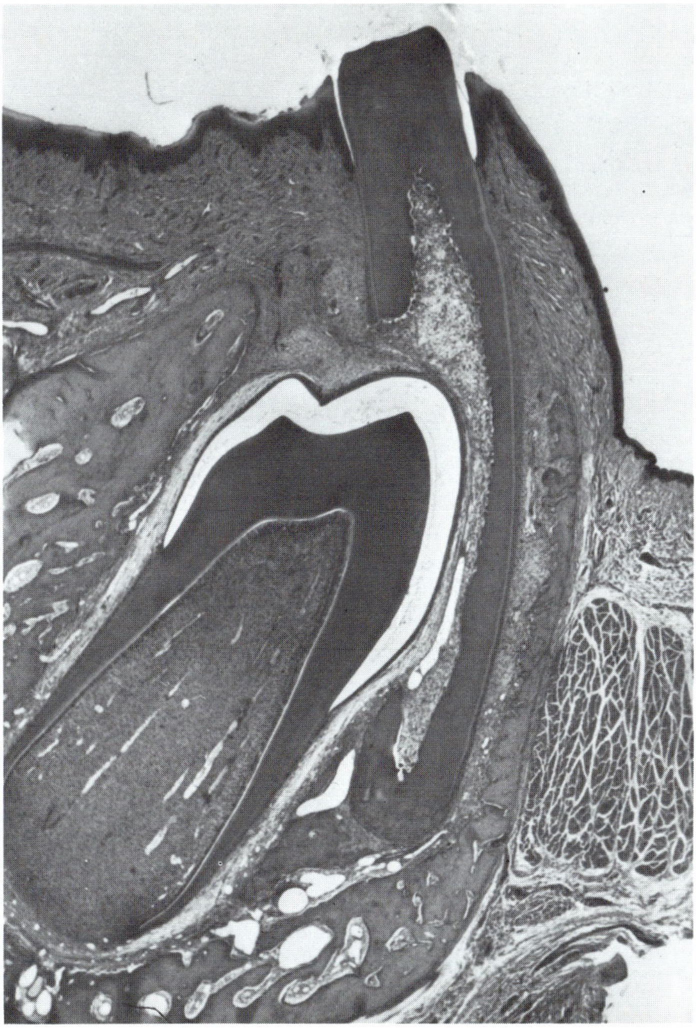

Fig. 9.4. A permanent tooth in a cat awaiting eruption beneath the deciduous predecessor (by kind permission of Mr J. Cunningham, School of Dental Surgery, University of Liverpool).

There is a wide range in the time of emergence of any particular tooth, in some cases as much as 5 years, that is ± 2.5 years from the mean.

The normal sequence of eruption is $M^1$, $I^1$, $I^2$, $Pm^1$, C, $Pm^2$, $M^2$, $M^3$ in the upper jaw, and this may be varied in the lower jaw by the first incisor being before the first molar and the canine being earlier than the first premolar. However, there are variations in sequences and these may have a genetic basis as has been found, for example, in orders such as $Pm_2$, $M_2$ and $M_2$, $Pm_2$. In

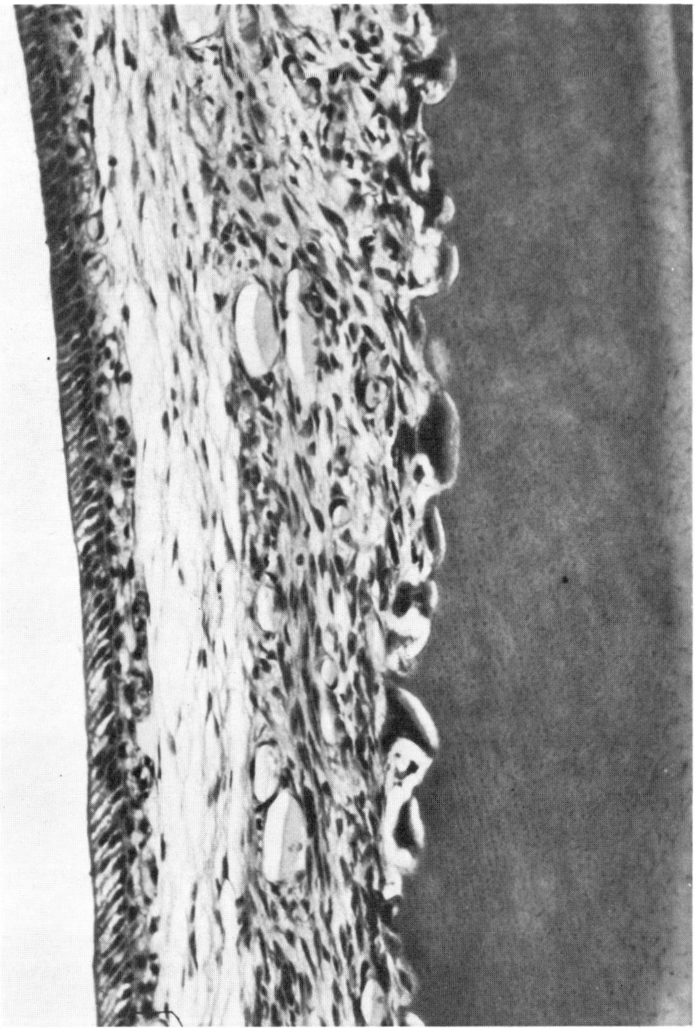

Fig. 9.5. Higher magnification of Fig. 9.4 showing giant cells and resorption (by kind permission of Mr J. Cunningham, School of Dental Surgery, University of Liverpool).

addition, there is evidence of overall control of eruption with respect both to sides and jaws (Garn and Smith 1980).

Dental emergence is earlier in black children in the U.S.A. compared with white, and also in African blacks compared with Europeans. The same appears to be true of certain Asiatic groups too, so that it is evident that former white standards will not be applicable to these other racial types.

There is clearly too much tooth material to accommodate in the jaws of a

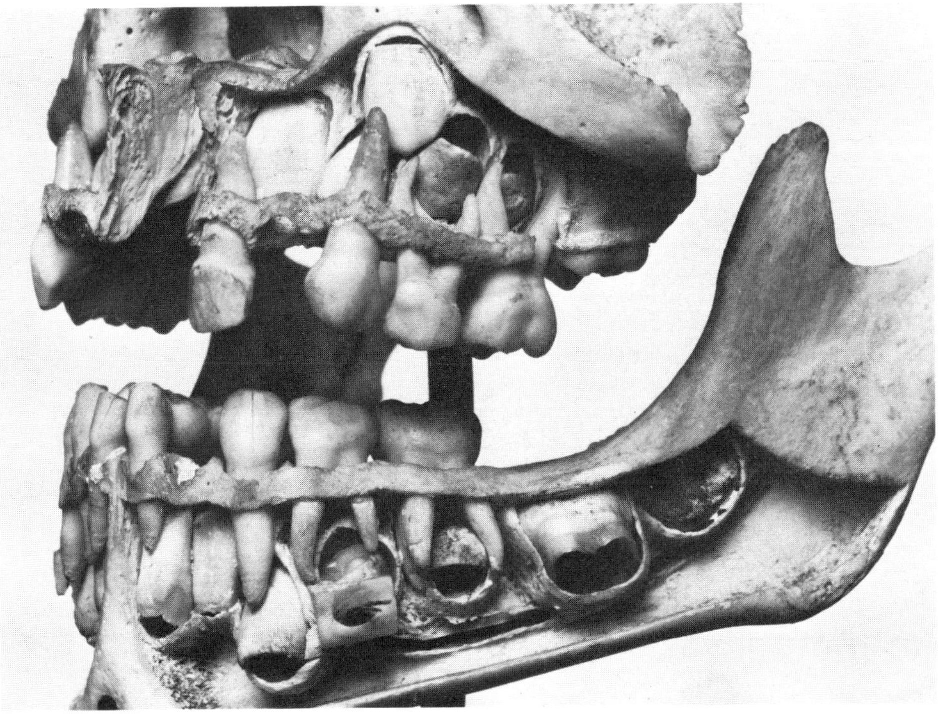

Fig. 9.6. Jaws of a child of about 5 years. Note the upright position of the deciduous incisors, the forming premolars between the roots of the deciduous molars and the high position of the permanent maxillary canine.

young child as the teeth are full sized and the jaws still growing. One of the problems of development then is to adjust the available space to meet the requirements of teeth present at any time in the mouth. Thus the relationship of tooth material to arch size is important and, unfortunately, in modern man is often ill matched. However, before dealing with that it will be as well to discuss the number of teeth as this too is relevant to the problem.

## TOOTH NUMBER

The normal number of deciduous teeth is 20 and of the permanent teeth 32, including the wisdom teeth which erupt rather after childhood. However, numbers may vary from being too many, supernumerary or supplemental teeth, to too few, oligodontia or hypodontia. The extreme case of virtually no teeth at all is usually referred to as anodontia and may be associated with other epithelial defects such as lack of sweat glands (Fig. 9.8).

Ectodermal dysplasia

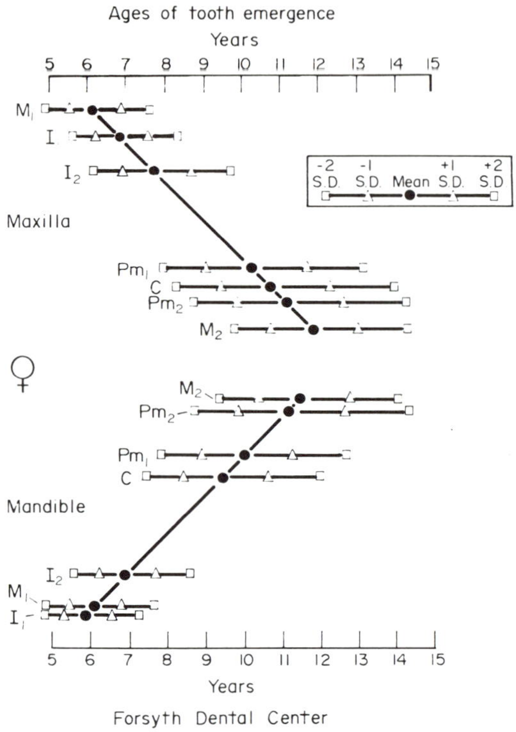


Fig. 9.7. Ages of tooth emergence of girls in the U.S.A. (In *Biology of Occlusal Development* (1977), by kind permission of Professor C. F. A. Moorrees, Forsyth Dental Institute, Boston and Dr. J. A. McNamara, Jr., Center for Human Growth and Development, University of Michigan).

### Supernumerary Teeth

A distinction is sometimes made between supplemental teeth with a normal morphology and supernumerary ones which are simplified in form.

There are certain pathological conditions such as cleidocranial dysostosis in which there are very many extra teeth which normally remain unerupted. However, in the more common case there may be one or two extra teeth and these are most often found in the maxilla either in the incisor or molar regions. If situated in the midline related to the incisors, they are referred to as mesiodens.

The frequency of occurrence in the permanent dentition varies in different surveys being between 1 and 3 per cent of individuals and is considered to be higher in males than females.

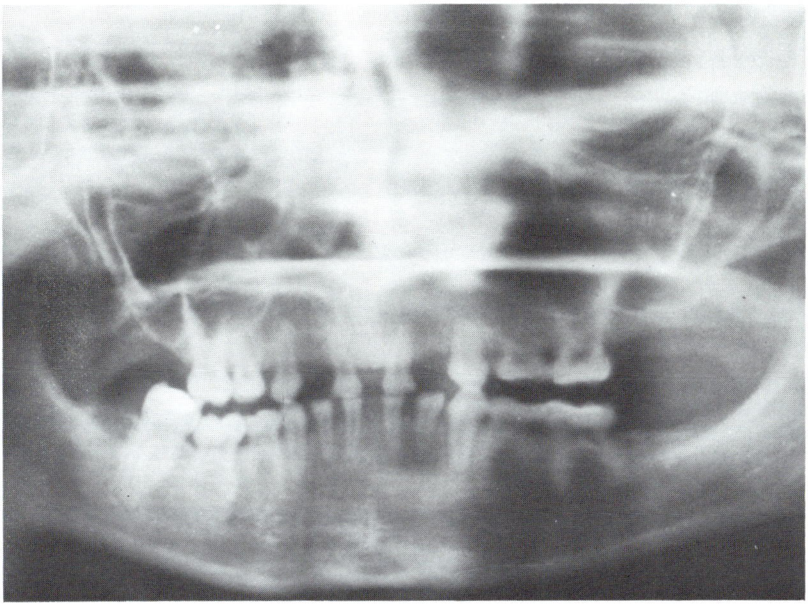

Fig. 9.8. Radiograph of boy of 12 years suffering from anodontia. The only permanent tooth present is the lower right first molar. The deciduous upper lateral incisors are also missing.

**Oligodontia (or Hypodontia)**

People with missing teeth are quite common, the third molars being absent for example in 7-26 per cent of white populations. Of the other teeth, individuals showing oligodontia in the permanent dentition in different investigations range from 2 to 10 per cent. The most commonly missing teeth after the wisdoms are the second premolars, followed by maxillary lateral incisors. There may be a correlation with lack of teeth in the deciduous dentition.

It is apparent that the common missing teeth are the end ones of each series, the second incisors, second premolars and third molars, and this is, no doubt, due to the lack of stability of these teeth during the evolutionary process.

It has been postulated that individuals with missing third molars have a significantly higher incidence of other missing teeth and also reduction in the size of the remaining teeth and delayed tooth formation. However, not all investigators have found a relationship between missing third molars and other missing teeth. It is clear from twin and family studies that there is a strong hereditary component in tooth number, although it is unlikely to be a simple Mendelian system.

## DEVELOPMENT OF THE DENTAL ARCH

It has to be acknowledged that the dental arch is part of the facial complex and, of course, grows along with the rest of the face. However, it is convenient to look at it in relationship with the teeth, since this is the clinical view seen by dentists in their everyday work.

In addition it should be realized that the relationship between teeth and dental arches in modern man is far from satisfactory, that is to say there is often disharmony between the two. This may result in overcrowding of the teeth and in some cases even preventing the emergence of certain teeth altogether.

The reasons for this are probably complex, but there are two obvious ones which can be mentioned here. If a Saxon or Medieval skull is looked at, it will be observed that there is much attrition, or wearing away, of the teeth even in relatively young persons. This is not only on the occlusal surface of the teeth but also between, on approximal surfaces. Therefore the teeth in an adult from these periods will be smaller mesiodistally than when they emerged into the mouth. The amount of space gained hereby on each side is something like half the width of a premolar tooth and thus it can be seen that any minor overcrowding could be accommodated by forward movement of the posterior teeth. In modern man attrition is very minimal and gives virtually no space in this way.

The second point to note is that the teeth develop and grow in sheltered positions in the jaws and are not normally affected much by adverse environmental factors, except for occasional interference with mineralization as shown, for example, by enamel hypoplasias. This is indicated by the high correlations between parents and offspring with respect to tooth size, showing that hereditary factors are paramount.

However, jaws have a much longer period of growth, at least up until puberty, if not later, and this leaves them much more susceptible to environmental factors in the shape of illnesses, malnutrition and early dental extractions, all of which may prevent them reaching their full genetic potential. This is indicated by the low correlations found for dental arches between parents and offspring compared with those of tooth size (Bowden and Goose 1968).

The process of growth of the dental arches is, of course, a continuous one from before birth up until the teens, but it will be convenient to look at certain obvious stages in more detail for clarity

### At Birth

The gum pads have already been referred to, so it is only necessary here to indicate the state of development of the unerupted teeth at this point (Fig. 9.9). About two-thirds of the crowns of the deciduous incisors are mineralized, one-third of the canines and the first deciduous molar usually has its occlusal surface completed. The second deciduous molar still only has the cusps mineralized but not joined up, and the first permanent molar may show the tips of one or two cusps. There is not enough room normally to accommodate the teeth within the gum pads, and therefore crowding shows in the incisor region at this stage.

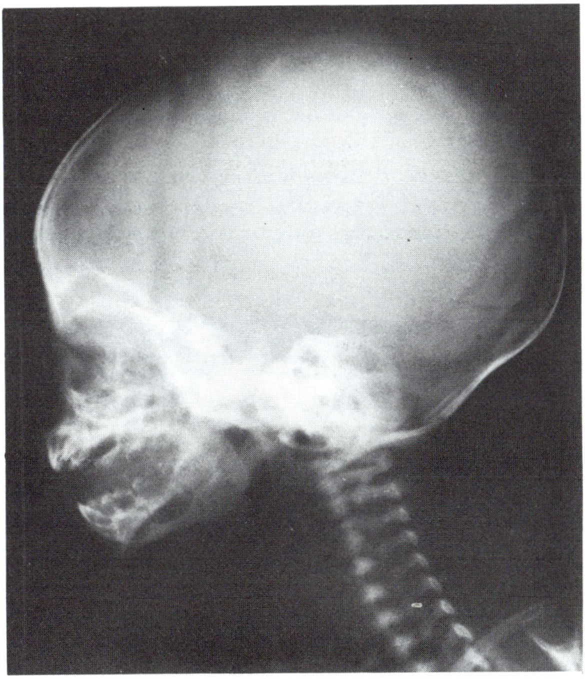

Fig. 9.9. Radiograph of newborn child. The partial mineralization of the deciduous teeth can be seen, the incisors being in advance of the others (by kind permission of Dr. H. M-L. Carty, Department of Radiodiagnosis, University of Liverpool).

### Thirty Months

By this time the deciduous dentition is usually completely in occlusion. The deciduous incisor roots are complete and the canines and molars almost so (Fig. 9.10). The permanent incisor crowns are about two-thirds complete and the canines nearly one-half. The first permanent molars crowns are nearly complete and in the maxilla the occlusal surfaces are facing downwards and backwards. In the lower ones the occlusal surfaces may face inwards or outwards as well as upwards and forwards and this reminds us that the space available in the jaws at this time is not adequate to allow the crowns of the permanent teeth to occupy the positions they will, when erupted.

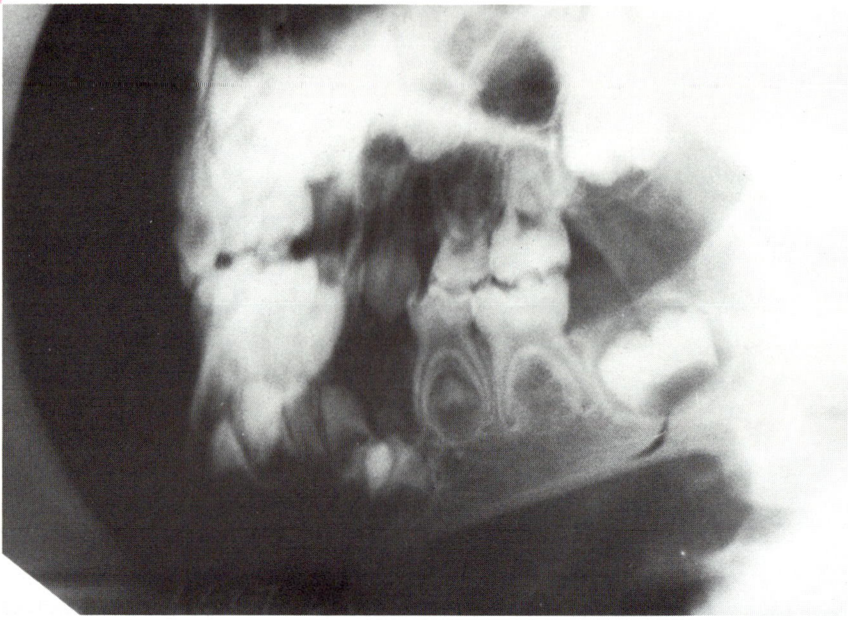

Fig. 9.10. Radiograph of a 30-month-old child (by kind permission of Mr P. D. Bird, Liverpool A. H. A. (T)).

It should be noted that the orientation of the long axes of the deciduous teeth in the arches is upright, which contrasts with those of the permanent ones to come.

Often there is spacing between the deciduous teeth when erupting or soon afterwards and this space is considered necessary if crowding of the permanent dentition is not to occur later. Further development of the crowns of the permanent teeth and their position with respect to their deciduous predecessors can be seen in Fig. 9.6 in a child about 5 years of age.

### Six-Seven Years of Age

This period is characterized by the emergence of the first permanent molars coming into place behind the second deciduous molars and their roots are more than half-formed (Fig. 9.11). The crowns of the premolars which started mineralizing at about 2-3 years and the canines are now almost fully formed and the former are seen lying between the roots of the deciduous molars. The maxillary canine is high up at this stage related to nasal cavity and maxillary sinus.

The incisors have about half of their roots formed and are in a position to erupt as resorption of the deciduous incisors is occurring. At this period there is an increase in width between the deciduous canines, helping to make space

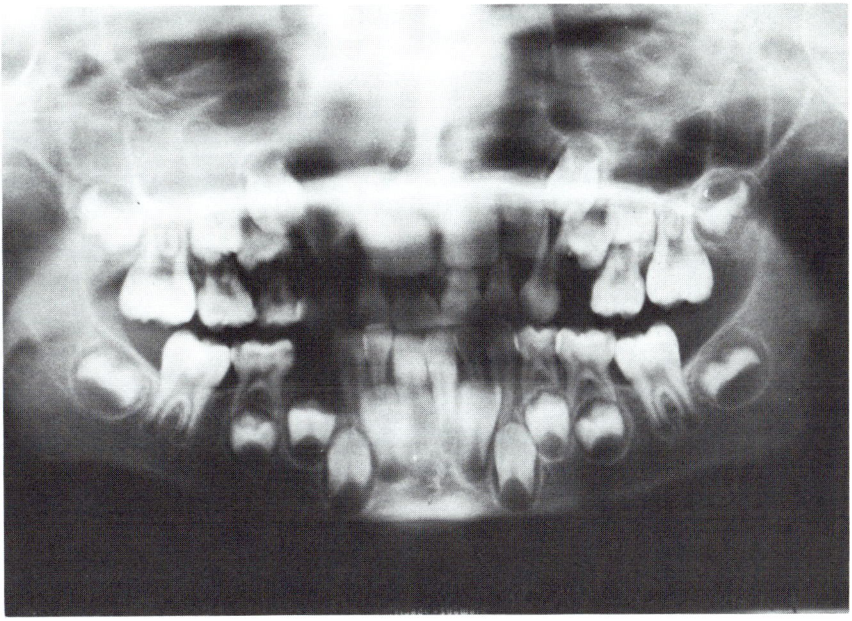

Fig. 9.11. Radiograph of a child of about 6 years of age.

for the eruption of the permanent incisors which are considerably larger than their predecessors. Also in the upper jaw, particularly, further space is made available by the fact that the permanent incisors erupt with their long axis inclined forward and therefore lie in front of where the deciduous incisors used to be. However, there is often some overcrowding at this age, particularly in the lowers which may be regarded as normal, since further growth of the arches has yet to take place.

The second permanent molar crown is almost complete and it lies behind the first molar with the upper inclined backwards and the lower forwards rather as did the first molar at an earlier stage.

When the first permanent molars erupt, the distal surface of the mandibular second deciduous molar is on much the same level as the maxillary one, thus the first permanent molars are unable to interdigitate in the way they do later in the adult.

### Ten-Eleven Years of Age

The permanent incisors are fully erupted and usually their roots finished or nearly finished forming, the laterals being a little later than the centrals (Fig. 9.12).

The deciduous canines will usually have commenced to resorb and the permanent canines will be moving towards emergence. The premolars have

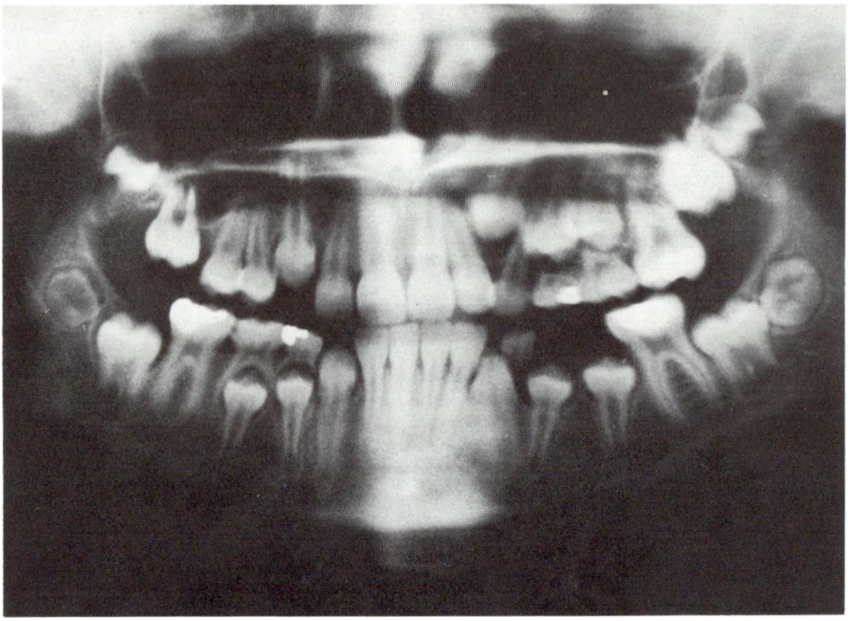

Fig. 9.12. Radiograph of a child of about 11 years of age.

started to erupt, the lowers first, and will be replacing the deciduous molars.

It is necessary to realize that the combined mesiodistal dimension of the permanent canine and two premolars is less than that of the deciduous canine and molars by 2-4 mm and this additional space (leeway space) may help to accommodate the emerging permanent canines. In the lower arch there is more space available as the mandibular deciduous molars are relatively larger and this allows the mandibular first permanent molar to move forward more and therefore come into the normal adult type of relationship with the upper. However, as correlations between the mesiodistal widths of permanent and deciduous teeth are not especially high (about 0.4), it is not easy to predict, in any individual case, the size of the permanent successors from the deciduous molars.

The normal sequence of eruption, as has been stated before, is earlier in the mandibular than the maxillary arch. In the upper the usual sequence is first premolar, canine and then second premolar. However, the canine may sometimes be very late and cause problems clinically by erupting in a bad position or sometimes not at all.

In the lower, the canine often precedes the first premolar with the second premolar coming last but, again, variability is present.

The crown of the second molar is complete and the root formation taking place. Its eruption is usually about 12 years of age.

At about this stage it is usual to be able to see radiographically whether the third molars are present or not, but in some cases the crypts only are visible. The eruption time and position of the wisdom teeth are exceedingly variable, resulting often in the inability of these teeth to erupt at all.

## THE SIZE AND SHAPE OF THE DENTAL ARCH

The form of the developing arches has been described in a variety of ways such as parabolic, ellipsoid, U-shaped, V-shaped or catenary. However, none of these have proved very fruitful for further analysis and since it is obvious there is great variability there may be little point in pursuing the subject. Clearly someone with a broad face is likely to have a broad dental arch and one with a thin face a more narrow arch.

New computer-based studies, however, have made it possible to summarize a series of two- or even three-dimensional coordinates of the dental arch and thus to compare different shapes including assymetrical ones more accurately than before, and further interesting findings may emerge from this development.

There have been a number of studies of size changes in the dental arch, but it has to be realized that there are difficulties in providing satisfactory information about arch size for several reasons, the most important one being the great variability shown between children. Some investigators have attempted to reduce some of this variability by comparing children at the same dental, rather than chronological, age.

Another factor is the representativeness of the material. If only good occlusions are chosen, one is ignoring the large variation that is around this, for example children with overcrowded jaws.

Finally, in a longitudinal survey numbers are, of necessity, small and the results of a study in one part of the world will not necessarily be applicable to those elsewhere, even apart from obvious factors such as race.

Table 9.1 taken from Lundström (1969) shows the changes found in arch dimensions from 3 to 6 years of age. The arch width is normally measured between the deciduous canine tips or the central fossae of the second deciduous molars. Arch length is measured from between the deciduous first incisors to a line drawn tangential to the posterior surfaces of the second deciduous molars.

It may be seen that in general there is an increase of arch width during this period and a slight decrease in arch length presumably due to the closure of interdental spaces.

During the mixed dentition, meaningful figures are hard to come by due to the different times of shedding and erupting teeth and also lack of fixity of measuring points. However, Figs. 9.13 and 9.14 show the findings from a

TABLE 9.1

Changes in Arch Dimensions with Age in the Complete Deciduous Dentition (mm) (After Lundströr in Dental Practitioner 1969)

| STUDY | Material | | Arch width (c-c) | | Arch width (e-e) | | Arch length (e-e to a-a) | |
|---|---|---|---|---|---|---|---|---|
| | No. of subjects | Follow-up period | Upper | Lower | Upper | Lower | Upper | Lowe |
| Lewis and Lehman (1929) | 170[a] | 3-6½ | +0.2 | +0.3 | +0.7 | +0.4 | | |
| Goldstein and Stanton (1935) | 94-69[b] | 3-6 | +1.5 | +1.2 | +1.4 | +0.6 | -0.5 | -0.7 |
| Cohen (1940) | 15F<br>13M | 3½-6½ | +1.0<br>+2.0 | +1.5<br>+1.7 | +0.9<br>+0.6 | +0.4<br>+1.2 | | |
| Holcomb and Meredith (1956) | 50F<br>50M | | +0.8<br>+0.6 | +1.0<br>+0.8 | | | | |
| Meredith and Hopp (1956) | 40F<br>37M | 4-6 | | | +1.1<br>+0.9 | +0.7<br>+0.6 | | |
| Moorrees (1959) | 70-78[c] | 4-6 | +0.2<br>+0.4 | +0.7<br>+0.8 | +0.2<br>+0.3 | 0.0<br>+0.7 | -0.8<br>-0.7 | -0.3<br>-0.5 |
| Sillman (1964) | 65 | 3-6 | +1 [d]<br>+1 | +1<br>+1 | +2<br>+2 | +1<br>+1 | -1<br>-1 | -0.5<br>0 |

[a] Whole material: at ages 3-6½ years the number varied between 25 and 52 individuals.
[b] Material of 300 children studied between 1 and 11 years of age.
[c] Whole material comprised 184 North American white children, from whom 78 upper and 70 lowe arches were selected as having a full complement of teeth in normal position at the end of the exam nation (17-19 years). Between ages 4 and 6 years the number varied between 20 and 59 in each ag and sex group.
[d] Approximate figures obtained from growth curves.

longitudinal study of Moorrees (1958) which was obtained from serial dental casts of 184 North American White Children who had normal dentitions at 17-19 years of age.

Between 5 and 10 years, during the eruption of the permanent incisors, the mean intercanine distance increased approximately 3 mm. Arch length, however, although increasing at first, especially in the upper due to the greater labial inclination of the permanent incisors, from about 10 until 14 years decreases and this has already been commented on in connection with the "leeway space". The maxillary intercanine distance increases in this later period by about 2 mm, but in the mandible decreases. However, again there is much variability.

After 14 years little change occurred in either width or length in this study, which may be due partly to the particular selection of the subjects referred to

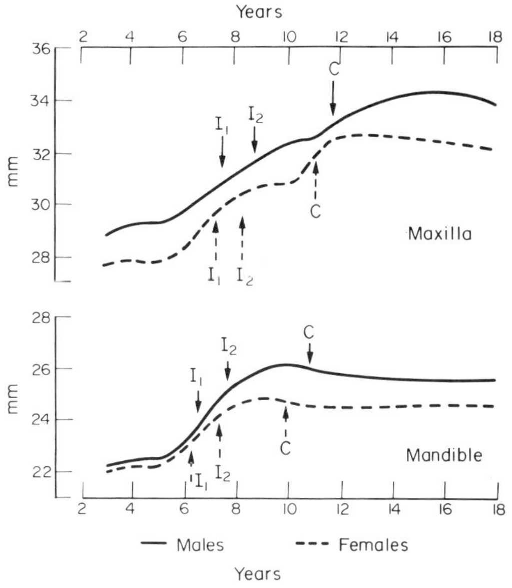


Fig. 9.13. Changes in dental arch width with age (by kind permission of Professor C. F. A. Moorrees, Forsyth Dental Institute, Boston, and the editor of the *Journal of the Canadian Dental Association*). The arrows indicated are calculated from data by Hurme (1948).

earlier.

In a later paper Moorrees and Reed (1965) showed that more meaningful results were obtained by relating these findings to dental age. In general the mean trends then showed greater steepness and sharper inflections than in the previous curves which were more smoothed out.

## ARCH RELATIONSHIPS

The arches have for convenience been considered separately so far, but of course they are related to each other as well. In infancy, this relationship as has been seen is somewhat loose and one of the reasons for the presence of the teeth, no doubt, is to stabilize it. Thus ever since the eruption of the deciduous incisors a sensory feedback mechanism is added to the already existing neurological control of the jaws. This is mediated by sensors in the periodontal ligament which arrest the contraction of closing muscles before the force on teeth becomes excessive.

The earlier obsession of anatomists and orthodontists with the minutiae of details of occlusion is now seen to have been somewhat misplaced, as the principal function of the developing dentition is to guide the dental arches into a suitable position wherewith to carry out their normal functions. In earlier populations such as the Saxons, soon after the teeth were in position, attrition

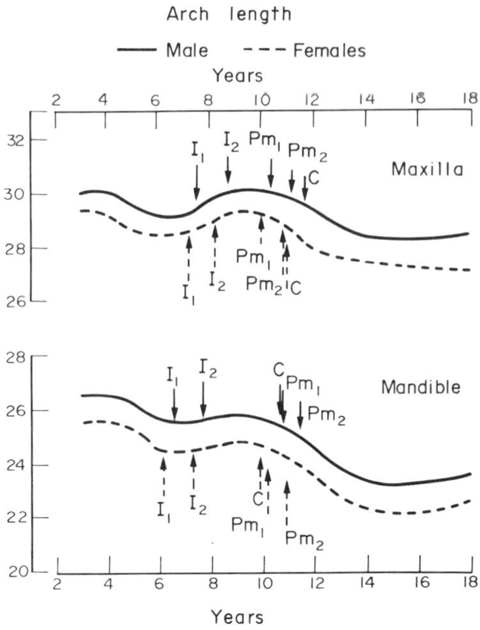


Fig. 9.14. Changes in dental arch length with age (by kind permission of Professor C. F. A. Moorrees, Forsyth Dental Institute, Boston, and the editor of the *Journal of the Canadian Dental Association*). The arrows indicated are calculated from data by Hurme (1948).

rapidly wore away cusps and the modern pattern of interdigitation of teeth did not exist as the occlusal surfaces became almost flat.

However, in modern populations it is possible to see in general terms how the various teeth occlude together and Fig. 9.15 shows these details for the cheek teeth. It has long been agreed that the first permanent molars represent an important "keystone" of the arch and the conventional classification of the relationship between these teeth was given by Angle at the end of the last century.

*Class I*

The lower first molars are in normal anteroposterior relationship to the uppers, that is the mesiobuccal cusp of the upper first molar in the buccal groove of the lower. With this will usually be associated the tips of the maxillary canines, being in the same vertical plane as the distal edge of the lower canines in occlusion and corresponding interdigitation of the other buccal teeth. This is customarily regarded as normal, but other relationships are fairly common* and so cannot all be regarded as necessarily pathological and may well be merely part of the wide spectrum of variability present in mankind.

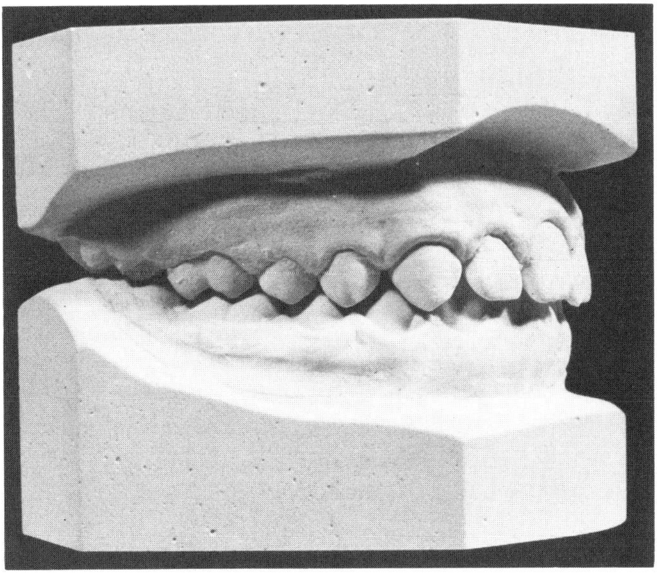

Fig. 9.15. Lateral view of models showing normal (Class I) occlusion in a 14-year-old child.

*Class II*

The lower first molars occlude at least half a cusp in distal relationship to the uppers or the mesiobuccal cusps of maxillary first molars lie in the embrasures between the mandibular second premolars and the first molar. The lower dental arch is, therefore, posterior or "postnormal" to the upper. Customarily there are two main subdivisions:

Class II, Division 1 — Maxillary incisors usually proclined.
Division 2 — Maxillary central incisors retroclined, but laterals may be proclined.

*Class III*

The lower first molars are in mesial relationship to the uppers, or the mesiobuccal cusps of maxillary first molars lie in the embrasures between the first and second lower molars. The lower dental arch is "prenormal" to the upper, again usually by at least half a cusp.

* About one-third in a recent survey of 13,000 schoolchildren in the United Kingdom did not conform to this norm (Todd 1975).

It is important to realize that Angles' classification refers only to the dental occlusion and does not take into account the various forces which bring about occlusion. These include skeletal and neuromuscular interaction, inherited factors relating to tooth/tissue ratio and environmental causes such as early loss of deciduous teeth.

There are racial differences in these types of occlusion. Those having a dolicocephalic tendency, for example in North-west Europe, have a higher proportion of Class II occlusion, particularly division 1, that is proclined maxillary incisors. Those with a more brachycephalic headform such as the Chinese have more of a tendency towards Class III occlusions.

The amount the upper teeth overlap the lower teeth in a horizontal plane is known as the overjet and has been measured by various investigators and in the United Kingdom tends to be around a mean of about 3.5 mm. However, it can range from a negative amount (in Class III cases, since the upper incisors are behind the lowers) to about 10 mm. Obviously it will be highest in Class II division 1 cases and so there may be racial differences noticed on this account. Table 9.2 shows a frequency distribution of overjet as shown in the U.K. survey (Todd 1975), the mean is 3.33 mm in this example for 14-year-olds.

TABLE 9.2

Frequency Distribution of Over-jet Measurement for Upper Left Central Incisors in mm (Todd 1975)

| 14-year-olds* | Present |
|---|---|
| -1 or less | 1 |
| Zero | 3 |
| +1 | 19 |
| +2 | 28 |
| +3 | 22 |
| +4 | 11 |
| +5 | 8 |
| +6 | 3 |
| +7 | 2 |
| +8 | 1 |
| +9 | 1 |
| +10 | 1 |
| +11 or more | - |
| Total number | 923 |

* Negative implies Class III occlusion

The vertical overlap of the incisors is known as the overbite, and it is difficult to measure this quantitatively so it is usually expressed as the proportion of the crown of the lower incisors which is overlapped by the uppers. In the majority of cases in the United Kingdom it is within the middle third of the crown of the mandibular incisors, but again can be quite variable.

So far we have considered the occlusion as though it was static but, of course during function movements occur in all directions. There is thus considerable development from infancy where function was more or less limited to sucking movements.

## BIBLIOGRAPHY

BeGOLE, E. A. (1980) Application of the cubic spline function in the description of dental arch form, *J. Dent. Res.* **59,** 1549.

BERKOVITZ, B. K. B. (1976) Theories of tooth eruption, in *Eruption and Occlusion of Teeth,* ed. D. F. G. Poole and M. V. Stack, Colston Papers No. 27, Butterworths, London.

BOWDEN, D. E. J. and D. H. GOOSE (1968) Inheritance of palatal arch width in human families, *Arch. oral Biol.* **13,** 1293.

BROTHWELL, D. R., V. M. CARBONELL, and D. H. GOOSE (1963) Congenital absence of teeth in human populations, in *Dental Anthropology,* ed. D. R. Brothwell, Pergamon Press, Oxford.

DORIS, J. M., B. W. BERNARD and M. M. KUFTINEC (1981) A Biometric study of tooth size and dental crowding, *Am. J. ortho.* **79,** 326.

FALKNER, F. (1957) Deciduous tooth eruption, *Arch. Dis. Child.* **32,** 386.

FINNEY, D. J. (1951) *Probit Analysis,* 2nd ed., Camb. Univ. Press, Cambridge.

GARN, S. M. (1977) Genetics of dental development, in *The Biology of Occlusal Development,* ed. J. A. McNamara, Jr., Center for Human Growth and Development, Univ. Michigan, Ann Arbor.

GARN, S. M. and B. H. SMITH (1980) Eruption sequence similarities in the maxilla and mandible, *J. dent. Res.* **59,** 1534.

GOOSE, D. H. (1971) The inheritance of tooth size in British families, in *Dental Morphology and Evolution,* ed. A. A. Dahlberg, Univ. Chicago Press, Chicago.

GRAHNEN, H. (1956) Hypodontia in the permanent dentition, *Odont. Revy.* **7,** Suppl. 3.

GRAHNEN, H. and B. LINDAHL (1960) Supernumerary teeth in the permanent dentition, *Odont. Revy.* **12,** 290.

HURME, V. O. (1948) Standards of variation in the eruption of the first six permanent teeth, *Child. Develop.* **19,** 213.

LAVELLE, C. L. B. (1979) The time of tooth emergence in four population samples, *J. Dent. for Child.* **46,** 114.

LEIGHTON, B. C. (1977) Early recognition of normal occlusion, in *The Biology of Occlusal Development,* ed. J. A. McNamara, Jr., Center for Human Growth and Development, Univ. Michigan, Ann Arbor.

LUNDSTROM, A. (1968-9) Changes in crowding and spacing of teeth with age, *Dent. Practit.* **19,** 218.

MANSON, J. D. (1967) Bone changes associated with tooth eruption, in *The Mechanism of Tooth Support, A Symposium,* J. Wright, Bristol.

MELCHER, A. H. and W. BEETSEN (1977) The physiology of tooth eruption, in *Biology of Occlusal Development,* ed. J. A. McNamara, Jr., Center for Human Growth and Development, Univ. Michigan, Ann Arbor.

MOORREES, C. F. A. (1958) Growth changes of the dental arches—a longitudinal study, *J. Canad. Dent. Ass.* **24,** 449.

MOORREES, C. F. A. and R. B. REED (1965) Changes in dental arch dimensions expressed on the basis of tooth eruption as a measure of biologic age, *J. dent. Res.* **44,** 129.

MOORREES, C. F. A. and R. L. KENT, Jr. (1977) Patterns of dental maturation, in *The Biology of Occlusal Development,* ed. J. A. McNamara, Jr., Center for Human Growth and Develop ment, Univ. Michigan, Ann Arbor.

SCOTT, J. H. (1957) The shape of the dental arches, *J. dent. Res.* **36,** 996.

SHAH, R. M. and M. A. BOYD (1979) The relationship between presence and absence of third molars and hypodontia of other teeth, *J. dent. Res.* **58,** 544.

SILLMAN, J. H. (1964) Dimensional changes of dental arches: longitudinal study from birth to

25 years, *Am. J. Ortho.* **50,** 824.
TODD, J. E. (1975) *Children's Dental Health in England and Wales, 1973,* H.M.S.O., London.
VAN HASSEL, H. J. and R. G. McMINN (1972) Pressure differential favouring tooth eruption in the dog, *Arch. oral. Biol.* **17,** 183.

# *Statistical Appendix*

## MEANS AND STANDARD DEVIATIONS

### The Mean Value

A measure of fundamental importance in statistics is the average. If a set of values are taken such as the height of a group of men, the price of a jar of coffee at a number of supermarkets, or the number of goals scored at a selection of football matches, then the average value for that set possesses the attribute of being particularly representative of the set. There are three different types of average, all of which are representative of the set of values from which they are calculated, but tend to be used in different situations. They may have the same value for a particular set of values, but in general do not.

The types of average are known as the mean, the mode, and the median. The mean, which is the measure most widely used, is further subdivided into the arithmetic mean, geometric mean and harmonic mean, although we shall only be concerned with the arithmetic mean here.

The difference between these types of average can be illustrated by a simple example. Supposing 15 dental students took an examination and their marks out of 20 for the paper were:

5 9 10 12 7 13 13 18 10 11 12 15 12 17 8

*Arithmetic mean.* This aims to give some measure of the centre of the set of values and is defined as

$$\text{Arithmetic mean} = \frac{\text{Sum of the values}}{\text{Number of values}}$$

In this case the mean is $\frac{172}{15}$ or 11 (to the nearest whole number).

*Mode.* This is simply the most frequently occurring value in the data and is used when most of the data tends to cluster around one particular value. In this case it is 12.

*Median.* This is the central value in terms of magnitude and can be obtained by ordering the data in ascending value and choosing the central one. (If there is an even number of values in the set, the middle two are chosen and a value halfway between the two is calculated.) Its particular use is that it not only provides a representative value of the set but also divides the values equally in two halves. In the above example the ordered values become:

5 7 8 9 10 10 11 <u>12</u> 12 12 13 13 15 17 18

so the value of the median is also 12.

The arithmetic mean is the type of average which is most generally used and will be the one referred to subsequently.

Care should be exercised when drawing conclusions from a mean calculated from a set of data. In the above example the mean provided a meaningful representative value by which to summarize the group of examination marks. However, supposing three people make the following deposits in a Building Society: £10, £30, £1,000. The mean size of the deposit is £347, but clearly this is of no use as a representative value for this set of data, since no one has made a deposit anywhere near this size. This example illustrates two important points which should be considered when calculating means.

(a) The mean on its own may not tell us all we need to know about the data, and some measure of the spread of values is also important.
(b) In general, it is advisable to use as many values as possible in calculating the mean; that is, to ensure the sample of data is large enough to be able to draw valid conclusions from it. Both these points will be discussed in a little more detail later.

### Measures of Spread—the Standard Deviation

The mean has been discussed above as a single summary statistic for a group of values and it has been stressed that it is usually necessary also to give some idea of the spread of values in the data to obtain a full picture.

The simplest measure of the spread of a set of data is the range or the difference between the largest and smallest value. This is a useful measure only if there are no extreme values in the data, which are not representative of the data as a whole.

A more reliable and widely accepted measure is the standard deviation. Its significance is difficult to interpret at first sight, but if our data is normally distributed (see later), then 68.27 per cent of the values are expected to be within one standard deviation either way of the mean value. The formula for the calculation of standard deviation is:

$$\sqrt{\sum_{i=1}^{n} \frac{(x_i-\bar{x})^2}{n}}$$

where $n$ is the number of values in our data.

$$\sum_{i=1}^{n} (x_i - \bar{x})^2$$

is the sum of the squares of the difference between each value and the mean. *Note:* the symbol $\sum_{i=1}^{n} x_i$ indicates the sum of all values of $x$ in a particular set when there are $n$ values in the set. It is often abbreviated to $\Sigma x_i$ for simplicity of writing. (For theoretical reasons $n$-1 is used in practical examples instead of $n$.)

## FREQUENCY DISTRIBUTIONS

A useful way to get an overall idea how the data is distributed before any statistics are calculated is to plot what is known as a frequency distribution. This is done by grouping the data into classes or categories and determining the number of values belonging to each category. In the case of the examination marks given above, the categories would be ranges or bands of marks. The bands should be chosen so that they are wide enough for a clear pattern in the data to be discernible, but not so wide that all the detail in the data is lost. Using the example of the examination marks, frequency distributions have been plotted using three different band widths: 1 mark, 2 marks and 5 marks. These types of distributions are more generally known as histograms (Fig. A.1).

In histogram (i) the band width is too small for an overall pattern to show up, while in histogram (iii) some of the fine detail is lost. Histogram (ii) is about right and gives a good feel where the centre of the distribution is and how the values are distributed about the centre.

It can be seen that the frequencies in this distribution have a peak at the centre and tail off towards either extreme. This is a typical shape found in statistics and will be discussed later.

It is often useful to talk of the *relative frequency* of the bands, which is defined as the frequency of that band divided by the total frequency over all bands. In the example using a band width of 2 marks, the relative frequencies are:

| No. marks | 5-6 | 7-8 | 9-10 | 11-12 | 13-14 | 15-16 | 17-18 | 19-20 |
|---|---|---|---|---|---|---|---|---|
| Rel. frequency | 1/15 | 2/15 | 3/15 | 4/15 | 2/15 | 1/15 | 2/15 | 0 |

It can be seen that the relative frequency gives an idea of the probability that a student picked out at random will obtain a mark in each of the bands.

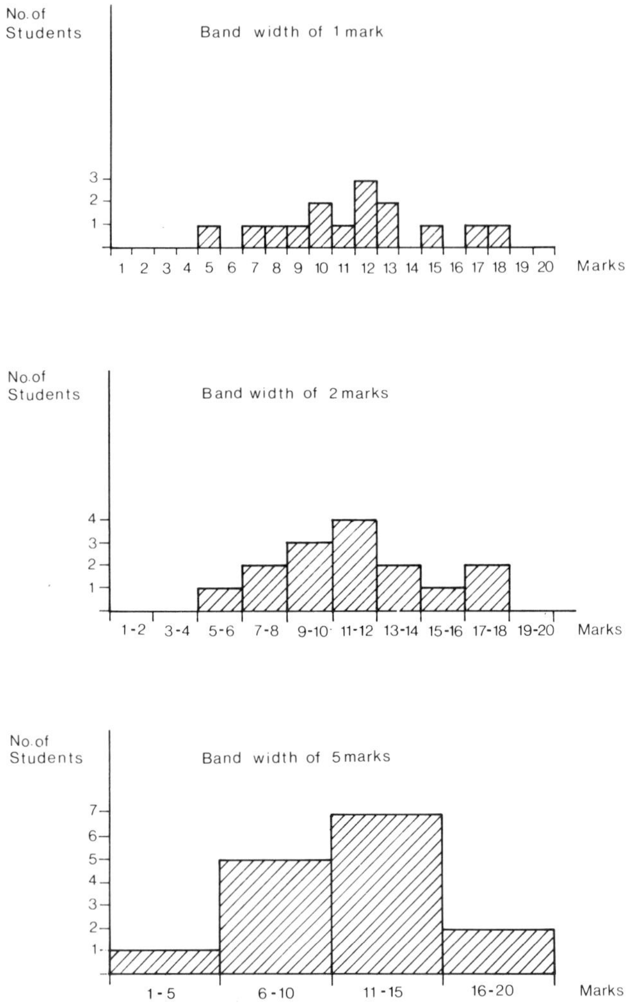


Fig. A.1. Histograms of students' marks with different band widths. The top one is 1 mark, the middle 2 marks and the lower one 5 marks.

An important feature of the relative frequencies is that they add up to 1.

The type of frequency distribution shown above is known as a discrete distribution, which is one in which the values can only take on certain distinct values—in this case only integers.

If we assumed that the students above could obtain fractional marks and there were enough students taking the examination, the band width could be successively reduced, making the rectangles thinner and thinner until we would obtain what is known as a continuous distribution, which is generally plotted as a curve. It is often useful to assume for analytical purposes that our discrete distribution approximates to a continuous one. The reason this is done is that continuous curves can be described in mathematical terms and have properties which enable us to draw statistical conclusions about our original data which we would otherwise not be able to do.

### Normal Distribution

There are a number of theoretical continuous distributions which can be used, the most common of which is known as the normal distribution. The shape of the normal curve is bell-shaped as shown in Fig. A.2 and it can be seen that if a curve were drawn by eye through any of the histograms in Fig. A.1, the resulting continuous distribution would be a similar shape to the normal.

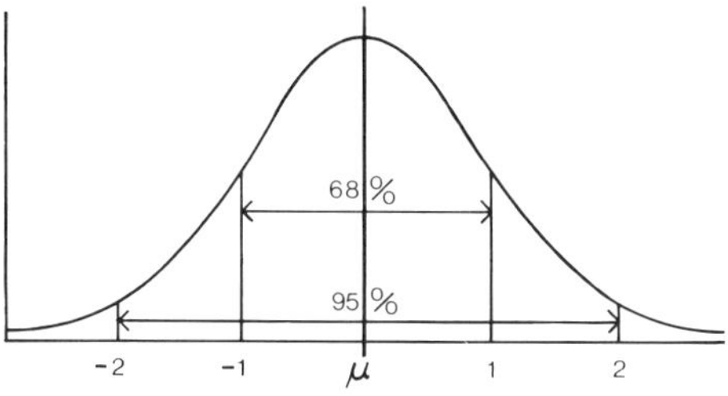


Fig. A.2. Normal distribution showing magnitude of ± 1 and ± 2 standard deviations.

Of the two axes $x$ and $y$, $x$ represents the value of the particular quantity we are concerned with (such as examination marks in the example) while $y$ is known as the *probability density*. Some idea of what probability density means in practice can be obtained by referring back to the idea of relative frequency mentioned earlier in connection with discrete distributions. It was stated then that the relative frequency gave the probability of a value occurring in a particular range and that the sum of relative frequencies is 1. Now in the continuous case it is not meaningful to talk about the probability of one particular value occurring. This is because in a continuous distribution there are an infinitely large number of possible values which could occur and so the probability of any single one occurring is infinitely small.

Instead we consider the probability of a value occurring in a particular range, as in the discrete case, and for a continuous distribution this is defined as the area under the curve over that range. Again, referring to the discrete case where we noted that the sum of relative frequencies was 1, for the continuous case the total area under the curve is 1, that is we are 100 per cent certain that a value picked at random will fall somewhere within the boundaries defined by the curve.

In the case of the normal distribution, the bell-like shape means that the probability density is highest near the centre of the distribution. In other words, if we divided the $x$ axis up into equal ranges, the area under the curve would be the greatest at the centre of the distribution, meaning that a random value has the highest probability of falling within that range. The single value at the centre of the normal distribution is the mean value, usually given the symbol $\mu$ (or $\bar{x}$ for sample mean, see next section). A possible way of dividing the normal distribution up into ranges is to choose the standard deviation as the band width. For the normal distribution this is given the mathematical symbol $\sigma$ and a particular property of this distribution is that about 68 per cent of the total area is contained between $\pm$ 1 standard deviation of the mean, or that there is a 0.68 probability of a value occurring within this range of the distribution. Similarly, about 95 per cent of the area is within $\pm$ 2 $\sigma$ of the mean and 99.73 per cent within $\pm$ 3 $\sigma$. This is illustrated in Fig. A.2. The tails of a normal curve extend to infinity on either side of the mean so there is a finite, but very small, chance of values further out than 3 $\sigma$ from the mean.

The mathmatical equation of the normal curve is:

$$y = \frac{1}{\sigma\sqrt{2\pi}}\, e^{-\frac{(x-\mu)^2}{2\sigma^2}}$$

For any particular normal distribution, the only varying quantities in this expression are $y$ and $x$. $\mu$ and $\sigma$ define the position (relative to zero) and the shape of the distribution and are known as its parameters. Given the same mean ($\mu$), the standard deviation is responsible for the shape of the normal distribution, a larger $\sigma$ giving more spread and a flatter distribution. This effect is shown in Fig. A.3.

## SAMPLING

It is often desired to obtain a particular piece of information about a group or population such as the number of people who clean their teeth more than twice a day or the average length of metal strips in a particular batch of an industrial process. It is clearly not possible to send a questionnaire to every person in England asking how many times a day they clean their teeth and it may also be impractical and expensive for a factory inspector to measure every metal strip. However, by choosing a representative sample of the population and testing that, it may be possible to draw conclusions about the population from which the sample came. The reason the last sentence contains an element of doubt about the ability to draw conclusions is that the sample must be very carefully chosen if the right conclusions are to be drawn about the population.

The three key points to bear in mind about the sample chosen are:

(i) It must be large enough.
(ii) It must be representative.
(iii) It should be randomly chosen.

The question of how large the sample should be will be enlarged on later, but intuitively it can be seen that, for example, no reliable information will be forthcoming about the tooth-brushing habits of people in England if only two people are asked. There are also penalties for making the sample too large, but these tend to be ones of expense and the statistical conclusions are generally more reliable the larger the sample.

It is also very important to try and make the sample as representative as possible. It should be attempted to try and eliminate any systematic bias towards particular areas of the population. In the case of the measurement of metal strips, for example, take a batch as being 1 day's production from a particular machine. If the first 100 strips coming off the line were inspected and the mean length calculated to be 10.53 cm, it would not be valid to assume that this would be the average length over the whole day's production, as the machine might gradually slip out of adjustment and produce shorter strips throughout the day. Clearly, to draw valid conclusions about the batch of strips, a full day's production should be available and the sample chosen from them.

Finally, the sample chosen should be random. This is a condition which must be satisfied for the mathematical laws of probability to be applied to the sampling variabilities. In practice, this means that the sample should be chosen so that each member of the population has an equal chance of being chosen. This can be intuitively understood by taking a rather extreme example of the batch of metal strips. Supposing, instead of choosing the strips at random, a strip was chosen every 50 strips coming off the line and the mean length was found to be 10.34 cm; this would be assumed to be a reasonable estimate for the mean of the whole batch. However, supposing the machine producing the strips had developed a systematic fault which meant that every tenth strip was 0.2 cm shorter than the others; this would mean that only the shorter strips would have been sampled and the wrong conclusions about the batch would have been drawn.

In the case of the strips, physically picking out strips at random would ensure the randomness necessary, but in the case of a sample of people a common method used is to number each member of the population and pick out those selected by generating random numbers, for example by using tables of random numbers or by a computer program.

The measure most usually of interest from a sample is its mean value, known as the *sample mean.* It has been found that in the large majority of cases the sample means of a number of different random samples are normally distributed and that the mean of the sample means is the population mean.

Referring back to the section on the normal distribution, it can be seen that if we knew something about the standard deviation of the sample this would give some indication as to the reliability of using the sample mean as an estimate for the population mean. Figure A.2 shows about 95 per cent of the area of the normal distribution lies within $\pm$ 2 standard deviations of the mean or that there is about a 0.95 probability of a value chosen at random from the distribution falling within $\pm 2\ \sigma$. Therefore, we can say that there is a 0.95 chance of the population mean lying within $\pm$ 2 standard deviations of the sample mean.

It can be shown mathematically that the standard deviation of the distribution of sample means (known as the *standard error*) is given by

$$\text{Standard error of the mean} = \frac{\sigma}{\sqrt{n}}$$

where $\sigma$ is the standard deviation of the population and $n$ is the number of items in the sample.

It is clear statistically why it is desirable to have as large a sample as possible, because as $n$ increases the standard error of the mean goes down, and as there is roughly a 0.95 probability of the population mean lying within 2 standard errors, the smaller the standard error the more accurate the estimate of the population mean becomes.

In practice, the population standard deviation $\sigma$ is usually not known and an estimate in the form of the standard deviation of the sample mean is used.

Confusion must not arise between the standard error of the mean, which is the standard deviation of sample means about the population mean, and the standard deviation of the sample mean which is a measure of the spread of values in the sample about the sample mean.

## CONFIDENCE INTERVALS

As explained above, the purpose of sampling is to obtain a sample estimate of one of the parameters of the population. If the population is normally distributed, then the two parameters of interest are the population mean $\mu$ and the standard deviation $\sigma$ (more usually expressed as the variance which is the square of the standard deviation, $\sigma^2$).

Thus if we take a sample and find its mean $\bar{x}$, this gives us some information about the population. As mentioned in the previous section, the sample means will be normally distributed about the population mean so it is possible that if we were particularly lucky the sample mean would coincide with the population mean. However, it is more likely to be a little high or low and therefore we cannot make a precise statement of the whereabouts of the population mean on the basis of our sample mean. As a result we usually have to say that the population mean is likely to lie within a certain range of values defined by what is known as a *confidence interval.*

The confidence interval is so-called because its width depends on the confidence that we have in the population mean lying within it. The most commonly used confidence level is 95 per cent, which means that if 100 samples were taken we would expect the sample means of 95 of them to be within the unshaded region in Fig. A.4. As the normal distribution is symmetrical, we can conversely say that there is a 0.025 probability of a sample mean being in each of the "tails" of the distribution. Thus if a statistician takes a number of samples and calculates the mean and confidence intervals he might find them spread about the true population mean as in Fig. A.4. The confidence intervals shown all contain the population mean except the fourth one down. Since we have chosen a 95 per cent confidence level, in this case we would expect the 95 out of 100 or 19 in 20 confidence intervals to include the population mean.

Obviously a 95 per cent confidence level is not the only one which could be chosen, and if we wanted to be more cautious and be more sure that the population mean lay within our confidence interval then we could choose a 99 per cent level. However, by being more sure that the confidence limit contains the population mean, a wider interval has to be specified, because for a 99 per cent confidence level we have to have less of the probability in the tails and the confidence interval becomes less precise.

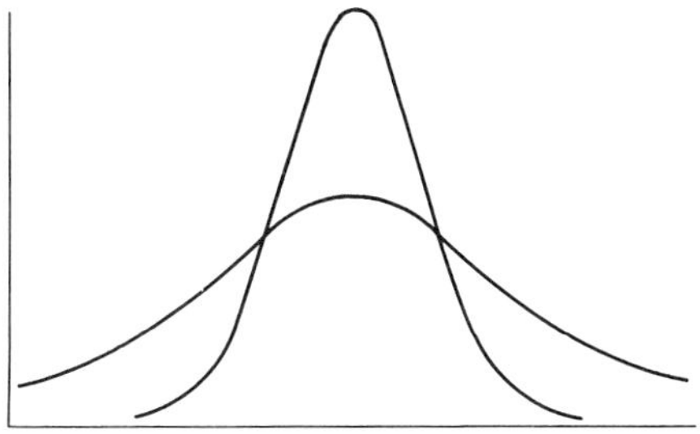

Fig. A.3. Two normal distributions: the flatter one, with more spread, has a larger standard deviation.

## HYPOTHESIS TESTING

Generally speaking, the statistician is concerned about whether it is reasonable to believe in the truth of a certain statement about a situation. Hypothesis testing is a systematic way of drawing conclusions from statistical results.

An example of the sort of situation in which hypothesis testing would be useful is in the comparison between the average heights of two samples of men. The statistician obtains two mean values and finds that the mean value for the height of one is greater than that of the other. This is a result he would expect intuitively, but he would be concerned to know whether the difference was a real one or whether it could have arisen purely by chance. This is where hypothesis testing comes in, and the general procedure used is as follows.

A *null hypothesis* is adopted which is to assume that there is no statistical difference between the mean heights in the two samples. In general the null hypothesis assumes the opposite of what the statistician is trying to prove in the experiments, and here he is hoping to prove that there is a difference between the heights of the two samples of men, so he adopts the null hypothesis that there is no difference.

When a difference occurs which is very unlikely to have arisen by chance, it is generally referred to as statistically significant. The degree of significance is chosen on the basis of the confidence we have in the reality of the difference, that is on the probability levels chosen. We normally refer to a result as significant at the 1 per cent level, for example, which means that our result would have only a 0.01 probability of occurring by chance.

The way the analysis could be carried out in practice for the example above would be to adopt the null hypothesis that both the samples came from the same population, or that there is no significant difference between their means.

To enable the comparison to be carried out, another probability distribution needs to be introduced which is known as the *t*-distribution where, in general, *t* is defined as

$$t = \frac{\bar{x} - \mu}{S/\sqrt{n}} = \frac{\text{Error in mean}}{\text{Standard error of mean}}$$

where $\bar{x}$ is the sample mean,

$\mu$ is the population mean,

$s$ is the sample estimate of the population standard deviation, $\sigma$,

$n$ is the sample size.

The *t*-distribution rather than the normal is used here, as we have no prior knowledge of the true population standard error, but have to make an estimate of it from our sample data which introduces a little more uncertainty into the distribution. Therefore the *t*-distribution is similar in shape to the normal (bell-shaped), but has a slightly wider spread.

Supposing we have the following results for the actual heights in inches of two groups of men; for example, American and Japanese:

| | | | | | | | | | | | | |
|---|---|---|---|---|---|---|---|---|---|---|---|---|
| height of American | 65 | 72 | 68 | 64 | 69 | 71 | 66 | 73 | 68 | 70 | | |
| height of Japanese | 66 | 64 | 63 | 70 | 68 | 66 | 67 | 60 | 61 | 65 | 67 | 62 |

Now if our null hypothesis is true, and there is no difference between the heights of the two groups of men, we would expect $\bar{x}_1 - \bar{x}_2$ to have a mean value of zero ($\bar{x}_1$ is the sample mean height of Americans, $\bar{x}_2$ sample mean height of Japanese). It can also be shown mathematically that the standard error of this combined distribution is

$$Sp\sqrt{\frac{1}{n_1} + \frac{1}{n_2}}$$

where $n_1$, $n_2$ are the numbers in the two samples.

The expression for $t$ in this case is then

$$t = \frac{\text{Error in mean}}{\text{Standard error of mean}} = \frac{(\bar{x}_1 - \bar{x}_2) - 0}{Sp\sqrt{\frac{1}{n_1} + \frac{1}{n_2}}}$$

The expression for $Sp$ (known as the pooled sample variance) is as follows:

$$Sp^2 = \frac{1}{(n_1 + n_2 - 2)} \left[ \sum_{i=1}^{n_1} (x_{1i} - \bar{x}_1)^2 + \sum_{i=1}^{n_2} (x_{2i} - \bar{x}_2)^2 \right]$$

Using the data above, $\bar{x}_1 = 68.6$

$\bar{x}_2 = 64.9$

$Sp = \sqrt{\frac{80.4 + 98.9}{10 + 12 - 2}} = 2.99.$

So we calculate $t$ as $\frac{68.6 - 64.9}{2.99\sqrt{\frac{1}{10} + \frac{1}{12}}} = 2.89.$

We need to compare this value of $t$ with the critical value of $t$ at the significance level chosen. If we choose the 5 per cent probability level we can look up a value of $t$ from standard statistical tables. In order to do this we need to know the number of degrees of freedom which in this case is $n_1 + n_2 - 2 = 20$. The $t$-value we eventually obtain from these tables is 2.086.

Since the $t$-value obtained from our data exceeds this, there is less than 5 per cent chance that we would obtain a $t$-value as high as this by chance, and so we can safely assume that that the null hypothesis is false, the two means do not come from the same population and there is a statistical difference between the heights of American and Japanese men (the former being taller). We generally say this result is significant at the 5 per cent level.

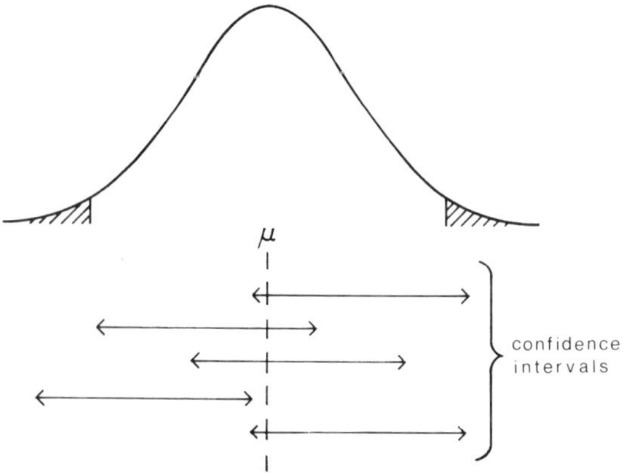


Fig. A.4. Distribution of sample means around the population mean. The confidence intervals all contain the population mean except the fourth one down.

## CORRELATION

If two quantities vary in such a way that movements in one are accompanied by movements in the other, then they are said to be correlated.

There are many examples of correlation occurring in everyday life. An increase in the temperature will be accompanied by an increase in the sale of cold drinks; an increase in the sales of cassette tapes is accompanied by a decrease in the sales of LP records; people in higher socio-economic groups tend to take more holidays abroad.

It can be seen from the examples above that it is possible for an increase in the first quantity to be accompanied by either an increase or a decrease in the second quantity. In the first case, where an increase in the first quantity was accompanied by an increase in the second, we say that the quantities are positively correlated, while in the second case we say they are negatively correlated, as in the case of the sales of cassettes and LPs.

An important point to note is that if two quantities are correlated, it does not necessarily mean that there is a causal relationship between them, that is that a change in one actually causes a change in the other. The changes that do occur in the two quantities may be actually due to a separate cause. Thus the number of road accidents may be correlated to the sales of wing mirrors. However, it would be expected that the trend towards drivers having wing mirrors would lead to better visibility and reduced number of accidents. In reality the situation is simply that the sales of cars have increased, leading to an increase in the number of accidents *and* the sales of wing mirrors.

It is also possible that a correlation may be found where there is no connection whatsoever between the two quantities. For example, it was found that there was a strong correlation between the number of births in the United

Kingdom and the stork population in Scandinavia! These sorts of correlations are normally referred to as "nonsense correlations".

Therefore, although a mathematical correlation may exist between two quantities, care should be taken when drawing any conclusions about the nature of the relationship between the quantities. It should be always borne in mind that a correlation is not necessarily evidence of a causal relationship.

### Correlation Coefficient

This is a measure of the degree of correlation between the variables under consideration. It varies between +1 and -1, the sign indicating whether the correlation is positive or negative. The nearer the correlation coefficient to ±1, the stronger the correlation is said to be and the stronger the relationship between the two variables is. In the case of perfect correlation when the coefficient is actually ±1, if the value of one variable is known, the value of the other can be calculated with certainty. In practice, perfect correlation would occur when the relationship between the two variables is governed by a physical law. Thus with a given voltage it is always possible to calculate the electric current exactly if the resistance is known.

The nearer to 0 a correlation coefficient is, the weaker the relationship between the two variables until at 0 there is no relationship (in this sense we mean there is no linear relationship, although a relationship of a higher order, such as quadratic, may exist).

The correlation coefficient for a particular population is defined to be

$$\varrho = \frac{\sigma_{xy}}{\sigma_x \sigma_y}$$

where $\sigma_x$ is the standard deviation of population $x$,
$\sigma_y$ the standard deviation of population $y$,
$\sigma_{xy}$ the standard deviation of the "joint distribution" of $x$ and $y$.

Remember that previously the population mean and standard deviation were not generally known and have to be estimated by taking samples. In the same way we are unlikely to have full knowledge of the population of $x$ and $y$ and so will only be able to obtain an estimate of $\varrho$, usually given the symbol of $r$ and known as the *sample correlation.*

This can be calculated from the following expression.

$$r = \frac{\Sigma(x_i-\bar{x})\,(y_i-\bar{y})}{\sqrt{[\Sigma(x_i-\bar{x})^2]\,[\Sigma(y_i-\bar{y})^2]}}$$

### Scatter Diagrams

The usual first step taken when deciding whether there is any relationship between two variables is to draw a scattergram where the values of one variable ($y$) are plotted against the other variable ($x$). If there is a strong correlation, there will be an obvious straight-line relationship apparent with little "scatter", while the weaker the relationship the more the scatter increases, until there is no obvious relationship at all (Fig. A.5).

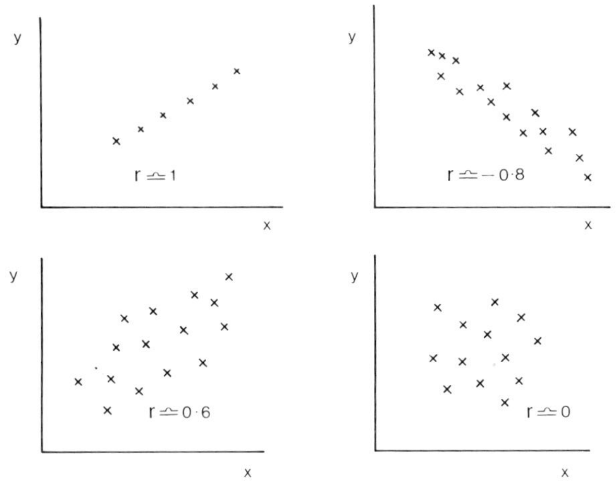


Fig. A.5. Scatter diagrams for different values of the correlation coefficient $r$.

## REGRESSION ANALYSIS

In the previous section it was shown how correlation could give the strength of the relationship (if any) which exists between two variables. What correlation does not do, however, is to give any indication of what that relationship is quantitatively.

A technique which is very widely used in statistics and defines the nature of a relationship between two (or more) variables is known as regression. Regression is a more powerful tool than correlation and hence it is proposed to go into a little more depth into this than was done with correlation. Although correlation is a less powerful technique, the two are closely related mathematically and correlation can be a useful aid in interpreting regression analysis.

Regression is concerned with defining mathematically a linear relationship between a particular dependent variable and one or more independent variables. The most elementary case is that of simple regression which has the form $y = mx + c$ giving a straight line; $m$ is the gradient of the line and $c$ its intercept on the $y$-axis. The independent variable is the one which corresponds to $x$ and is the quantity from which $y$ (the dependent variable) is measured. Another point to note about this equation is that it is linear, that is it contains no squared or higher powers of $x$.

As an example of the way in which simple linear regression might be used, consider the case of the amount of savings by families of particular incomes. It would be expected that families with higher incomes would be able to save more in general and thus it might be reasonable to expect a linear relationship between the savings and income.

The first thing to do in a case where any sort of relationship between quantities is expected is to plot the data on a graph. Suppose the incomes and savings of five families were examined and found to be as follows:

| Family | Income (£) | Savings (£) |
|---|---|---|
| A | 7000 | 700 |
| B | 13000 | 1400 |
| C | 10000 | 1100 |
| D | 5000 | 600 |
| E | 5000 | 300 |

Since the savings is the variable of interest, this is the dependent variable while the income is the variable which the savings depend on (the independent variable). This data has been plotted on a graph in Fig. A.6.

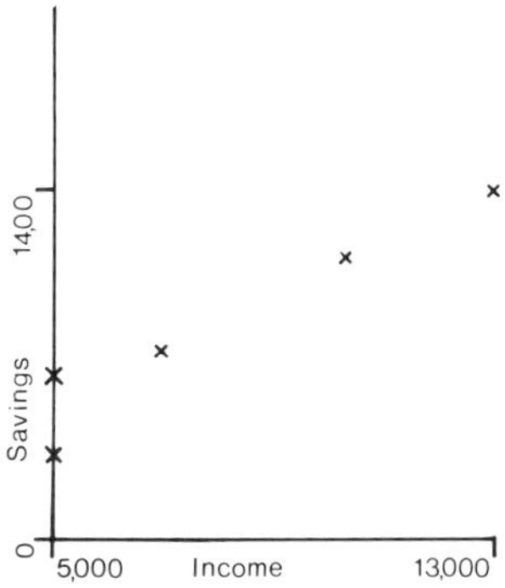


Fig. A.6. Relationship of savings with income.

It can be seen from the graph that the results do not fall on a perfect straight line, although there seems to be a definite linear trend. The problem is that if we accept that there is an underlying linear relationship between savings and income, how do we estimate what it is? A possible approach is to plot the best straight line through the points by eye, find the point at which the line cuts the $y$-axis (the intercept) and calculate the gradient. This might lead to reasonable results in certain circumstances, but is liable to cause bias and will not lead to consistent results—different people would probably plot slightly different lines.

What is needed is a more systematic approach and various criteria have been suggested for fitting "best" lines through a set of points. The criterion most usually used is to minimize the sum of squares of the errors. If the value of the fitted line is $\hat{y}_i$ for data item $i$, then we can say that this criterion minimizes the following expression (for $n$ data points):

$$\sum_{i=1}^{n} (y_i - \hat{y}_i)^2$$

Figure A.7 shows the distance of three data points from a fitted line and each of these distances are equivalent to $y_i - \hat{y}_i$, two being negative in value (below the fitted line), the third being positive (above the line).

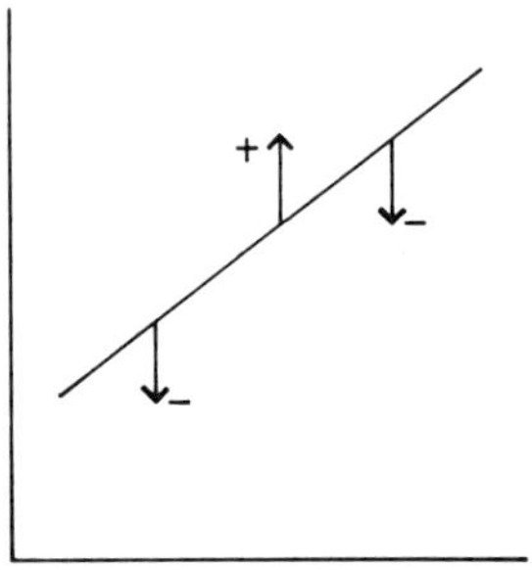


Fig. A.7. Fitting a line by the least squares method.

The reason why the square of the distances of the points from the line is minimized is twofold.

(i) Squaring overcomes the problem of sign, making all the errors positive.

(ii) Squaring emphasizes the large errors and in trying to satisfy the "least squares" criterion a big weight is given to trying to reduce the large errors.

The usual notation used for a regression equation is of the form

$$y = a + bx$$

where $a$ is the intercept on the $y$-axis and $b$ the gradient. In order to calculate the parameters of the regression equation $a$ and $b$ from the data it is necessary to solve the following simultaneous equations which are obtained mathematically from a least squares analysis;

$$\Sigma y = b\Sigma x + na$$
$$\Sigma xy = b\Sigma x^2 + a\Sigma x$$

Taking the data above on savings and incomes, the simplest way to approach this is to draw up a table of calculations as follows, remembering that $x_1$ are the incomes, $y_i$ the savings.

Results shown in £1000s are as follows:

| | $x_i$ | $y_i$ | $x_i^2$ | $x_i y_i$ |
|---|---|---|---|---|
| | 7 | 0.7 | 49 | 4.9 |
| | 13 | 1.4 | 169 | 18.2 |
| | 10 | 1.1 | 100 | 11.0 |
| | 5 | 0.6 | 25 | 3.0 |
| | 5 | 0.3 | 25 | 1.5 |
| Totals | 40 | 4.1 | 368 | 38.6 |

So $\Sigma x_i = 40$, $\Sigma y_i = 4.1$, $\Sigma x_i^2 = 368$, $\Sigma x_i y_i = 38.6$.

Substituting in the pair of simultaneous equations above we obtain:

$$4.1 = 40b + 5a \ (1)$$
$$38.6 = 368b + 40a \ (2)$$

If we multiply (1) by 8 and subtract from (2) we obtain:

$$5.8 = 48b \text{ or } b = 0.120.$$

Substituting for $b$ in equation (1) gives:

$$-0.7 = 5a \text{ or } a = -0.140.$$

Before quoting the final regression equation, $a$ must be multiplied by 1000, as we have expressed the incomes in terms of £1000s for ease of calculation.

Thus the regression equation for savings against income is

$$\text{Savings} - 0.120 \times \text{Income} - 140.$$

**The Regression Model**

So far all we have done is to fit the best line through a set of data points using the least squares method. What a regression analysis tries to do in statistical terms is to estimate the underlying true relationship between the two variables we are considering. In this sense we are trying to do the same thing as in sampling, where attempts are made to draw conclusions about a population by taking a limited sample of data from that population. In the example above we were just looking at a sample of families and trying to discover what the true relationship between income and saving is by finding the best relationship from the data we have at our disposal. As explained before in the case of sampling, we can never be sure that the conclusions we draw from our analysis are the correct ones, but only that the true result has a certain probability of lying within a certain range. In the same way as the estimation of the sample mean of a population, $\bar{x}$ is only an approximation to the mean $\mu$, so the values of $a$ and $b$ are only estimates of the "true" parameters of the regression which are normally referred to as $\alpha$ and $\beta$.

We normally postulate what is known as a regression model, which in the case of simple linear regression is of the form:

$$y_i = \alpha + \beta x_i + e_i.$$

We then use our data to estimate $\alpha$ and $\beta$, bearing in mind that the resulting line will only be an approximation to the true line.

An extra term appears in this equation which is $e_i$, the error term. This is a random error or disturbance and has a normal distribution with mean zero. This error arises through causes which the statistician has no control over such as, for example, measurement of the data. In the savings case above, no error of this type would arise. However, if a regression model were being used in a scientific experiment, for example, to examine the relationship between yield and temperature for a particular process, then the data would be subject to a certain amount of experimental error in the measurement.

A second and more important contribution to the error term is that the underlying relationship between the two variables is not a perfect one and perhaps there are other outside variables having an effect on the values of the dependent variable which are not accounted for in the model.

The error term, in fact, is reflected in the scatter of points around a straight line. In the absence of random error, a particular value $x_i$ would give rise to a value of $y_i$ which would lie on the true regression line, but this value is reduced or increased as a result of random error. The larger the amount of scatter, the larger part the error term plays in the equation until there arrives a point at which there can be said to be no valid relationship between the two variables. There are statistical tests to decide on the validity of a particular regression model, but these are outside the scope of this discussion. In essence, these tests examine the significance of the gradient term $b$ being different from zero. If $b$ is found not to be significantly different from zero, then no relationship of the form postulated is likely to exist.

Assuming that we have calculated the coefficients $a$ and $b$ and found that a relationship does exist between the variables considered, then what use could this regression equation be put to? One of the most frequent uses is in prediction, where we have an $x$ value and wish to predict what the $y$ value would be. Such an example from Chapter 1 could be the prediction of adult height from a child's height. When this is done an equation of the form

$$y_i = a + bx_i$$

is used. Obviously we cannot include the random error term since, by its nature, we do not know how big it will be or whether it will have a negative or positive effect. When a prediction is made then, it is made in the knowledge that the value is likely to be different from the actual value as a result of random error.

We do not know what the exact difference will be, but it is possible to obtain some knowledge of whether the error term is likely to be large or not. This comes from a consideration of the correlation coefficient and this is where the two techniques of correlation and regression link together. The correlation coefficient indicates the strength of the relationship and a stronger relationship will have less random error. This also shows up on the scatter diagram as less scatter. In practice, good predictions will not be obtained for a correlation coefficient of less than about $\pm$ 0.8.

**Multiple Regression**

It was stated above that one possible reason for the random error term being large in a particular regression was that the relationship postulated between the two variables may not be a good one and there is a large amount of scatter when the data for these variables are plotted on a graph. It may be that the reason for this is that another variable (or variables) is also affecting the situation. For instance, consider our example of the savings and incomes of various families. When the results were plotted on the graph in Fig. A.6, the points did not fall on a perfect straight line, that is there was some scatter. One possible reason for this is that there is another important variable which affects the savings of a family apart from income.

A possible variable which might have a bearing on this is the number of children in the family. Looking back at the data, we see that families D and E had incomes of £5000 but D saved £600, whereas E saved only £300 and it may well be that the explanation for this is that family E have more children. This approach is merely an extension of simple linear regression known as multiple linear regression, and the usual form of a multiple regression model is:

$$y_i = \alpha + \beta_1 x_{1i} + \beta_2 x_{2i} + \beta_3 x_{3i} + e_i.$$

Theoretically the statistician is at liberty to carry on adding new variables to the equation *ad infinitum*. However, there are statistical tests to see if the new variable added significantly improves the regression model and there will be a point at which no further improvement is possible. Generally speaking a multiple regression model will not contain more than about 5-10 variables, but there are exceptions, particularly in the area of economic modelling. For example, the Government Economic Model, which is a sophisticated multiple regression model, will contain many more.

It is possible to extend regression analysis to include relationships between variables which are non-linear, and this is known as polynomial regression.

## MULTIVARIATE ANALYSIS

Multivariate analysis moves away from the idea of looking at one variable or the relationship between one variable and another. It is more concerned with grouping or classification of particular objects. In general there will be a set of objects, each of which will have the same set of variables associated with it which describe the object in some way. Consider the following example: a study was carried out to assess the feasibility of classifying old people into a number of groups ranging through fit healthy married couples living in their own home to those who are seriously ill in hospital. The people then are the "objects" under consideration here, and the types of variables chosen to describe the people were: Marital status, Mobility score, Type and quality of home, Income and age. Given such a set of data, there are a number of ways in which it can be studied before any conclusions are drawn:

(i) To see if the data collected is too complex to represent the situation. For example, it might be found that too many variables were being used to describe the objects of study and they could be adequately represented by a smaller set.

(ii) Whether the objects fall naturally into groups and how many groups would be necessary to classify the objects.

(iii) It may be of interest to see if the variables also fall into distinct groups as well as the objects.

(iv) To examine the interdependence of variables to see which variables are independent of each other (correlation coefficient of zero) and which variables are related to others. This could have implications for (i), as if two variables are strongly correlated, then only one of them is necessary to classify the object.

### Cluster Analysis

This is the analysis of whether objects fall into distinct groups or clusters according to measurements of a set of variables describing the objects. In the example quoted above concerned with the grouping of old people, the analysis used was a cluster analysis. The groups that are used are defined by the statistician who sets up the experiment.

### Discriminant Analysis

This analysis has been developed to cope with the problem of allocating an object to one of an existing number of groups which are not defined by the statistician. Therefore, a sample of observations are taken from each group with the purpose of defining rules by which any new objects may be allocated to a particular group.

The sort of situation in which this type of analysis could be used is, for example, when a recently discovered fossil skull is required to be put in one of two or more existing categories of fossils.

### Principal Component Analysis

This is a technique designed to reduce a matrix of correlated variables to a smaller set of uncorrelated linear combinations. Thus, the first component will account for the greatest amount of variation and the second, uncorrelated with the first, will account for the next greatest amount of variation. Others follow in a similar way, but the importance of them soon tails off.

Such a technique can be particularly useful for generating hypotheses which may then be tested with other data.

# *Index*